CACHE LEVEL

2

◆ Maria Ferreiro Peteiro
◆ Elizabeth Rasheed
◆ Bev Saunder

Extended Diploma in
Health &
Social Care

cache
Endorsed

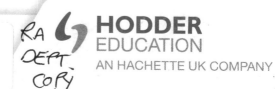

HODDER
EDUCATION
AN HACHETTE UK COMPANY

Upon successful completion of this qualification, learners will be awarded the NCFE CACHE Level 2 Extended Diploma in Health & Social Care 601 / 8855 / 8. This CACHE branded qualification is certified by the Awarding Organisation, NCFE.

Hachette UK's policy is to use papers that are natural, renewable and recyclable products and made from wood grown in well-managed forests and other controlled sources. The logging and manufacturing processes are expected to conform to the environmental regulations of the country of origin.

Orders: please contact Hachette UK Distribution, Hely Hutchinson Centre, Milton Road, Didcot, Oxfordshire, OX11 7HH. Telephone: +44 (0)1235 827827. Email education@hachette.co.uk Lines are open from 9 a.m. to 5 p.m., Monday to Friday. You can also order through our website: www.hoddereducation.co.uk

ISBN: 978 1 5104 7167 2

© Maria Ferreiro Peteiro, Elizabeth Rasheed and Bev Saunder 2019

First published in 2019 by

Hodder Education,

An Hachette UK Company

Carmelite House

50 Victoria Embankment

London EC4Y 0DZ

www.hoddereducation.co.uk

Impression number 10 9 8 7 6 5 4 3

Year   2023 2022 2021

Cover photo © adamkaz/E+/Getty Images

Illustrations by Aptara Inc., India

Typeset by Aptara Inc., India

Printed in India

A catalogue record for this title is available from the British Library.

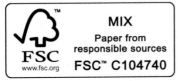

MIX
Paper from
responsible sources
FSC™ C104740

Contents

Answers available online at www.hoddereducation.co.uk/product/9781510471672

How to use this book

Key features of the book

How will I be graded?

The table below shows what learners must do to achieve each grading criterion. Learners must achieve all the criteria for a grade to be awarded. A higher grade may not be awarded before a lower grade has been achieved, although component criteria of a higher grade may have been achieved.

Grade	Assessment Criteria number	Assessment Criteria/What you need to show
D1	1.1	Outline the life stages of human growth and development. Provide information to outline each of the stages of human growth and development: • infancy • childhood • adolescence • early, middle, late adulthood.
D2	1.2	Outline social, emotional, cognitive and physical development within one (1) life stage. Information must relate to social, emotional, cognitive and physical development within one (1) life stage.

The table shows what learners must do to achieve each grading criterion.

✔ Check your understanding

1 What does the term 'inclusion' mean?
2 Name two pieces of legislation that promote equality, diversity and inclusion in care.
3 Give two examples of how an individual's rights can be promoted in care.

Questions at the end of each learning objective, to revise key points at every stage.

Key term

Person-centred care involves the health and social care practitioner placing the individual at the centre of their working practices. They must always act in the individual's best interests to ensure that the individual remains in control of their care and support.

Definitions of terms that are used in health and social care practice.

Define Activity

Produce a leaflet that defines the terms: equality, diversity, inclusion. Include examples that support the meaning of each of these terms.

Activities linked to specific command words in the specification.

Case scenario

Shannon has been working as a respite worker for over 20 years and does not believe that she needs much CPD because she is very experienced and mentors new respite workers. Shannon also believes that as she attends all the mandatory training provided, she is fully kept up to date with current best practice.

If you were Shannon's manager, what would you say to her in relation to the importance of CPD?

An example of a scenario, with questions for the learner.

Activity

Research one piece of legislation from Table 1. You may find it useful to use the government's website: www.gov.uk. Create a poster that outlines how it supports equality, diversity and inclusion in the health and social care sector.

An activity that helps consolidate learning.

Read about it

Equality and Human Rights Commission – (information about types of discrimination) www.equalityhumanrights.com/en/adviceand-guidance/age-discrimination

Government Equalities Office – (information about equality legislation and policy) www.gov.uk/government/organisations/governmentequalities-office

Skills for Care – (information about the Code of Conduct for Healthcare Support Workers and Adult Social Care Workers in England) www.skillsforcare.org.uk/Documents/Standardslegislation/Code-of-Conduct/Code-of-Conduct.pdf

Further resources and links to useful websites at the end of every unit.

Classroom Discussion

Discuss the importance of person-centred practice when providing care and support to individuals. Give examples of the benefits of person-centred practice to individuals.

Areas for discussion in the classroom.

Acknowledgements

Maria Ferreiro Peteiro

Thank you to the Hodder Education and CACHE teams for all their ideas, support and enthusiasm working on this book with me. Another BIG thank you goes to my husband, family and Simba, without whom relaxation and fun in between writing wouldn't have been possible. You all kept me motivated and on track.

Elizabeth Rasheed

I would like to thank my family for their support and encouragement while writing this book, and to thank the Open University for providing opportunities for all to develop their potential.

Bev Saunder

A huge thank you to Gemma at Hodder Education for giving me the opportunity to branch out as an author in Health and Social Care.

A special thank you to Simon whose endless support and constant supply of food and beverages kept me going during the writing process.

The Publishers would like to thank the following for permission to reproduce copyright material.

Photo credits

Unit opener pages 7, 38, 73, 107, 139, 172, 197, 228 © naphtalina/iStockphoto; page 10: © Monkey Business Images/Fotolia.com; page 16: © Barabas Attila/Fotolia.com; page 21: © Syda Productions/stock.Adobe.com; page 22: © Monkey Business/stock.Adobe.com; page 28: © deanm1974/Fotolia.com; page 30: © Tyler Olson/stock.Adobe.com; page 33: © deanm1974/Fotolia.com; page 78: © Rawpixel.com/stock.Adobe.com; page 84: belahoche – stock.adobe.com; page 90: Jacob Lund – stock.adobe.com; page 94: © Robert Kneschke/stock.Adobe.com; page 95: © Photographee.eu – stock.adobe.com; page 99: © Paul Maguire – Fotolia.com; page 111: 4.3 © poco_bw – Fotolia.com; 4.4 © Wordley Calvo Stock/stock.Adobe.com; page 114: © The Makaton Charity; page 117: © WavebreakmediaMicro/stock.Adobe.com; page 148: © godfer – stock.adobe.com; page 153: © Katarzyna Białasiewicz – 123RF.com; page 159: © rocketclips/stock.Adobe.com; page 161: © Noam – Fotolia.com; page 163: © gewitterkind/stock.Adobe.com; page 165: © jovannig/stock.Adobe.com; page 167: © Monkey Business/stock.Adobe.com; page 170: © Monkey Business/stock.Adobe.com; page 179: © Rawpixel.com – Shutterstock.com; page 181: © Panitan/stock.Adobe.com; page 190: © Monkey Business/stock.Adobe.com; page 200: © United States Marine Corps/Wikipedia Commons (Public Domain); page 207: © dundanim – Fotolia.com; page 213 © Igor Dutina – Fotolia.com; page 220: © DenisProduction.com/stock.Adobe.com; page 231: top © Africa Studio – Fotolia; middle © Multiart – iStock via Thinkstock/Getty Images; bottom © Image Source/Alamy; page 232: 8.1 © AlinaMD – iStock via Thinkstock/Getty Images; 8.2 © photocrew – Fotolia; page 236: © Crown copyright 2016. Public Health England in association with the Welsh Government, Food Standards Scotland and the Food Standards Agency in Northern Ireland; page 237: © British Nutrition Foundation; page 238: © BVDC – Fotolia; page 239: © pkproject/stock.Adobe.com; page 241: © Zilotis – Fotolia.com; page 245: © Noam – Fotolia; page 250: © lzf – iStock via Thinkstock/Getty Images; page 255: © Zsolt Bota Finna – Fotolia

Every effort has been made to trace all copyright holders, but if any have been inadvertently overlooked, the Publishers will be pleased to make the necessary arrangements at the first opportunity.

Although every effort has been made to ensure that website addresses are correct at time of going to press, Hodder Education cannot be held responsible for the content of any website mentioned in this book. It is sometimes possible to find a relocated web page by typing in the address of the home page for a website in the URL window of your browser.

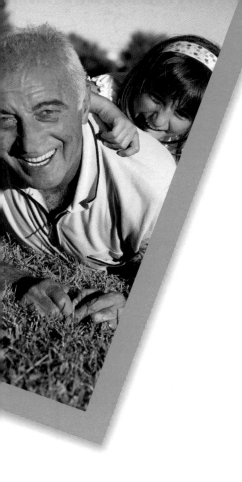

Equality, diversity and rights in health and social care

About this unit

Equality, diversity and inclusion underpin all person-centred practice. They are essential for delivering high-quality care and support. In this unit, you will learn more about what these terms mean in relation to health and social care and why they are important. You will also find out about relevant legislation and inclusive ways of working.

You will develop your understanding of how discrimination can happen and the different ways it can be challenged. Your learning will also include considering how health and social care practitioners' values, beliefs and experiences can influence their delivery of care.

Finally, you will explore the concept of person-centred practice, its benefits and how it is used to support individuals. Ethical dilemmas may arise when health and social care practitioners balance individuals' rights with their duty of care. You will develop your understanding of such dilemmas to help you manage these situations.

Learning Outcomes

LO1: Understand equality, diversity and inclusion in health and social care.

1.1. The terms:
- equality
- diversity
- inclusion.

1.2. Legislation, policies, procedures and codes of practice in relation to equality, diversity and inclusion:
- Care Act 2014
- Health and Social Care Act 2012
- The Equality Act 2010
- Human Rights Act 1998
- United Nations Convention on the Rights of the Child 1989
- related policies and procedures
- codes of practice relevant to the sector
- current legislation as relevant to Home Nation.

1.3. How the health and social care practitioner contributes to inclusive practice:
- knowledge of individuals' beliefs, culture, values, needs and preferences
- promote rights
- value diversity
- person-centred practice
- access to services
- information and advice
- manage risk.

LO2: Understand discrimination.

2.1. Types of discrimination in relation to:

- direct
- indirect.

2.2. Approaches to challenge discrimination:

- strategy
- communication
- reporting
- whistleblowing
- modelling
- training.

2.3. How the health and social care practitioner's own values, beliefs and experiences can influence delivery of care:

- self-awareness
- acknowledging belief systems, attitudes and behaviours
- influence of others on own belief system, attitudes and behaviours to include: media, family and peer pressure
- professional versus personal
- respect and value diversity.

LO3: Understand person-centred practice.

3.1. The concept of person-centred practice:

- individual central
- individual in control.

3.2. How person-centred practice is used to support individuals:

- informed choices
- dignity and respect
- care planning
- tailored communication
- consent
- risk management.

3.3. Impacts of person-centred practice on individuals:

- meets individual needs (social, emotional, cognitive and physical)
- individual rights
- independence
- decision-making and confidence
- health and well-being.

3.4. Ethical dilemmas that may arise when balancing individuals' rights and duty of care:

- confidentiality
- managing values and beliefs
- risk taking
- rights versus responsibilities.

LO1 Understand equality, diversity and inclusion in health and social care

1.1 The terms equality, diversity, inclusion

What is equality?

Equality is very important for maintaining people's rights and ensuring that everyone feels valued and safe. Imagine how you would feel if you were being treated unfairly by someone you knew. Perhaps you would feel angry, upset, frightened or devalued?

Equality is not about treating everyone the same. Equality means:

- treating every person fairly with dignity and respect. You should find out how they want to be treated rather than how you think they should be treated.

- valuing every person as an individual. You should respect people's differences and individual needs by not treating people the same.

- supporting every person's rights, such as their rights to privacy; to make their own choices; and to be independent.

- providing every person with equal life opportunities, such as access to education and work, and to develop and maintain relationships.

It is important to understand what equality means if you want to ensure that you are supporting and respecting the rights of the **individuals** and **others** you work with, such as individuals' families and your colleagues. If you did not support or respect the rights of individuals and others you work with, you would be treating them unfairly and breaking the laws. Laws are in place to protect people's rights to not be **discriminated** against. For example, The Equality Act 2010 sets out the different types of discrimination that exist. You will learn more about the Act and other relevant laws in AC1.2.

What is diversity?

Diversity is very important for being able to recognise people's differences and ensuring that everyone is treated as an individual. People are different in a variety of ways: for example, their physical appearance (i.e. hair colour, weight, height, how they dress, etc.), age, sex, **ethnic group** and where they live. It is these differences that make each person unique.

Diversity means:

- respecting every person's differences (e.g. by finding out their likes and dislikes; meeting their individual preferences such as the way they dress or the food they eat).
- valuing every person as a unique individual, learning more about their **values**, **beliefs** and customs, and their personal experiences.
- supporting every person's differences by sharing and discussing different or new ideas, such as in relation to work and day-to-day activities.
- supporting every person's choices by encouraging people to make their own choices in line with their individual preferences, views and beliefs.

It is important to understand what diversity means to ensure that you recognise and value people as individuals. Understanding and respecting diversity means that you will be contributing to a positive environment. This is because people from different backgrounds and beliefs will feel valued and that they belong.

What is inclusion?

Inclusion is very important for ensuring every person has a meaningful role in the group, community or society that they live in. Imagine how you would feel if you were unable to be in control of your life or your care and support.

Inclusion does not just mean 'being involved'. Inclusion means:

- respecting every person's right to realise their potential by enabling them to work towards their life goals and to access the support they require.
- valuing every person's right to have a meaningful role by finding out what role they would like and supporting them to achieve it, such as a parent, partner, employee, member of a group.
- supporting every person's strengths by enabling the individual to recognise their abilities and developing their confidence, **self-esteem** and respect.
- supporting every person's **active participation** by enabling the individual to participate in new and different activities. This includes opportunities to socialise and develop relationships with others.

It is important to understand what inclusion means when supporting individuals to develop a positive sense of **well-being**. Understanding and supporting inclusion means that you will provide support to individuals to be in control of their own care and support. This will enable them to meet their own unique needs and lead fulfilling lives.

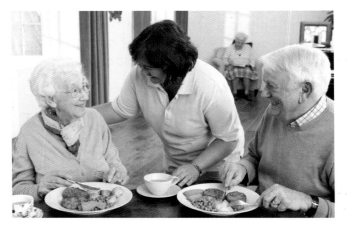

Figure 1.1 How do you support individuals' rights for inclusion?

Define Activity

Produce a leaflet that defines the terms: equality, diversity, inclusion. Include examples that support the meaning of each of these terms.

1.2 Legislation, policies, procedures and codes of practice in relation to equality, diversity and inclusion

Current legislation

All health and social care practitioners' ways of working are based on current UK and international **legislation**. The legislation outlined in **Table 1.1** promotes people's rights, such as being:

- treated equally
- respected for their differences
- able to realise their potential
- protected from unlawful and unfair treatment.

For further information, you will find the 'Read about it' section at the end of this unit useful.

 Key terms

Active participation refers to an individual's involvement in all aspects of their own life, care and support.

Beliefs are opinions that an individual accepts as true; not necessarily based on fact.

Discrimination is the unfair or unequal treatment of an individual or a group.

Ethnic group refers to a group of people who share a common cultural background, such as the country they come from or the language they speak.

Individuals are persons accessing health and social care services.

Legislation refers to laws that must be followed, for example Acts of Parliament, as well as

regulations, such as the General Data Protection Regulations (GDPR).

Others are parents/carers, family, friends, colleagues, external partners and health and social care practitioners.

Self-esteem is the value or confidence a person places upon themselves.

Values are standards based on moral principles or beliefs that are important to the person.

Well-being refers to how a person thinks and feels about themselves, physically, mentally and emotionally. It may include aspects that are social, cultural, spiritual, intellectual and economic.

Table 1.1 Legislation

Legislation	How it relates to equality, diversity and inclusion
Care Act 2014	Promotes the: ● well-being of individuals who require care and support and their carers ● rights of individuals and their carers to be in control of their care and support, meeting their unique needs and preferences.
Health and Social Care Act 2012	Promotes the rights of individuals to: ● high-quality health and social care and support ● have care and support that is fair, inclusive, safe and meets their diverse needs.
The Equality Act 2010	Ensures that individuals are not treated unfairly because of their differences in relation to their: ● age ● disability ● sex, sexual orientation or gender reassignment ● marriage and civil partnership ● pregnancy and maternity rights ● **race** ● religion. The four main types of discrimination are unlawful: ● **direct** ● **indirect** ● **harassment** ● **victimisation.** (You will learn more about types of discrimination in LO2 of this unit.)
Human Rights Act 1998	Promotes the rights and freedoms that every UK citizen has, such as: ● respect for private and family life ● liberty ● to not be discriminated against. Public organisations (such as the government, police and local councils) work together to uphold people's rights to being treated fairly, with dignity and respect.
United Nations Convention on the Rights of the Child (UNCRC) 1989	Ensures that: ● the rights of all children are upheld, such as being listened to, respected and protected from abuse ● adults and organisations work together to promote and uphold children's rights.
European Convention on Human Rights 1950	Ensures that: ● people's basic human rights are upheld, such as being treated fairly and with dignity ● people have access to the European Court of Human Rights if an individual's rights have not been upheld.
The Mental Capacity Act 2005	Establishes the: ● rights of individuals who lack **mental capacity**. It ensures that decisions that concern them are made in line with their unique needs, views and preferences ● use of **Independent Mental Capacity Advocate (IMCA) services.**

Key terms

Direct discrimination is when someone is treated unfairly because of a **protected characteristic** they, or someone they know, has or appears to have.

Harassment refers to unwanted, intimidating or aggressive behaviour related to a protected characteristic.

Independent Mental Capacity Advocate (IMCA) services represents a person where there is no one independent of services, such as a family member or friend, who can represent them. The service is available in England to support individuals and their carers who wish to make a complaint about their NHS treatment or care.

Indirect discrimination is when a practice or system is applied without taking into account an individual's protected characteristic.

Mental capacity refers to an individual's ability to make their own decisions.

Policies are statements of how an organisation works based on legislation, such as a safeguarding policy. They outline the organisation's aims and how it works. Policies refer to an organisation's commitment, for example to data protection.

Procedures are step-by-step guides of how to put a policy into practice.

Protected characteristic refers to the nine characteristics protected from discrimination under the Equality Act.

Race refers to the common physical qualities or characteristics associated with a group of people from the same culture and/or shared history, for example skin colour, ethnic origin, national origin and nationality.

Victimisation is when someone is singled out or treated unfairly. For example, for supporting or speaking up for an individual with a protected characteristic.

Activity

Research one piece of legislation from Table 1.1 You may find it useful to use the government's website: **www.gov.uk**. Create a poster that outlines how it supports equality, diversity and inclusion in the health and social care sector.

Related policies and procedures

In the health and social care sector, organisations use and comply with the legislation you have learned about so far to ensure they uphold individuals' rights relating to equality, diversity and inclusion. Organisations have **policies** in place that state how they aim to work and **procedures** that detail how they put their aims into practice.

Below are some examples of the policies and procedures related to equality, diversity and inclusion that health and social care organisations may have. How do these compare to those of organisations you know about?

- **Policies** – set out an organisation's commitment to promote equality, diversity and inclusion and prevent discrimination in the workplace, for example an Equality, Diversity and Inclusion Policy.

- **Procedures** – set out how an organisation will promote equality, diversity and inclusion: for example, by meeting the needs of individuals who have protected characteristics and tackling discrimination, through a Promoting Equality, Diversity and Inclusion At Work policy.

Codes of practice relevant to the sector

Codes of practice are useful guides for health and social care practitioners. They outline how the values or principles of equality, diversity and inclusion must be applied in day-to-day working practices. Some organisations have their own codes of practice but there are some that are especially relevant to the health and social care sector. Below are two examples you may have come across:

1 **The Code of Conduct for Healthcare Support Workers and Adult Social Care Workers in England**

- Overseen by **Skills for Health** and **Skills for Care**.
- Sets out a number of principles that health and social care practitioners are expected to follow, such as promoting and upholding individuals' and their carers' rights to:
  - privacy
  - dignity
  - confidentiality
  - well-being
  - promoting equality, diversity and inclusion in their working practices.

2 **The Mental Capacity Code of Practice**

- Supports the Mental Capacity Act 2005.
- Sets out how the principles of the Act should be applied for those who work with individuals who lack capacity.
- Outlines the support that can be provided to an individual who is unable to make a decision, what information should be provided to individuals, and how.

Legislation, organisations' policies, procedures and codes of practices are all linked and together they enable health and social care practitioners to understand and promote equality, diversity and inclusion when providing care and support to individuals and others.

Current legislation as relevant to Home Nations

You have learned about the equality and diversity legislation that applies to adults in England. Other pieces of legislation are relevant to Northern Ireland, Scotland and Wales, for example:

- **Northern Ireland** – The Equality Act 2010 does not apply to Northern Ireland; it only applies to England, Scotland and Wales. Examples of legislation relevant to equality and diversity include The Employment Equality (Repeal of Retirement Age Provisions) Regulations (Northern Ireland) 2011, which protects the rights of people of retirement age, and the Autism Act (Northern Ireland) 2011, which protects the rights of individuals with autism, their families and carers.
- **Scotland** – The Criminal Justice (Scotland) Act 2003 and the Offences (Aggravation by Prejudice) (Scotland) Act 2009 promote the rights of people to not be victimised or harassed through violent or distressing behaviour.
- **Wales** – The Equality Act 2010 (Statutory Duties) (Wales) Regulations 2011 promotes equality, diversity and inclusion.

🔑 Key terms

Codes of practice set out the standards or values that health and social care practitioners must follow to provide high-quality, safe, compassionate and effective care and support.

Skills for Care is the sector skills council for people working in social work and social care for adults and children in the UK, as well as for workers in early years, children and young people's services. It sets standards and develops qualifications for those working in health and social care.

Skills for Health is the sector skills council for people working in healthcare in the UK. It sets out standards and develops qualifications for those working in healthcare.

1.3 How the health and social care practitioner contributes to inclusive practice

As you will have learned in AC1.2, **inclusive practice** involves health and social care practitioners working in ways that respond to individuals' unique needs and preferences. They should support individuals so that they have a meaningful role in society and develop a sense of well-being. Inclusive practice enables health and social care practitioners to provide high-quality care and support that is unique to the individual, safe and effective.

Knowledge of individuals' beliefs, culture, values, needs and preferences

Everyone is entitled to their own beliefs, culture, values, needs and preferences.

- Beliefs are strong principles that influence how we live. For example, they may affect what you wear, what you eat, or the religion you practise.
- Culture refers to the traditions or customs we share with other people from one country or group. For example, you may share customs with other people who originate from another country.

- Values are what we consider to be important in our lives, such as our family, friends, our health, having a home and our rights.
- Needs refer to the areas where we require support and this will vary from person to person. These may be, for example, in relation to finding a job, learning a new skill or improving how we communicate with others.
- Preferences refer to our likes and our own personal choices. For example, they may relate to the activities we enjoy, the food we like to eat or the clothes we like to wear.

Health and social care practitioners can develop a good knowledge of individuals in order to ensure that inclusive practice is being upheld. This knowledge informs the care and support provided to meet the individuals' unique beliefs, culture, values, needs and preferences. Examples of how to get to know an individual include:

- Discussion with individuals
- Spending time with individuals
- Observation
- Reading an individual's **care or support plan**
- Collecting information from others who know them well, for example family, friends, an advocate or a colleague who has worked with them over a period of time.

Table 1.2 Developing knowledge of individuals' beliefs, culture, values, needs and preferences

Inclusive practice knowledge	Examples
Knowledge of individuals' beliefs - This knowledge is essential for understanding and respecting individuals' needs and promoting their well-being. - Individuals' religious beliefs may influence how their care and support are provided.	- Hinduism – those from this faith may believe that cleanliness can only be observed by using running water for washing in. So, a shower may have to be provided rather than a bath (or the availability for them to wash by pouring water over themselves). - Judaism – those from this faith may believe that they must only eat **kosher** food. They may not eat pork or consume meat and milk at the same meal.

Inclusive practice knowledge	Examples
Knowledge of individuals' culture ● Being aware of individuals' cultural customs and traditions will give individuals a sense of belonging. It will also make them feel valued and respected.	In some cultures: ● typically, the eldest member of the family is the person who makes the decisions. Health and social care practitioners will need to work with this person in relation to an individual's care to avoid showing any disrespect. ● individuals may find it difficult to question or challenge decisions made by health and social care practitioners. Health and social care practitioners should practise person-centred care to ensure that individuals are central to all decision making, as appropriate.
Knowledge of individuals' values ● This knowledge of what is important to an individual can be used as the basis of all care and support provided. ● When contributing to inclusive practice, the health and social care practitioner must not allow their own values to influence individuals. This is so that the individual remains in control of their care and support.	● An individual may value the time to sit quietly on their own without any distractions when they return from college. Respecting this will promote a sense of well-being. ● An individual may value being independent when going out shopping. Asking the individual how best to support them to do this is another way to contribute to working in inclusive ways.
Knowledge of individuals' needs ● This knowledge is essential for treating individuals as unique, ensuring that the care and support provided is focused on their needs.	● An individual might use facial expressions and eye contact to communicate. It is important that their communication needs are met so that they can express what they are thinking and feeling, interact with others and make their own choices and decisions. ● An individual's social needs might mean that they like to meet and socialise regularly. It is important to provide them with opportunities so that their social needs are being considered.
Knowledge of individuals' preferences ● This knowledge is required to understand personal likes and dislikes, providing care and support that **empowers** the individual.	● An individual might prefer to have a hot snack at lunch rather than a sandwich. Meeting their preferences will mean that they will be more likely to be involved in making it and look forward to it. ● An individual might prefer to have a bath rather than a shower in the mornings. Meeting their preferences will contribute to their well-being and support their empowerment.

Key terms

Care or support plan is a personalised plan for the care and support of an individual, identifying all those involved and their responsibilities.

Empower refers to enabling and supporting individuals to be in control of their lives.

Inclusive practice refers to working in ways that involve individuals in their own care and support so that they are in control of their lives.

Kosher refers to the way food is prepared, cooked and eaten under Jewish law. A food is permitted to be eaten because it is considered to be 'clean' in the Jewish religion.

Description Activity

Build a picture of an individual by describing their likes, dislikes, needs, beliefs, culture, values and preferences. Include details with examples of each.

Promote rights

Promoting individuals' rights underpins inclusive ways of working used by health and social care practitioners. All individuals who access services have rights that are supported by the promotion of equality, diversity and inclusion. **Table 1.3** provides you with some examples of the different rights individuals have and how these can be promoted by the health and social care practitioner to contribute to inclusive practice.

Table 1.3 Individuals' rights and inclusive practice

Rights	Examples of how to promote
Privacy	• Knocking on an individual's closed door before entering their room. • Providing an individual with access to a private room when discussing their care or support.
Dignity	• Supporting an individual to change their clothes if they have dropped food or drink on themselves. • Placing a towel around an individual if they are getting out of the bath.
Choice	• Asking an individual what they would like to wear. • Providing an individual with different options about the activities they could participate in.
Respect	• Addressing an individual by their preferred name. • Speaking to an individual calmly and politely.
Independence	• Enabling an individual to prepare their own lunch. • Supporting an individual to make arrangements for what they would like to do at the weekend.
Effective communication	• Speaking clearly when communicating with an individual who has hearing loss. • Speaking in short phrases when communicating with an individual who has **dementia**.
Be involved in their own care and support	• Empowering an individual to organise a meeting to discuss their own care and support. • Asking an individual what improvements they would like to be made to their care and support.
Be protected from danger, harm and abuse	• Identifying, reporting and recording potential and actual dangers when they occur, such as a faulty plug socket, worn or loose carpet, or changes in an individual's behaviour when they are visited by a family member.

Promoting individuals' rights contributes to inclusive ways of working because doing so makes individuals feel valued and respected and therefore improves the quality of the care and support provided. It also influences the working relationship between the health and social care practitioner by developing mutual respect, trust and understanding.

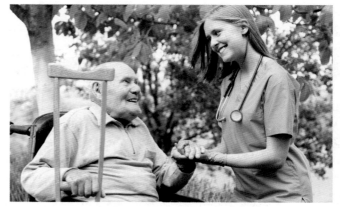

Figure 1.2 What rights do individuals with care and support needs have?

Key term

Dementia is a disorder of the mental processes caused by brain disease or injury. Examples of symptoms include memory loss and/or difficulties with thinking, problem-solving or language.

Value diversity

Valuing diversity contributes to working inclusively. By doing this, it means that the health and social care practitioner recognises that every individual they work with is their own, unique person. Valuing diversity also contributes to inclusive practice, because it involves:

- respecting individuals' differences (e.g. by supporting an individual to practise their faith, or to eat a vegan diet)
- understanding individuals' differences (e.g. by finding out how an individual would like to be moved from one position to another, or what service(s) an individual would like to access when recovering at home from a fall)
- ensuring individuals remain at the centre of their own care and support (e.g. by encouraging an individual to focus on their abilities, or empowering an individual to express what care and support they would like to have).

Person-centred practice

Person-centred practice involves the health and social care practitioner placing the individual at the centre of their working practices. They must always act in the individual's **best interests** to ensure that the individual remains in control of their own care and support. You will learn more about the concept of person-centred practice and how it is used to support individuals in LO3 in this unit. The diagram below provides details of how person-centred practice contributes to working in inclusive ways.

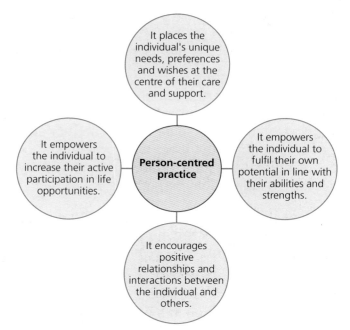

Figure 1.3 Person-centred practice

Access to services

When individuals plan their care and support, the health and social care practitioner can contribute to inclusive practice by sharing their knowledge of the services that are available. For example, the health and social care practitioner may have had experience of supporting other individuals to access different leisure services in the local area. They may have gathered useful information about the facilities each service provides, how much they cost, and their strengths and weaknesses. This information could then be shared with the individual, who can then be empowered to make an **informed choice**.

In addition, the health and social care practitioner can show inclusive ways of working when they are providing individuals with access to the care and support they require to meet their unique needs, views and preferences. You might find it useful to recap your previous learning on inclusive practice in AC1.2.

Information and advice

Information and advice is required in health and social care for many different reasons. For example, getting to know individuals, working with others, planning individuals' care, and providing consistent care and support. Health and social care practitioners can also contribute to inclusive practice by ensuring that the information and advice they provide to individuals and others is:

- **Accessible** – provided in a format that can be understood by the individual and others. For example, this may involve using verbal and/or written language that is clear and free from **jargon**.

- **Suitable** – provided in a way that meets the needs of the individual and others. For example, this may involve using sign language when advising an individual who is deaf, or a formal writing style when emailing an individual's relative about an aspect of their care.

- **Impartial** – provided in a way that does not influence the individual. For example, this might involve explaining the pros and cons of a range of activities that are available for individuals to access. This will help them to make their own informed choices regarding which activity they would like to participate in.

- **Up-to-date** – provided in a way that is timely and current. For example, when an individual's physical needs change, this needs to be documented clearly and immediately. This is so that the care and support provided to the individual reflects their change in needs.

Manage risk

Health and social care practitioners have an important role to make sure that when individuals who access services take risks, they do so positively. For example, an individual who is prone to falling when walking could be supported to use a mobility aid such as

Key terms

Best interests refers to considering an individual's circumstances and preferences before making a decision or choice on their behalf.

Impartial refers to being fair and objective.

Informed choice means having all the necessary information including the options available to make choices and decisions.

Jargon is the use of technical language or terms and abbreviations that are difficult for those not in the group or profession to understand.

a walking frame so that they can mobilise independently. This is because it enables individuals to make their own choices and remain in control. Inclusive practice when supporting individuals to manage risks involves:

- **Informing** individuals to understand what the risks and dangers are. For example, an individual who has recently had a hip operation could fall and injure themselves if they want to go for a walk because they might have reduced mobility.

- **Supporting** individuals to understand how risks and dangers can be managed so that they stay safe. For example, suggesting that the individual asks a member of staff to accompany them when they want to go out for a walk. This will provide them with additional support while walking and minimise the risk of falling over.

- **Encouraging** individuals to take risks. For example, suggesting that a member of staff could accompany the individual when they go for a walk if they feel nervous or frightened of falling over. This will increase the individual's confidence and enable them with independence to continue to do the things they enjoy.

Managing risks is part of inclusive practice because individuals feel valued when their choices are respected. This can help to create opportunities for individuals to learn new skills and develop new interests. You will learn more about how person-centred practice is used to support individuals with risk management in LO3: AC3.2 of this unit.

Check your understanding 1

1 What does the term 'inclusion' mean?
2 Name two pieces of legislation that promote equality, diversity and inclusion in care.
3 Give two examples of how an individual's rights can be promoted in care.

LO2 Understand discrimination

2.1 Types of discrimination

As you will know from learning about The Equality Act 2010 and other legislation relevant to equality, diversity and inclusion, the term 'discrimination' refers to treating a person or groups of people unfairly due to factors such as their gender, sexuality or religious beliefs. Discrimination prevents inclusive practice and can lead to disempowerment, because when individuals are discriminated against, they do not have access to the same opportunities as everyone else. Therefore, this can negatively impact their confidence and well-being. For example, imagine if you went to the cinema with your friends and were refused entry because you use a wheelchair and there was no suitable access for you to enter the building. How would you feel? How would this affect your well-being and your social expectations? Perhaps you would feel upset or angry that you were not allowed in with your friends. Discrimination does not only happen in social situations but also in education, employment and when accessing services.

There are different types of discrimination that are recognised in law but unlike

equality, diversity and inclusion, all types of discrimination are negative and for this reason must not be tolerated. You will learn about useful approaches to challenge discrimination in AC2.2 of this unit.

- **Direct discrimination** occurs deliberately and involves treating an individual with a protective characteristic unfairly. For example, an older adult is not asked if they want to participate in a social activity because of their age; a male individual is excluded from a cookery course because of their gender; or an individual from a Christian background is denied a job opportunity because of their religious beliefs.

- **Indirect discrimination** occurs unintentionally and involves applying a practice or system that appears to treat a group of individuals equally, but leads to individuals who have a protected characteristic being treated unfairly. For example, a health and social care organisation that has a policy in place expecting staff to work full-time may exclude staff who have family commitments, including caring for relatives or children. Another example is a social club that will only accept a driver's licence as proof of identification, which may exclude individuals with disabilities who cannot drive; or information about a health group that is only available in English may exclude individuals who do not speak or read English.

Summarise Activity

Take it in turns to summarise the different types of discrimination you know about. Include brief details about each type.

2.2 Approaches to challenge discrimination

Discrimination can have a negative impact on people because it can result in a lack of confidence and self-esteem, as well as reduce life opportunities and expectations. It is therefore essential to have approaches to challenge discrimination in place, as they are everyone's responsibility in health and social care.

Strategy

One approach to challenge discrimination is having a plan in place, and ensuring everyone understands it and works together to put it into practice. In health and social care organisations, policies and procedures will be in place that detail their commitment to challenging discrimination and how to do so. A health and social care practitioner will be expected to follow their employer's procedures if they become aware that discrimination has or may have occurred. The employer's procedure may include the steps to take, such as:

- not ignoring the discriminatory behaviour
- how and when to report and record what has occurred
- maintaining **confidentiality**.

You will learn more about reporting discrimination later in this section.

Communication

Communicating effectively when challenging discrimination includes using positive approaches. This involves communicating verbally, non-verbally and in writing. Positive approaches will ensure that the information provided is understood and received in the way that it was intended. For example, when a health and social care practitioner recognises that discrimination has or is taking place, they should say this to the person carrying out the discrimination or to a more senior person, such as their manager or employer.

When a health and social care practitioner communicates their concerns, they must do so by:

- using language that is free from jargon (so that it can be understood)

- speaking in a medium **tone** and **pitch**
- ensuring that their **body language** is respectful.

This will mean that the communication comes across as assertive, positive, and will be more likely to be listened to by others.

Effective written communication is also very important when challenging discrimination because it provides a clear message and avoids misunderstandings. For example, when a health and social care practitioner records that discrimination has taken place, they must only write down accurate and factual information rather than their personal opinions. It must also be free from jargon and be completed fully, i.e. with all the relevant information, date, time, their signature. This will mean that the communication is valid, respectful and professional.

Key terms

Body language is a form of non-verbal communication in which thoughts, feelings and intentions are expressed through the movement and position of the body.

Confidentiality refers to keeping something private, such as an individual's personal information. It means protecting an individual's personal, sensitive or restricted information and only disclosing it with those who need to know.

Pitch refers to the quality of a vocal sound made by a person in a communication (e.g. low, high).

Tone refers to the strength of a vocal sound made by a person in a communication (e.g. quiet, loud).

Reporting

When discrimination has occurred, it is the responsibility of all health and social care practitioners to report it at the time it occurred. This ensures that the person is made aware of their discriminatory behaviour quickly, so that they can then stop doing it and **reflect** on their actions. Reporting discrimination at the time it occurs is important because it will minimise the harm it is causing and enable actions to be taken to address it. For example, the person showing the discriminatory behaviour could be **disciplined**, have their work supervised by a senior staff member, or be asked to attend further training.

All health and social care practitioners must follow their work setting's procedure for reporting discrimination. The manager or employer will then ensure that the person(s) being discriminated against are safeguarded from any further harm taking place. They will also notify the relevant authorities, such as the **Care Quality Commission (CQC)**.

Whistleblowing

All health and social care practitioners have a **duty of care** to report all unsafe and illegal practices, including discrimination. If discrimination is reported at work and no action is taken by the manager or employer (or their actions are unsatisfactory) then their concerns can be reported to someone more senior in the organisation, such as a Director or the Care Quality Commission. All information shared will be treated as confidential.

Legislation is in place to protect whistleblowers' rights to not be discriminated against in the workplace. This is so that they will not be negatively affected as a result of reporting discrimination. Health and social care

practitioners must follow their organisation's procedures for **whistleblowing**.

Modelling

The working approaches and practices that health and social care practitioners use can have a huge impact on the likelihood of discrimination occurring again. For example, health and social care practitioners can model good practice to others they work with through positive behaviours that are fair, non-discriminatory and that value and respect individuals' rights and differences. As you will have already learned in this section of the unit, modelling positive approaches is also necessary when health and social care practitioners respond to discrimination. This is so that others will understand that discrimination will always be challenged and never tolerated. Modelling good practice is essential so that everyone is treated fairly and equally regardless of their differences.

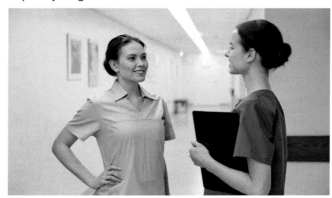

Figure 1.4 How can you be a good role model?

Key terms

Agreed ways of working are the working practices that are followed in a work setting, including policies and procedures.

Care Quality Commission (CQC) is the regulator of all health and social care services in England.

Disciplined refers to the action taken by an employer against an employee when their behaviour and/or work does not meet expected standards.

Duty of care refers to the health and social care practitioner's legal obligation to ensure the safety and well-being of individuals and others, such as their colleagues and visitors, while providing care and support.

Reflect refers to when a person evaluates their experiences, which can relate to their personal life and/or work to improve and change how they act, think and behave.

Whistleblowing refers to reporting any information or activity that is deemed illegal or unethical, such as unsafe practices or abuse.

Training

Training courses on equality, diversity and inclusion raise people's awareness, developing their understanding of behaviours and how these impact on others, including how to change them. Training also provides useful information about, for example, the legislation in place for challenging discrimination. It provides opportunities for having discussions with others and reflecting on occasions when discrimination has been challenged, as well as the approaches that were used and which ones were effective. Training may also include reviewing and discussing with colleagues **agreed ways of working** and relevant policies and procedures that are in place

Description Activity

Select one type of discrimination that you have learned about. Describe two different approaches you could use to challenge this type of discrimination positively.

2.3 How the health and social care practitioner's own values, beliefs and experiences can influence delivery of care

Health and social care practitioners have their own values, beliefs and experiences that will form part of who they are, and may therefore affect how they carry out their job roles. Health and social care practitioners work with many different people who will also have their own values, beliefs and experiences that may be similar or different to theirs. It is for this reason that they need to be aware of how their own values, beliefs and experiences can impact on their working practices, so that they do not obstruct the quality of the work, care and support that they provide.

Self-awareness

It is very important for health and social care practitioners to be aware of their own values, beliefs and experiences and how these may affect their work practices. This

is to ensure that they do not have a negative impact on the delivery of care and support. Self-awareness involves health and social care practitioners being:

- **honest** about their own values, beliefs and experiences
- **willing** to recognise their own prejudices
- **understanding** of how their own values, beliefs and experiences may impact on the delivery of care.

Self-awareness can be increased through the reflection process, discussing with individuals and others they work with, and meeting with their manager or employer. For example, a health and social care practitioner may have completed an apprenticeship as part of their training and value this type of study more than a university education. As part of the reflection process, they may consider how this might affect how they work with individuals. For example, an individual in their care might need support when choosing a university they would like to go to. What could the health and social care practitioner do to stop their values and experience from affecting the support they provide to the individual? Perhaps they might not share their own values and experience of an apprenticeship with the individual, so that they do not influence the individual's views about going to university. They might also make sure they present all of the relevant information about university courses in an impartial way, so that the individual can make their own informed choices.

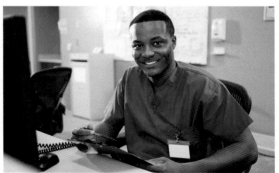

Figure 1.5 How honest are you about how your beliefs impact on others?

Acknowledging belief systems, attitudes and behaviours

Recognising that health and social care practitioners' belief systems, **attitudes** and **behaviours** may be different to those of individuals will allow them to value and respect individuals' differences and take these into account when providing care and support. They may agree or disagree with others' beliefs, but it is important that they accept that others are entitled to hold those beliefs just as they are entitled to their own. Acknowledging belief systems, attitudes and behaviours therefore involves health and social care practitioners being:

- aware of their own **prejudices**
- able to reflect on their own prejudices
- accepting of individuals' unique differences that are the basis of how they live their lives (even if they are different to their own)
- understanding of individuals' rights to hold their own belief systems, attitudes and behaviours.

Key terms

Attitudes are the ways an individual expresses what they think or believe through what they say or do.

Behaviours are the ways in which an individual acts physically and emotionally, for example self-harming or not eating, including when interacting with others.

Prejudices are the negative opinions that you may have of someone, which are not based on experience of interaction.

Acknowledging belief systems, attitudes and behaviours is not always easy. This requires being able to reflect on feedback received from others, for example:

- A health and social care practitioner may be vegan and might openly discuss the benefits of being vegan as a lifestyle choice, since they do not harm or exploit any animals.

- Talking about their personal beliefs may make individuals who are not vegan feel uncomfortable about eating meat or wearing leather when the health and social care practitioner is present.

- It is therefore important for the health and social care practitioner to acknowledge how their own beliefs may influence others in a negative way. They should reflect on how they could take steps to avoid doing so. For example, they could not talk about their beliefs at work and think carefully about how and what they say, so that individuals do not feel awkward or under pressure when they are around them.

- They could also reflect on the positive and negative feelings they have about different groups of people and think about how these could affect their work. They could discuss these with their manager so that the care and support provided is of a high quality and any prejudices can be addressed.

Influence of factors on own belief system, attitudes and behaviours

Our belief systems, attitudes and behaviours are formed throughout our lives from early childhood to late adulthood. They can be influenced by factors, such as:

The media

What we see on the television, hear on the radio and read about online or in newspapers can influence our beliefs, attitudes and behaviours. For example:

- If you watch a television documentary about how individuals who live alone may be more vulnerable to abuse, then you might be more aware of any neighbours you have who are living on their own, ensuring that you are more vigilant.

- If you hear on the radio that there has been an increase in the number of burglaries in a particular area, then you may believe that the area is unsafe. You might decide to avoid the area and recommend to others that they do the same.

- If you read in an online article that a group of people who live in your area have raised money to keep the local library open, then you might be more likely to visit the library and tell others to do so too.

Family

Family members can be very important to us, especially when influencing our beliefs, attitudes and behaviours. For example, if a close family member believes that eating well and exercising regularly helps them to stay healthy, then this may influence the lifestyle choices that you make.

If you are surrounded by people who behave positively, then this will influence how you think about yourself and others. For example, you may find that you believe in your own potential and are not afraid to share your ideas and opinions with others.

Similarly, if you are surrounded by people who show negative behaviours, then this may also influence your thoughts and attitudes towards others. You may, for example, not trust others or behave in an unfair way towards them.

Peer pressure

Your peers are those who you relate to and who know you well. They might also influence your beliefs, attitudes and behaviours because you may feel under pressure to be like them or remain part of the peer group. For example, you may believe in following a healthy lifestyle that includes not drinking alcohol. However, if all your peers drink alcohol when you go out together, you may feel under pressure to do so too. What you think, say and feel may also be affected by your peers. For example, if your peers at work talk about the positive effects that person-centred ways of working can have on individuals' lives, then you may be more

likely to practise these when you provide care and support.

Being aware of how your beliefs, attitudes and behaviours are formed can affect the way you think, feel and behave towards others. It will enable you to ensure that they do not have a negative impact on the care and support you provide to individuals.

Professional versus personal

All health and social care practitioners are professionals. Therefore, they have important **responsibilities** and sets of behaviours that they are expected to follow. These are essential for providing safe, consistent and high-quality care and support and may include, for example, supporting individuals to make their own choices and respecting their rights.

Sometimes, there may be a conflict between the set of behaviours health and social care practitioners are expected to follow and their own beliefs and behaviours. For example, there may be an individual who is obese and has care and support needs. As a professional, a health and social care practitioner must respect the individual's choice to live their life how they want to. So, if the individual chooses not to follow a healthier lifestyle after being informed about the potential consequences on their health, then the health and social care practitioner must respect this. This may be very difficult to do, especially if the health and social care practitioner believes that following a healthy lifestyle is important and essential for well-being. Perhaps the health and social care practitioner believes this because they have experienced the negative impact this had on a close family member.

To ensure this does not impact negatively on the care provided, the health and social care practitioner must:

- be aware of the differences between their own professional and personal values, beliefs and experiences

- be aware of the professional and personal values, beliefs and experiences of others
- respect the values, beliefs and experiences of others, even if they are different to their own.

Key term

Responsibilities are obligations that are required when carrying out your duties and care at work.

Respect and value diversity

As you will have learned, a health and social care practitioner's day-to-day practices are influenced by their own values, beliefs and experiences and you have been able to consider the importance of appreciating such influences in order to work professionally. The legal and organisational requirements that are in place mean that health and social care practitioners must always treat individuals with dignity and respect when providing care and support. For example, they can do this by treating individuals fairly, respecting their privacy and promoting their independence. Other examples of the ways that health and social care practitioners can show that they recognise, value and respect diversity, include:

- valuing the differences individuals have by encouraging individuals to be their own unique person
- respecting individuals' rights to make their own choices by providing the individual with the information they need
- treating individuals with dignity by valuing their beliefs and preferences while being respectful towards them.

It is important that health and social care practitioners can work in ways that show respect and value diversity, because it is essential for:

- providing safe, compassionate and high-quality care and support
- developing good working relationships with individuals that are based on trust

- developing a good understanding of individuals' differences and person-centred care.

Explain Activity

Identify the values, beliefs and experiences that a health and social care practitioner may have. Explain how these may have been formed using examples. Explain, using examples, the different ways that these can influence the provision of care to individuals in positive ways.

Check your understanding 2

1 Give one example of direct discrimination.
2 Describe how whistleblowing can be used to challenge discrimination.
3 Describe how others can influence a health and social care practitioner's beliefs.

LO3 Understand person-centred practice

3.1 The concept of person-centred practice

Your values are unique to you and contribute to what makes you different to others, such as your family and friends. Because your values are important to you, they will also influence the day-to-day choices and decisions you make.

The care and support you provide will also be underpinned by a set of values that are commonly referred to as 'person-centred values'. Applying these values to your practice will ensure that the care and support you provide is high quality and personalised to each individual. You will learn more about these in AC3.2.

Individual central

Person-centred practice involves placing the individual you care for or support at the centre of everything you do. You can do this by focusing the care and support you provide on the individual's:

- **Strengths** – find out what a person is good at or their unique personality traits in order to respect their individual differences. For example, you may find out that they have a keen interest in sports or observe that they have a very enthusiastic personality. Therefore, you could encourage them to participate in new or alternative sports-based activities and provide opportunities for them to meet other people.

- **Abilities** – focus on what an individual can do rather than what they can't. This will help to empower them and feel in control of their care and support, as they can then lead on their day-to-day decisions. For example, an individual is able to get dressed without any support or can walk for longer distances by using a walking frame. Therefore, you could encourage the individual to continue to get dressed independently or support them to use their walking frame.

- **Needs** – find out what an individual's needs are by asking them and/or those who know them well, such as their family and friends. This means you can support an individual based on their needs, rather than on what you *think* they may need. For example, an individual might say they don't feel confident cooking on their own. Therefore, you could support them by helping them and demonstrating different ways to follow a recipe, so they feel more confident doing this independently.

- **Wishes** – find out what an individual's hopes and wishes are to enable them to feel understood as a person. For example, you could support the individual by helping them to use the internet to book their holiday online and to research the facilities available in the country they wish to travel to, such as disabled access at the airport and at the hotel. Therefore, you could discuss with the individual what support they need in order to plan, carry out and achieve their wishes.

- **Preferences** – find out what an individual's preferences are so you can tailor your care and support to that specific individual. For example, they might ask you what you think they should wear because they don't think they can make good choices on their own. Therefore, you could ask the individual what clothes they like to wear and why, whether they have any favourite items of clothing and if there are any colours in particular they like.

Individual in control

Person-centred practice not only keeps the individual at the centre of their own care and support but also involves supporting the individual to be in control of their life. This also relates to the decisions they make on a day-to-day basis. Imagine how you would feel if others made your decisions for you, or if others ignored your views and opinions. How would this make you feel? Why?

You can ensure that the care and support you provide enables individuals to:

- live as independently as possible and to do as much for themselves as they can. Not doing so denies individuals their right to make their own choices and live their lives the way they want to.

- understand their rights and the support they are entitled to. Not doing so prevents individuals from being in control of their care and support. This might potentially lead to them being discriminated against by being treated unfairly.

- assess the risks they may face. Not doing so prevents individuals from living as independently as possible. You will learn more about how to support individuals to manage risks safely in AC3.2.

- feel that they are respected and valued. Not doing so prevents individuals from developing feelings of self-worth and self-respect that are essential for being in control of their lives.

Working in person-centred ways means that you can contribute to an individual's care and support positively, focusing on their unique needs, wishes and preferences.

Define Activity

Create a poster that defines the concept of person-centred practice. Include examples that support the meaning of person-centred practice.

3.2 How person-centred practice is used to support individuals

Informed choices

You will already know that person-centred practice involves respecting individuals' choices and decisions. To do so, you must provide the individual with the information they need in order to understand the choices and decisions they are making. This information must be presented in a format that they understand. You can only do this if you know the individual's communication needs, i.e. using pictures, speaking in short phrases, etc. You will learn more about how to support individuals with tailored communication later on in this section.

You should also provide individuals with sufficient information about their options when making choices, including the benefits and drawbacks, so that they fully understand the consequences of their decisions. This is referred to as making 'informed choices'.

For example, you can support an individual who wants to go out one evening to make informed choices by discussing with the individual:

- where they want to go out (e.g. to a place they know, or somewhere different or new)
- what they want to do (e.g. go out for a meal, to the cinema, etc.)
- when they want to go out (e.g. morning, afternoon, early or late evening)
- how they want to get there (e.g. taxi or public transport)
- the benefits of going somewhere they know (e.g. they will know how to get there; they will be in familiar surroundings, etc.) and the drawbacks (e.g. they might get bored; the surroundings may have changed since they last went there, etc.)
- the benefits of going somewhere new or different (e.g. it's an opportunity to meet new people or do something different) and the drawbacks (e.g. they might find it uncomfortable to go somewhere different or not like it at all)
- the benefits of using different transport methods (e.g. a taxi means they will arrive at the destination safely; public transport is cheap) and the drawbacks (e.g. a taxi has to be booked for a specific time; public transport may not be as reliable).
- the risks of going somewhere new and how to manage them (e.g. letting someone know where you are, knowing public transport times, etc.). You will learn more about how to support individuals to manage risks later on in this section.

Dignity and respect

Person-centred practice is used to support individuals' **dignity** and respect. This way of working involves health and social care practitioners:

- treating individuals well (i.e. speaking to an individual respectfully and treating them with care)
- showing respect (i.e. listening to and taking into account an individual's rights, views and wishes)
- valuing individuals (i.e. treating them as an individual person with their own needs and preferences)

- promoting individuals' sense of self-worth (i.e. enabling an individual to take risks
- empowering individuals to be in control (i.e. supporting an individual to take the lead and be actively involved in decisions about their care and support).

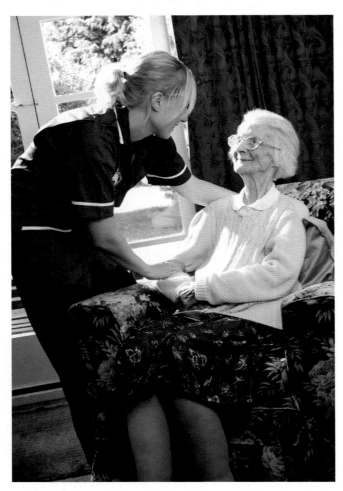

Figure 1.6 Do you know how to support an individual's dignity?

Care planning

Person-centred practice involves applying person-centred values when providing care and support to individuals. A care plan is also sometimes referred to as a support plan or individual plan. It includes information about an individual's specific preferences for their care and support. Care plans can be developed and updated by the individual along with others who know them well, such as a family member. Your manager will then look at the care plan, assess and approve it.

A care plan includes the following information about the individual:

- personal details (e.g. name, date of birth, address)
- their preferences (e.g. likes, dislikes, interests, wishes, hopes)
- their needs (e.g. care and support needs)
- their support network (e.g. the names and contact details of family, those providing care and support).

A care plan can be used to support individuals as part of person-centred practice. This is because it includes information about the individual's:

- ability to manage certain activities by themselves. It focuses on their strengths to encourage them to be as independent as possible.
- need for support. It enables the individual to be fully involved and lead their care and support to achieve what they want to do.
- unique needs, preferences and wishes so that their individuality can be fully supported.

 Case scenario

Kimberley has a learning and physical disability and requires support at meal times. Kimberley is worried about sharing a table with others at meal times, because she feels embarrassed that she needs support with both eating and drinking.

1. Describe how to promote Kimberley's dignity and respect.
2. Describe how to support Kimberley with making informed choices at meal times.
3. Explain how Kimberley's care plan can be used to support her at meal times.

Tailored communication

Good communication that is tailored to the individual is essential for providing person-centred care and support. It ensures that you can understand and value the individual for who they are as a person. This can help to build trust and respect, allowing the individual to feel at ease with you.

Health and social care practitioners can support individuals through tailored communication by first getting to know them so that they can build up a picture of who they are (e.g. by speaking with the individual and/or those who know them such as their family, advocate and other health and social care practitioners). In this way, they can find out about their:

- childhood experiences
- family and cultural background
- beliefs and values
- care and support required to meet their needs.

Collating all this information about the individual takes time. It may involve not only speaking to individuals and/or those who know them, but also reviewing other records such as individuals' care plans, communication records, photographs or images.

All individuals have different ways of communicating. Tailored communication enables health and social care practitioners to communicate with the individual in their preferred way that meets their communication and language needs, wishes and preferences. For example, you can use tailored communication with an individual with:

- a **hearing impairment** – for example, by using **British Sign Language (BSL)** or an **interpreter** to ensure the individual is fully involved in the communication, understands what is being communicated and is able to express what they want to communicate. In addition, the individual may use specialist equipment such as hearing aids or **hearing loops** to communicate with others.

- dementia – for example, by using short phrases, avoiding asking too many questions or using unfamiliar language that may confuse the individual or prevent them from understanding what you are communicating. In addition, the individual may benefit from you giving them sufficient time to respond to your communications, as they might process the information they're receiving from you slowly.

- a **learning disability –** for example, by communicating with them using their preferred language. Examples include **Makaton**, a language that uses a combination of signs, symbols and spoken language or the **Picture exchange communication system (PECS),** a non-verbal communication system that uses symbols and pictures.

Tailored communication also involves being able to communicate effectively with individuals in different situations by observing their responses. This is so that you can understand how they are feeling and communicate with them in a way that shows your support and **compassion.** For example, if an individual appears to be upset, then you can show your support and compassion by asking them if there is anything you can do to help. Similarly, if an individual appears angry, then you can show your support and compassion by communicating to them that you can see that they're angry. You could ask them whether they would like you to give them some time on their own to calm down. It is important to remember that every individual is a unique person and therefore their communication preferences will be personalised.

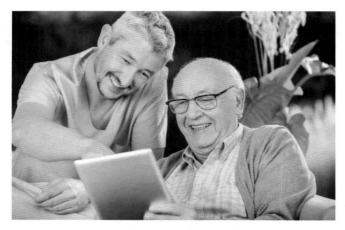

Figure 1.7 What does tailored communication look like?

Consent

When providing individuals with care and support, you must have their agreement to do so in order to comply with legislation such as the Mental Capacity Act 2005. You must provide them with the information required to ensure that they understand: this is referred to as 'informed **consent**'. Obtaining individuals' consent when providing care or support is important for working in a person-centred way, because it:

- respects individuals' rights by enabling them to make their own choices and decisions
- places individuals at the centre of their care and support by enabling them to be in control
- promotes individuals' dignity by allowing them to take and manage risks.

Key terms

British Sign Language (BSL) is the sign language used in the UK by individuals who have a hearing impairment. It uses a combination of hand gestures, facial expressions and body language. It is a different language to English with its own grammar and sentence construction.

Compassion refers to delivering care and support with kindness, consideration, dignity and respect.

Dignity involves respecting individuals' choices, views and decisions and not making assumptions about how they want to be treated.

Hearing impairment is a hearing loss that may occur in one or both ears. This can be partial (some loss) or a complete loss of hearing.

Hearing loops are the sound systems used by individuals who use hearing aids. They provide a wireless signal that is picked up directly by the hearing aid, thus minimising any unwanted background noise.

Interpreter is a professional who converts spoken/oral or sign language communication from one language to another. Interpreters must be good listeners and be able to process and memorise words and gestures while individuals are communicating.

Learning disability can be defined as a reduced ability to think and make decisions, along with difficulties coping with everyday activities, which affect a person for their whole life. For example, an individual with a learning disability may experience problems with budgeting, shopping and planning a train journey.

Makaton is a language programme to support spoken language. It is a method of communication using signs, symbols and speech, following the order of spoken words, that is used by individuals who have learning disabilities.

Person-centred practice refers to a way of working that takes into account the individual's whole person and focuses on their unique needs, abilities, preferences and wishes.

Picture exchange communication system (PECS) is a non-verbal method of communication using symbols and pictures.

For example, you can obtain the informed consent of an individual who requires support with eating and drinking by:

- asking the individual how they want to be supported. This could be in relation to preparing themselves to eat and drink (washing their hands); during eating and drinking (cutting food up into manageable pieces); and after eating and drinking (ensuring the area where they've been is left clean).

- discussing with the individual what the support will involve. This could involve responding to the individual's questions and concerns.

- supporting the individual to be in control. This involves supporting the individual to make their own choices and respecting their choices even if you disagree with them.

You may find it useful to review your previous learning in AC3.2 of this unit on what is involved in supporting individuals with informed choices and how this is part of informed consent. Sometimes, it may not be possible for an individual to give their consent because they **lack the capacity** to do so. In these circumstances, a representative such as an advocate may decide on the individual's behalf, providing they act in the individual's best interests. You should speak to the individual's advocate but, in the first instance, you must make every effort to consult the individual.

At other times, it may not be possible to establish consent with an individual. This might be because the individual is undecided or you cannot guarantee whether the individual has given their consent. If this occurs, then you could:

- have another discussion with the individual where you explain the process again. Discuss the benefits, drawbacks, risks and how to manage them.

- seek advice from a more senior colleague, your manager or employer. They may be able to provide further guidance as to what to do to promote good quality care and support.

- consult with the individual's representative where you can discuss your concerns. You will need to check with your manager or employer that this is possible, as this information about the individual is personal and therefore protected when shared with others.

If you still cannot establish consent with an individual, even after trying all these options, then you might have to accept that it is not possible. Your manager or employer may have to seek advice from external organisations such as the courts, who can provide legal clarification, and **Professional Councils** who can provide additional support.

🔑 Key terms

Consent refers to an informed agreement to an action or decision.

Lack the capacity refers to when an individual is unable to make a decision for themselves because of a learning disability or a condition, such as dementia, a mental health need or because they are unconscious.

Professional Councils are organisations that regulate professions, such as adult social care workers who work with adults in residential care homes, in day centres and who provide care in someone's home. They can provide advice and support around working with individuals who lack capacity to make decisions.

Risk management

Taking risks is part of day-to-day life. Individuals who have care and support needs will also have the same rights as everyone else to take risks. Supporting individuals to take risks is an essential part of person-centred practice because it can impact on individuals positively, helping them to fulfil their potential and live their life in the way that they want. You will learn more about the positive impacts of person-centred practice on individuals in AC3.3.

Health and social care practitioners can support individuals through person-centred practice to manage risks positively. They can do this by discussing the risks with the individual; explaining what the risks are; how they can be managed safely; and how not to cause any harm. It is also important for health and social care practitioners to empower individuals to take risks so that they can build their resilience and grow in confidence.

For example, an individual might enjoy going for walks but is at risk of falling. You can support them by:

- identifying the risks with the individual (e.g. falling over, slipping, tripping)
- managing the risks safely (e.g. ensuring they go out for walks only when supported by someone else or by using a walking aid)
- exploring the benefits of taking the risks (e.g. walking is good exercise, which is beneficial for their health and overall well-being)
- exploring the consequences of not taking the risks (e.g. their mobility may deteriorate over time).

Evidence Activity

Identify the needs of an individual who requires care and support: this can be a fictitious person or someone you know. Remember not to use any real names if it's someone you know to protect the individual's confidentiality.

Describe how person-centred practice is used to support the individual to make their own informed choices and manage risks safely.

3.3 Impacts of person-centred practice on individuals

Person-centred practice impacts positively on individuals and their lives and, for this reason, it underpins all high-quality care and support delivered by health and social care practitioners. **Table 1.4** includes some examples of the positive impacts of person-centred practice on individuals:

Table 1.4 Impacts of person-centred practice on individuals

Impacts of person-centred practice on individuals	Examples of the benefits
Meets individual needs (social, emotional, cognitive and physical)	- Social needs – individuals are encouraged to take an active part in their own care and support, which might include trying out new activities, going out to different places, meeting people, making friends or developing existing relationships. - Emotional needs – individuals are encouraged to express their views, preferences and what they are thinking and feeling. Individuals need to know that they are being listened to, taken seriously and have their emotional needs met. - Cognitive needs – person-centred practice supports individuals to develop their knowledge and understanding of their own ideas and thoughts, for example by providing them with opportunities to learn and think so that they are mentally stimulated. - Physical needs – person-centred practice encourages individuals to do as much for themselves as possible, for example by encouraging them to develop their mobility skills when performing everyday tasks, such as walking and sitting upright, and their hand skills when brushing their teeth and eating with a knife and fork.

Impacts of person-centred practice on individuals	Examples of the benefits
Individual rights	• Dignity – promote individuals' self-respect by enabling them to do as much for themselves as possible and be fully involved in all choices and decisions that impact their lives. • Respect – promote ways of working that are respectful, treating individuals as their own person with their unique strengths, beliefs, needs and preferences. • Fulfil their capacity – enable individuals to identify their strengths, abilities, needs and the support they require to live the lives they want and to achieve their hopes and wishes.
Independence	Person-centred practice: • enables individuals to become more reliant on themselves rather than on others, such as health and social care practitioners and their families. This is to reduce their dependency on others. • encourages individuals to focus on their own strengths and abilities and on what they can do rather than on what they can't. This helps the individual to increase their confidence and become more independent. • empowers individuals to learn new skills and have different experiences, accessing the support they require to become more independent.
Decision-making and confidence	• Making their own choices and decisions helps individuals to feel more in control of their lives and therefore more confident in their own abilities. • Person-centred practice helps to focus on the individual and their preferences, which underpins their overall well-being. • Individuals also learn how to take and manage risks, developing their self-esteem by increasing confidence in their own worth and abilities.
Health and well-being	Person-centred practice can: • lead to good health and overall well-being because it focuses on the person as a whole along with their individual traits. • impact positively on an individual's cultural requirements because it involves understanding their personal history and family background. Taking a genuine interest in who the individual is will increase their sense of self-worth and therefore promote their well-being. • impact positively on individuals' mental health and well-being because it is a way of working that supports individuals to think positively and develop helpful ways of managing risks and responding to their feelings as well as new and different situations.

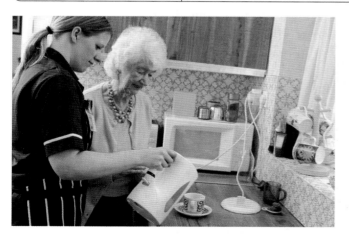

Figure 1.8 Do you know how to support an individual's independence?

> ### Classroom Discussion
>
> Discuss the importance of person-centred practice when providing care and support to individuals. Give examples of the benefits of person-centred practice to individuals.

3.4 Ethical dilemmas that may arise when balancing individuals' rights and duty of care

All health and social care practitioners are legally required to have a duty of care towards the individuals that they care for and support. This means that they must:

- always act in the best interests of individuals when carrying out their responsibilities. They must support an individual's rights to privacy, dignity and respect.

- make sure that individuals are not placed in any danger and are kept safe from harm. They must report any changes in an individual's behaviour that concerns them.

- always take action to prevent harm to individuals. Thy must discuss any risks with an individual, including the benefits and drawbacks of taking the risks.

- only carry out the work tasks that they are able to and have the required knowledge and skills to do so. They must be aware of their responsibilities and the agreed ways of working that must be followed.

Not maintaining the duty of care to individuals can have serious consequences, which **Figure 1.9** illustrates.

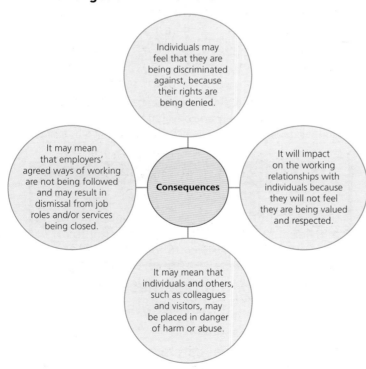

Figure 1.9 Consequences of health and social care practitioners not maintaining their duty of care

Sometimes, ethical dilemmas or conflicts may arise between the duty of care and individuals' rights because:

- health and social care practitioners' responsibility to fulfil their duty of care may be in direct conflict with an individual's rights

- individuals may not understand the duty of care health and social care practitioners have towards them and/or others

- individuals and health and social care practitioners may not be able to agree on how to manage a risk safely.

Confidentiality

Confidentiality is important for person-centred practice because health and social care practitioners must always respect individuals' personal information, their rights to privacy and only share individuals' personal information with others when there is a reason to do so. Sometimes, ethical dilemmas can arise because although individuals have the right to have all personal information held about them kept private, there may be occasions when the duty of care requires health and social care practitioners to share confidential information with others who need to know. This process is referred to as sharing confidential information on a '**need-to-know**' basis. For example, this may be when an individual requires hospital treatment or an individual discloses that they are being abused. In both these situations, not sharing confidential information may result in the individual's condition deteriorating and/or the individual continuing to be harmed.

Health and social care practitioners can ensure they follow person-centred practice when sharing individuals' confidential information by:

- informing the individual. In some cases, the individual's consent may also need to be obtained to ensure that their rights to dignity and respect are being maintained.

- informing the individual's representative when the individual lacks capacity and is unable to give their consent. This is to ensure that they are acting in the individual's best interests.

- checking the identity of those requesting confidential information and the purpose of their request. This is to ensure that only information that is necessary and relevant is shared.

- following their employer's agreed ways of working for confidentiality. This will include how, when and from whom to seek advice, in order to ensure they are complying with their responsibilities.

Key term

Need-to-know refers to the process of sharing confidential information with others who need it, i.e. when an individual discloses that they are being harmed.

Managing values and beliefs

Ethical dilemmas may also arise when individuals' values and beliefs conflict with health and social care practitioners' duty of care. For example, an individual may have a strong belief that a poor diet will not damage their health, because their father ate many processed foods and lived until he was 94 years of age. The individual is entitled to have their own beliefs and make their own choices, but at the same time, the health and social care practitioner is required to promote the individual's health and well-being. In this situation, the health and social care practitioner could state that they respect the individual's choices and beliefs, but still inform the individual of the potential negative effects of a poor diet on their health and provide them with information about the benefits of eating well.

Risk taking

Taking risks, although essential for person-centred practice, can also lead to ethical

dilemmas arising between health and social care practitioners' responsibilities to maintain individuals' safety while also promoting their right to take risks. For example, an individual with a learning disability may have considered all the potential benefits and drawbacks of going on holiday on their own. They might decide that they do want to go on their own and they have the capacity to make this decision. The health and social care practitioner must respect their right to make their own decisions and cannot prevent them from going on holiday alone. In this situation, the health and social care practitioner could fulfil their duty of care by suggesting different ways to stay safe, such as not meeting up with people who they don't know in an isolated place and only going to places that have been recommended by their tour guide.

Rights versus responsibilities

Supporting individuals' rights can at times conflict with the responsibilities that health and social care practitioners are required to carry out as part of their duty of care. For example, an individual who has early stages of dementia may want to continue to go shopping on their own. If they have the capacity to make this decision, then it is their right to maintain their independence for as long as they are able to and cannot be prevented from doing so. In this situation, the health and social care practitioner could explain to the individual their responsibility for ensuring their safety when going out. They could agree on measures that they could put in place together, such as the individual letting them know where they're going and how long they will be out for.

Overcoming ethical dilemmas that may arise between individuals' rights and the duty of care requires health and social care practitioners to be sensitive and skilful in using person-centred practice.

Description Activity

Identify a situation that may cause an ethical dilemma to arise when balancing an individual's rights and the duty of care.

Describe what the ethical dilemma is and outline the different ways to manage the individual's rights and the health and social care practitioner's responsibilities.

 ## Check your understanding 3

1 Give one example of how person-centred practice is used to support individuals.
2 Describe how person-centred practice can influence an individual's independence.
3 Describe an ethical dilemma that may arise between an individual's rights and the duty of care.

Read about it

Care Quality Commission [2018] 'Equally outstanding Equality and human rights – good practice resource', Care Quality Commission

Skills for Care [2018] 'Good and outstanding care guide – updated', Skills for Care

Care Quality Commission (CQC) – (information about the Mental Capacity Code of Practice) www.cqc.org.uk/sites/default/files/Mental%20Capacity%20Act%20Code%20of%20Practice.pdf

Care Quality Commission (CQC) – (information about whistleblowing) www.cqc.org.uk/contact-us/report-concern/report-concern-if-you-are-member-staff

Equality and Human Rights Commission – (information about the European Convention on Human Rights) www.equalityhumanrights.com/en/what-european-convention-human-rights

Equality and Human Rights Commission – (information about the Equality Act 2010) www.equalityhumanrights.com/en/equality-act-2010/what-equality-act

Equality and Human Rights Commission – (information about types of discrimination) www.equalityhumanrights.com/en/advice-and-guidance/age-discrimination

Government Equalities Office – (information about equality legislation and policy) www.gov.uk/government/organisations/government-equalities-office

Skills for Care – (information about the Code of Conduct for Healthcare Support Workers and Adult Social Care Workers in England) www.skillsforcare.org.uk/Documents/Standards-legislation/Code-of-Conduct/Code-of-Conduct.pdf

The British Institute of Human Rights – (information about the Human Rights Act 1998) www.bihr.org.uk/thehumanrightsact

UNICEF – (information about the United Nations Convention on the Rights of the Child 1989) www.unicef.org.uk/what-we-do/un-convention-child-rights/

How will I be graded?

The table below shows what learners must do to achieve each grading criterion. Learners must achieve all the criteria for a grade to be awarded. A higher grade may not be awarded before a lower grade has been achieved, although component criteria of a higher grade may have been achieved.

Grade	Assessment Criteria number	Assessment of learning/What you need to show
D1	1.1	The terms: • equality • diversity • inclusion. Examples may be used to support the definitions.
D2	1.2	Outline one (1) piece of legislation, policy, procedure or code of practice in relation to equality, diversity and inclusion.
D3	1.3	Describe how the health and social care practitioner contributes to inclusive practice. Examples may be used to support the description.
D4		A minimum of one (1) relevant and traceable reference must be included.
C1	2.1	Summarise types of discrimination. A minimum of three (3) types of discrimination must be summarised.
C2	2.2	Describe approaches to challenge discrimination. A minimum of two (2) approaches used to challenge discrimination must be described.
C3	3.1	Define the concept of person-centred practice. Examples must be used to support the definition.
B1	2.3	Explain how the health and social care practitioner's own values, beliefs and experiences can influence delivery of care.
B2	3.2	Describe how person-centred practice is used to support individuals.
B3		A minimum of two (2) relevant and traceable references must be included. A reference list must be included.
A1	3.3	Discuss impacts of person-centred practice on individuals. A minimum of four (4) impacts of person-centred practice on individuals must be discussed.
A*1	3.4	Describe ethical dilemmas that may arise when balancing individuals' rights and duty of care. A minimum of one (1) ethical dilemma that may arise when balancing an individual's rights and duty of care must be described.
A*2		References must be present throughout to show evidence of knowledge and understanding gained from wider reading. References must be relevant and traceable.
		Current legislation as relevant to Home Nation.

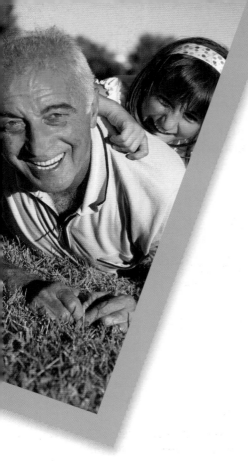

HSC M2
Human growth and development

About this unit

The human lifespan is a period of immense change. We start as helpless babies and depend on others for our survival. If we are fortunate, we go on to grow and develop through childhood and adolescence to become mature independent adults, capable of caring for ourselves and others until the ageing process takes its toll. In old age, we may again become dependent on others for our care. In this unit, you will learn about the stages of human growth and development and what influences them. You will look at some significant life events, from infancy to late adulthood, including the impact that these life events might have on the individual. Finally, you will learn how health and social care services in the UK support people throughout their lives.

Learning Outcomes

LO1: Understand human growth and development across the lifespan.

1.1 The life stages of human growth and development:

- infancy
- childhood
- adolescence
- early, middle, late adulthood.

1.2 Social, emotional, cognitive and physical development within each life stage:

- social – relationships, independence, cultural
- emotional – attachment, emotional resilience, self-image, self-esteem
- cognitive – language, memory, reasoning, thinking, problem-solving
- physical – early developments, physical health, puberty, ageing process.

1.3 Holistic development:

- interdependency of each developmental area: social, emotional, cognitive, physical.

LO2: Understand influences which impact upon human growth and development.

2.1 The nature versus nurture debate in relation to human growth and development:

- Nature: genetic, inherited characteristics and biological influences related to human development and behaviour.
- Nurture: environmental influences related to human development and behaviour.

2.2 The medical model of health and well-being:

- biological/physical, diagnosis, treatment, cure.

The social model of health and well-being:

- individual experience, social perception, equality, inclusion, participation.

→

2.3 Factors which impact upon human growth and development:

- biological
- lifestyle
- health
- education
- employment
- socio-economic
- culture
- environment
- relationships
- bullying
- aspirations.

2.4 The importance of recognising and responding to concerns regarding an individual's growth and development:

- intervention
- promote health and well-being
- meet individual needs
- meet the needs of others.

LO3: Understand significant life events across the lifespan.

3.1 Significant life events across the life stages:

- infancy — separation, nursery, weaning, toilet training
- childhood — school, siblings, moving home
- adolescence — puberty, relationships, leaving home
- early, middle, late adulthood — employment, co-habitation/marriage, parenthood, divorce, bereavement, retirement, age-related medical conditions, adapting to elderly care.

3.2 The impact that significant life events may have on an individual:

- emotion
- relationships
- independence
- health
- resilience.

LO4: Understand how health and social care services meet the care needs of individuals through the lifespan.

4.1 Care needs of individuals through the life stages:

- infancy
- childhood
- adolescence
- early, middle, late adulthood.

4.2 How health and social care services meet the care needs of individuals through the life stages:

- local authorities
- hospitals
- General Practitioner services
- day centres
- children's centres
- residential
- community
- rehabilitation
- counselling
- charities.

LO1 Understand human growth and development across the lifespan

Human **growth** refers to size, for example getting bigger or taller over time. Growth is stimulated or delayed by the amount of growth hormone produced by the pituitary gland in the centre of the skull at the base of the brain. Humans grow to varying sizes. However, it is possible to grow but not develop, for example a baby born with brain damage may grow into an adult, but not develop the skills needed to live independently and never learn how to walk or talk.

Development refers to gradually increasing ability in physical, social, **cognitive** and emotional skills and knowledge over time. A baby learns to walk, understand its first language, smile, talk, and love those who care for it. These are often called **developmental milestones**. It is possible to develop but not grow, for example some people have the genetic condition achondroplasia due to a faulty chromosome. This condition is also called restricted growth, or dwarfism. They do not physically grow to the usual adult height but can develop the skills needed to live independent, happy and fulfilling lives. Ellie Simmonds, the Paralympian Gold Medallist swimmer has achondroplasia, as does Warwick Davis, the actor and comedian.

1.1 The life stages of human growth and development

Life stages are the different phases of life that all individuals go through. These are infancy, childhood, adolescence and adulthood. Each stage is divided into smaller ones, for example early childhood and late childhood. These stages are not fixed and can vary from culture to culture. In some societies, puberty marks the start of adulthood and 65 years is considered to be very old. In other societies, adulthood is delayed until the early twenties, and people are expected to work until 67 years old.

Life begins with dependency. Babies depend on others for their survival. We gain more independence as we develop, and adulthood is the time when it is expected that we are independent. In old age, we may again become dependent on others.

Infancy

Infancy is from birth to two years. During this time the baby grows and develops a lot, using its senses to learn about the world. Infants cry to communicate their needs and parents soon learn the difference between cries of hunger and cries of boredom. During this stage, the infant is keen to explore the world, and becomes independently mobile, but does not understand the dangers of the

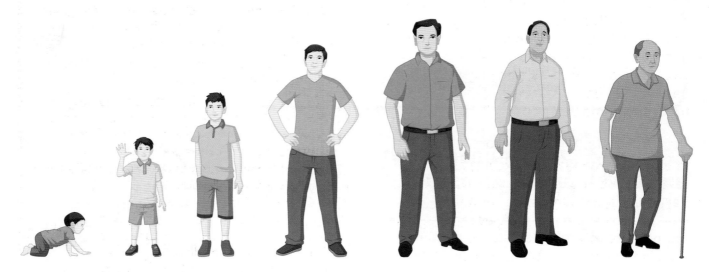

Figure 2.1 Human life stages

surrounding environment. For example, hot drinks left just within reach are a common cause of infants being scalded.

Childhood

Early childhood (from 3–5 years) is a period of intense cognitive development as the child learns to understand language and speak instead of crying to communicate needs. This is when children start to learn to read. Between the ages of three to five, they strive for independence and often express emotions in response to this, which reduces as they develop social skills. Physically, children learn fine motor skills, such as using a pencil to write. It is also a period of growth.

Late childhood (from 6–10 years) is when children consolidate their skills. Socially, they play more team games and rules become important. Children of seven or eight often say 'It's not fair' if someone breaks the rules.

Adolescence

Adolescence (11–17 years) is a time of physical and emotional upheaval, as the body produces hormones that change height, weight, and body shape. Physically, secondary sex characteristics develop. Breasts enlarge in girls. Boys develop facial hair and their voice deepens. Socially, adolescents may be awkward and insecure. It is a time for friendships and belonging.

Early, middle, late adulthood

In early adulthood (18–29 years) social relationships and careers are established. Early adulthood is the mark of fully-fledged independence and many life events may occur, for example moving out of home, getting married, new relationships, having children.

Middle adulthood (30–60 years) is a period of consolidation. Relationships may break down, careers change, family responsibilities may increase as children grow and as ageing older relatives require more support.

Late adulthood (60 years and older) is increasingly a time for providing support, perhaps babysitting grandchildren during school holidays, or caring for an ageing partner. In the later years, it is also a time for receiving support.

The UK population (66 million in 2017) is expected to reach 73 million by 2041. The population is ageing. A baby born between 2015 and 2017 can expect to live to 79 years if male, 83 years if female. Twenty-one per cent of all newborn boys and 32 per cent of all newborn girls will now live to be centenarians (**www.ons.gov.uk**). For many people, half their lives will be spent in mid or late adulthood and most health and social care will be needed for this sector of population.

Key terms

Cognitive refers to development of the mind and the process of acquiring knowledge and understanding through thoughts and experiences.

Developmental milestones are key events in development, such as a baby smiling for the first time or taking its first steps.

Growth refers to size, for example getting bigger or taller over time.

Life stages refer to the different phases in an individual's life. Often these are classified as infancy (0–2 years), childhood (3–10 years), adolescence (11–17 years), early adulthood (18–29 years), middle adulthood (30–60 years) and late adulthood (60+ years). Different areas of study focus on different stages; for example, child care practitioners may subdivide the stages of childhood to look at each stage in more detail. Those working with older people may subdivide late adulthood into 60–80 years and 80+ years.

1.2 Social, emotional, cognitive and physical development within each life stage

Throughout each life stage, there are a number of social, emotional, cognitive and physical developments that occur.

Social

Social development describes how we interact with other, learning the values, knowledge and skills that help us relate to others effectively and to contribute in positive ways to society. Learning to take turns is part of social development. Some key factors in social development include:

- **Relationships** are the means by which we develop socially. Children who are kept in isolation have difficulty developing social relationships: if no one speaks to them, they may not learn to speak. For example, Genie was locked in a room for 12 years by her abusive parents. When found, she could not speak and only after professional support, learned how to communicate in a limited way. Older people who are socially isolated, seeing no one for days, may sometimes lose their social skills because they have little interaction with others.

- **Independence**, i.e. learning to care for oneself, such as learning to dress and feed oneself, is part of social development. Being independent is valued and encouraged in British society. Children are proud of achievements such as dressing themselves. Loss of independence is seen as a matter of regret and even shame for some, for example when an older person can no longer manage to shower independently they may feel ashamed at having help.

- **Cultural** factors also influence social development. In some cultures, girls are expected to be obedient and submissive while boys are encouraged to be assertive or even aggressive.

Erik Erikson, a psychologist, developed a theory of psychosocial development through eight life stages to explain how we develop socially and emotionally through life. The ages for each stage are approximate. Different people reach each stage at different times but we all go through these eight stages. As times change and people live longer, the seventh stage may be prolonged and the eighth stage may start later for some.

Table 2.1 Erikson's stages of psychosocial development

Approximate age	Stage
Birth to 18 months	Trust v. mistrust
18 months to 3 years	Autonomy, striving for independence v. shame and doubt
3–5 years	Initiative v. guilt
6–12 years	Industry v. inferiority
13–18 years	Identity v. role confusion
18–40 years	Intimacy v. isolation
40–65 years	Generativity v. stagnation
65+ years	Ego integrity v. despair

Social development in each life stage

- Infancy is the stage when social bonds are formed. Babies form a close bond with their primary care giver, often their mother or father. By three months babies have learned to smile, recognise their care giver's face and respond to their voice. An infant who is loved and cared for feels emotionally secure and begins to explore their surroundings. By 18 months they can recognise themselves in a mirror. At around nine months they may develop a fear of strangers which may persist for a few months. It is a normal part of social development. The first two years of life are the most important for a child to form social bonds.

- From about 18 months to 3 years children learn to manage their feelings, getting over tantrums, and gaining confidence if they are encouraged and supported to be independent. If not loved and well supported they can feel shame and develop a low self-esteem.

- From 3–5 years children copy adults, make up stories and adventures, and experiment with what it means to be grown up. If encouraged at this stage they become confident in themselves. If discouraged they can feel guilty if they make a mistake. The family is the most important relationship for the child at this time in their life. The child absorbs cultural aspects, how to treat others, how to speak and behave.

- From 6–12 years children gain skills. They learn to read, write, play and develop a sense of industry (working hard). This is a very social stage of development and children compare themselves to others. If they feel inadequate compared to their peers they can have problems in terms of self-esteem.

- Adolescence, from around 13–18 years, is when a young person learns who they are. Up to this stage, social development is influenced by what others do. Now, for the first time, development is influenced by the person's own view of themselves as they model themselves on those they admire. This is the age when people become devoted to causes, become idealists or join fan clubs. They are especially vulnerable to being influenced as they try to fit in. Sometimes, adolescents question their role, whether to do with their gender, ethnicity or something else.

- From about 18–40 years is when people look for companionship and love. Key relationships at this stage are with marital partners and friends. Adults may set up home with another person and establish a family, passing on their cultural values to the next generation. If they do not, or if they experience relationship breakdown, they may become isolated.

- From about 40–65 years career or family responsibilities increase. Key relationships are family, work colleagues, and the local community. This too is a period when families change. Children may leave home, although increasingly many return to live with parents because of housing costs. Independence increases from birth through to middle age.

- Late adulthood, from 65, is when people look back on their lives with satisfaction or regret. Key relationships are family and friends. They may begin to lose independence because of poor health and may become socially isolated.

Emotional

Emotional development is about learning to recognise, understand, express and manage our feelings and to have empathy for others. It is closely bound up with social development, i.e. how we feel affects how we behave and interact with others.

Attachment is a key aspect of emotional development. John Bowlby, a British psychologist, discovered the importance of an infant's attachment to a **primary care giver**, usually the mother, in the first two years of life. This is a strong emotional bond forged over time. Michael Rutter, another psychologist, suggested the primary care giver could be the father or a grandparent, a sibling or a foster parent. Schaffer and Emerson suggested that by about 18 months, children may have several attachments, for example if they live in a large and loving family.

> ### 🔑 Key term
>
> **Primary care giver** refers to the person who has the greatest responsibility for the daily care and rearing of a child.

Emotional resilience is the ability not just to bounce back after a set-back, but to adapt to stress and changing circumstances while maintaining a stable mental well-being. It can be developed later in life but it is thought that children who have secure relationships and a supportive network in early life are more likely to have emotional resilience than those who are unsupported and insecure.

Self-image is the perception a person has of themselves. This usually comes from their own personal experiences or by internalising and accepting the judgements of others. Self-image is formed in childhood as we interact with others but becomes more important during adolescence when people struggle to find a balance between 'fitting in' and being their own person. Successfully negotiating this stage means a person has a positive understanding of who they are and can share this with others. They are more confident and able to mix with others without losing their own identity. If they do not develop a clear self-image they may be uncertain, and may become isolated.

Self-image is also important in early adulthood. For those with a positive self-image, forming friendships and achieving a balance between giving and receiving love and support helps in achieving intimacy. When someone has a poor self-image or lacks confidence, they can become needy and vulnerable or, alternatively, they can become distant, self-contained and isolated.

Self-esteem, i.e. how you value yourself, is linked with self-image and is very important from the early years. Children as young as three years old can have low self-esteem. As they interact more with others and gain skills, they can develop positive self-esteem. If, however, they do not develop positive self-esteem they may have a sense of inferiority, which undermines their ability to form relationships later in life.

Erikson's theory assigns different stages to different ages, but it is possible to become stuck in a stage, preventing further emotional development until the person has negotiated that stage.

Cognitive

Cognitive development relates to the way we think and understand the world around us. We develop thinking skills such as remembering, problem-solving, and decision-making. It also relates to information processing, conceptual resources, perceptual skill, and language learning. Jean Piaget, a Swiss psychologist, is known for his theory of cognitive development and describes how a child begins to understand the world, initially exploring it through the senses. By the age of two, most infants can say a few words and can name familiar objects. From about two to about seven years they develop more understanding of the world through play. They learn to use words in the right order and begin to understand numbers and time. From around eleven years they can understand abstract ideas such as 'goodness' and can work out problems in their head. Although Piaget's theory was later modified, it still gives an idea of how thinking develops. We are not born with the ability to think and reason — we develop it as we mature.

Language — babies are predisposed to learn language by listening to people around them and by associating a sound with an object. Noam Chomsky, an American linguist, suggested that there is an optimum (or 'best') time for young children to learn language and that the brain is programmed to acquire language by about 18 months. He suggested the brain has a **language acquisition device (LAD)**, which makes it easier for infants to learn language. He also suggested that if a child does not learn language at that time, it will be harder for them to pick it up later. Children who are born with severe hearing impairments and not treated, or children who are isolated and not spoken to in their early years, have delayed language development. Children learn to refine their use of language; for example instead of car, they can begin to identify different types of cars. Adolescents develop their own language using terms such as 'wicked', or abbreviations such as LOL. Their use of language is adapted for texting and social media. Adults develop specialist language associated with their work, for example a physicist may refer to fission and fusion, a biologist to mitosis. In late adulthood, ill-health may impact on language. A stroke may cause speech and recall problems and dementia may result in a person not being able to say what they want to say.

> ## 🔑 Key term
>
> **Language acquisition device (LAD)** refers to Chomsky's theory that there is a 'tool' in the brain that helps children to quickly learn and understand language.

Memory is another aspect of cognitive development. By about two years old, a child can remember where they put a toy. Memory strengthens with age and adolescents are expected to remember many things, especially for exams. As people age, memory can decline, but age alone does not cause memory loss. Illness, injury and psychoactive substances can all affect memory throughout any life stage. One of the biggest challenges facing health and care services is the increasing number of people, whether in middle or late adulthood, with memory loss associated with dementia.

Reasoning is a conscious, deliberate process. It requires logic and develops with maturity. Young children are not able to reason. Piaget suggested that reasoning develops only from around the age of seven, and even then, children may need real things to help work out abstract problems, for example sharing fifteen apples between five children. Although Piaget suggests abstract reasoning develops from eleven years onwards, children's development can vary. Reasoning is influenced by education. An adolescent and an adult who have been taught to consider different aspects of a situation may be able to reason logically. If they have not learned to reason logically they may be influenced by inappropriate role models. Reasoning is a skill that develops with practice and in the mature adult is not age-related. Sometimes reasoning can be affected by illness, for example a brain tumour may affect judgement. Psychoactive substances affect reasoning.

Thinking is a mental process and can be conscious or unconscious. Thinking is the overall description of mental processes that include reasoning and problem-solving. Thinking as a mental process develops gradually. A baby is hungry; unconsciously without being aware of the thought process, it cries to let adults know it is hungry. A child at school may be hungry but thinks consciously that soon it will be dinner time. Adolescents are expected to use thinking skills in school, college and in life. Adults use thinking skills in everything they do. Driving a car, working, shopping and cooking all require conscious and unconscious mental processes. Some adults have limited thinking skills, for example if they have learning disabilities or have acquired brain injury. They may then need support for daily living.

Problem-solving is one type of thinking, referring to a specific set of skills that begin by identifying the problem, exploring information and possible solutions, selecting the best idea, testing it and evaluating the results. Problem-solving is taught in schools at first with real situations and toys, then moving onto abstract ideas. Not everyone has well-developed problem-solving skills. Some adults do not use problem-solving skills,

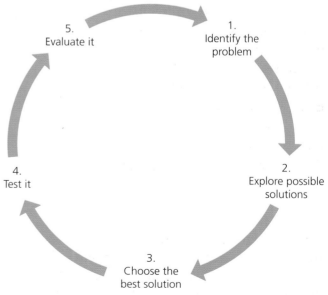

Figure 2.2 Problem-solving

and this can result in negative life choices, for example taking on more debt when they are short of money. Unfortunately, due to illnesses such as dementia, some people lose their problem-solving abilities.

Physical

Physical development relates to the growth and development of the body, including the brain, muscles and senses. It varies with the individual and is influenced by many things such as diet, exercise and health. Nevertheless, there are milestones which indicate the progress of physical development.

Table 2.2 Physical development from birth to three years old

Age	Physical development
At birth	Unable to support own head, responds to sudden sounds, closes eyes in bright light.
3 months	Can support own head but not yet able to sit without support, grasps objects, turns head to see things, can make eye contact.
6 months	Can sit with support, grasps objects and transfers them from hand to hand, rolls over. Interacts with others vocally and smiles at familiar people.
9 months	Sits unsupported, uses finger and thumb (pincer grip) to pick up objects, enjoys dropping them and looks for them. Can shuffle on bottom, or crawl.
1 year	Stands holding furniture, may be able to stand unsupported for a few moments and take a few steps.
1–2 years	Gross motor skills, i.e. stands without help, learns to walk and run. Climbs on furniture, begins to climb stairs using rail. Begins to throw a ball, starts to kick a ball. Fine motor skills, i.e. grasps a crayon with fist and begins to scribble, picks up small objects and puts them in containers, begins to turn pages of a book, stacks two blocks, begins to grasp spoon and tries to feed themselves. Can walk on tiptoe.
By end of 3 years	Can throw and catch a big ball, can stand on one foot, and watches others to see how things are done.

Early developments are closely monitored so that any delay can be spotted and action can be taken to prevent problems. For example, if a baby does not respond to sound they may have hearing problems. This will prevent them learning to speak. If action is taken, for example fitting a hearing device, their language development will be less affected.

Infancy is a time of rapid physical development. Babies begin learning to control what their arms and legs do. This is **gross motor control** (gross meaning 'big'). Once they have learned to control arms and legs, they begin to learn to control fingers (**fine motor control**) and pick up objects with finger and thumb, grasp a crayon and hold a spoon.

Childhood is a time of refining physical control. A baby may kick a ball and fall over, whereas a seven-year-old may be able to dribble a ball from one end of a playground to the other. Some children learn to play the violin from the age of two or three and develop exceptionally fine motor control.

Between 4–5 years old, a child is stable in sitting in a small chair at a table. Using gross motor skills, they walk easily on a narrow line, can climb ladders, stand on one leg for 8–10 seconds and can hop on either foot a short distance. They can walk on heels, skip on alternate feet, bend and touch toes with straight legs. They are skilful in climbing, sliding, swinging, digging. They can play ball games and move to music. Refinement of fine motor skills means they can hold a pencil or cut a triangle and can copy a square. They learn to form letters and write. They can dress themselves and fasten buttons.

🔑 Key terms

Fine motor control refers to the co-ordination of small muscles with the eyes, such as in movements using the hands and fingers, for example eating, cutting with scissors, buttoning clothing, etc.

Gross motor control refers to larger movements made by the arms, legs, feet or entire body, for example crawling, running, jumping, etc.

Table 2.3 NHS guidelines for exercise adapted from **www.nhs.uk/live-well/exercise**

Babies	Encourage physical activity during daily routines, and during supervised floor play, including tummy time.
Toddlers	Physically active every day for at least 180 minutes spread throughout the day, indoors or outside.
Under 5s	Should only be inactive when asleep. Watching TV, travelling, being strapped into a buggy for long periods is harmful to health. Energetic activity can include dance and gymnastics, or just riding a bike, swimming, climbing a tree.
5–18-year-olds	At least 60 minutes of physical activity daily, ranging from moderate activity, such as cycling and playground activities, to vigorous activity that makes them out of breath, such as running and tennis. On three days a week, include activities for strong muscles and bones, swinging on playground equipment, hopping and skipping, gymnastics or tennis.
Adults aged 19 to 64	150 minutes of weekly physical activity, for example, 30 minutes on five days every week. Brisk walking, running, playing tennis or football, combined with exercise to strengthen muscles, such as yoga or Pilates, is recommended.
Over 65	At least 150 minutes of moderate aerobic activity such as cycling or walking every week and strength exercises on two or more days a week. If they are generally fit and have no health conditions that limit mobility they should try to be active daily. If they have balance problems, yoga or tai chi twice a week will improve balance and co-ordination.

Physical health is important at every life stage. Some physical health conditions, such as cystic fibrosis, are genetic and inherited from a parent's faulty gene. Research is discovering ways to counteract the effects of many genetic health problems. Other health conditions can be the result of lifestyle choices. Two of the biggest health problems facing people today are diabetes and heart disease. These are influenced by poor diet and lack of exercise.

Adolescence is a time of rapid physical development. **Puberty** can begin at any point from the ages of 8 to 14 and can take up to four years. The body grows physically more rapidly than the brain, leading to clumsiness as the brain adjusts. Adolescents need a lot of sleep during this time of change. For girls, puberty begins with breast changes, they develop pubic hair and begin to have periods. They grow on average about 2 to 3 inches a year during puberty. For boys, puberty begins when the penis and testicles grow and pubic hair develops. The voice breaks, they become more muscular and they grow around 3 inches

a year. Both boys and girls get acne. Hormones change and the 'emotional roller coaster' they experience can cause unexplained mood swings, low self-esteem, aggression or depression (**www.nhs.uk/live-well/sexual-health/stages-of-puberty-what-happens-to-boys-and-girls**).

Physical development reaches a peak during early adulthood — most men and women are at their strongest and their bodies' systems perform at their best. Beyond this age physical performance deteriorates. This is known as the ageing process. Genetic factors have some influence on how we age but the most important factors are lifestyle choices. Muscles weaken and bones lose density unless they are used. Regular physical exercise combined with a healthy diet is the best way to delay ageing. The NHS recommends least 150 minutes (2 hours and 30 minutes) of moderate-intensity aerobic activity, such as cycling or fast walking, every week to improve bone density and prevent osteoporosis, and muscle-strengthening activities on two or more days a week (**www.nhs.uk/conditions/osteoporosis**).

Exercise becomes especially important in middle and late adulthood as hormone levels change. From around the age of 30 to 40, male testosterone levels fall almost 2 per cent a year. (**www.nhs.uk/conditions/male-menopause**). Women experience the menopause as oestrogen levels fall, usually between 45 and 55 years of age. They experience hot flushes, low mood, difficulty sleeping, and loss of libido (**www.nhs.uk/conditions/menopause**).

In late adulthood, many people have multiple health problems. A diabetic person may develop heart problems, cannot exercise as much as they should and so lose more bone density, making them more vulnerable to fractures. Dementia, a disorder of the brain, is not an inevitable part of ageing but is an increasing problem in ageing societies. According to the Alzheimer's Society, one in six people over the age of 80 have dementia but there are over 40,000 people under 65 with it in the UK (**www.alzheimers.org.uk**).

1.3 Holistic development

We try to separate out social, emotional, cognitive and physical development for the purposes of learning but people do not function in just one area. We cannot care for just one aspect of the individual while ignoring other aspects: care must be **holistic** and all-inclusive, to be effective.

Interdependency of each developmental area: social, emotional, cognitive, physical

Interdependency means being dependent on each other and affecting each other. Emotional development influences our social, cognitive and physical development. Cognitive development influences our social development, for example an individual with autism, a cognitive impairment, may find it difficult to make friends. Our physical development is affected by emotional and social factors, for example babies who are neglected or abused may fail to thrive and not grow as well as expected.

Abraham Maslow, an American psychologist, explained this interdependency as a hierarchy of needs, i.e. what we need to grow and develop to achieve our potential.

 Key terms

Cognitive development is how we understand the world and process information, perceive things and people, and learn language.

Emotional development is about learning to recognise, understand, express and manage our feelings and to have empathy for others.

Holistic refers to an approach that acknowledges the whole person, rather than just one aspect of them. You should look at an individual holistically in order to meet their needs.

Interdependency means depends on each other, all aspects of development, whether physical, social, emotional or cognitive, influence each other.

Physical development is about how we grow and develop control over our bodies.

Puberty is the physical and emotional change that marks the beginning of adulthood.

Social development describes how we interact with other people, learning the values, knowledge and skills that help us relate to others effectively.

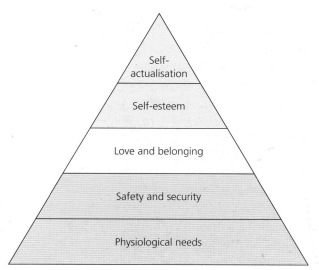

Figure 2.3 Maslow's Hierarchy of Needs

When physiological and safety needs are met, physical development occurs, for example a baby is hungry so cries, is given milk and held safely. Emotional development occurs when our need for love and belonging is met. Cognitive development and social development occur when we are valued by ourselves and others. All these factors are holistically linked. When needs are met, development occurs.

Activity

Create an information booklet for parents-to-be that outlines the life stages of human growth and development. Within the booklet, outline social, emotional, cognitive and physical development within one life stage.

In the booklet, describe holistic development. Use examples to support the description. Use and include at least one relevant and traceable reference.

 Check your understanding 1

1 Briefly describe three examples of life stages of human growth and development.
2 Give an example of each type of development: social, emotional, cognitive and physical.
3 Explain what is meant by 'holistic' development.
4 Give an example of how social, physical and cognitive factors are interdependent in early development.

L02 Understand influences which impact upon human growth and development

Humans grow and develop at different rates and several factors influence this process. Some influences are internal, for example our genes influence whether we have blue eyes or brown eyes. Some influences are external, for example whether we have food, get sick, or even whether we live in a safe place. In this section, we will examine some of the factors that influence human growth and development.

2.1 The nature versus nurture debate in relation to human growth and development

One important debate is whether human growth and development is influenced by our **nature** — what genes we are born with — or whether development is influenced by **nurture** — how we are raised.

Nature

Genetic inheritance is decided by the genes in our chromosomes. One way this has been studied is by comparing twins, for example the Minnesota Twin Study conducted by Thomas J. Bouchard in 1979. He studied twins who were separated at birth and brought up by different families, concluding that similarities between twins are due to genes, not environment. However, it is unethical to separate twins just to study the effects. Scientist study cases where twins have been separated due to adoption or some other mitigating circumstances.

Inherited characteristics and biological influences related to human development and behaviour

In a famous study of identical twins, called the Jim Twins, Jim Lewis and Jim Springer were separated at 4 weeks old and brought up by different families. They had no contact with each other until 1979 when they were 39. They found they both shared the same name, drove the same type of car and holidayed at the same place. They had even twice married women with the same first name. Dr Nancy Segal, a psychologist studying twins, found that social attitudes and life choices are often influenced by genes rather than by the way people have been nurtured. One set of separated twins had the same taste and were wearing exactly the same jewellery when they first met (**www.bbc.co.uk/news/ magazine-27188642**).

Inherited characteristics might include eye colour or dimples. Biological influences might include genetic conditions, such as inheriting a gene predisposing for breast cancer, cystic fibrosis or sickle cell anaemia.

Nurture

Nurture refers to how we are brought up and how the environment influences us, rather than the genes we inherit. Some people think that environment influences human development and behaviour, for example children whose parents read to them are more likely to learn to read early.

Increasingly, psychologists are realising that nature and nurture interact with each other. A person may have a genetic predisposition for depression, but if environmental factors do not trigger the depression, they will not become depressed.

Key terms

Genetic inheritance is the basic principle of genetics and explains how characteristics are passed from one generation to the next in the form of genetic material, i.e. DNA.

Nature refers to genetic, inherited characteristics and biological influences that relate to human development and behaviour.

Nurture refers to the environmental influences relating to human development and behaviour.

Activity

Prepare a transcript for a vlog in which you outline the nature versus nurture debate in relation to human growth and development.

2.2 The medical model of health and well-being

The **medical model of health** sees the body as a set of systems, for example the respiratory or circulatory system. It focuses on the biological or physical aspects of disease, such as infection, improper function of organs or joints and what might have gone wrong with a particular system. The emphasis is on diagnosis, i.e. deciding what the problem is, prescribing a treatment and finding a cure. The medical model of health assumes there is a 'pill for every ill' and that ill-health is physical and treatable. The weakness with this model of health is that it offers nothing for mental ill-health, incurable cancers or genetic disorders such as cystic fibrosis. The medical model of health is used in hospitals but is incorporated with a social model of health where possible.

The social model of health and well-being

The **social model of health** is holistic and looks at the whole person, including the social, physical, emotional, cultural and economic influences on their health. It values individual experience, for example understanding that homelessness can cause mental ill-health. The social model recognises the role of social perception, or how people form impressions of and make inferences about other people, in life chances and life choices. An example of social perception is when a young person is judged by how they speak, what they wear and where they live. They may be labelled as 'from the wrong part of town' and not given a job because of that view.

The social model of health focuses on:

- Equality of opportunity — giving people an equal chance in life

- Social inclusion — making sure everyone is included and their health needs considered
- Community participation — involving local communities in identifying health needs and planning to meet those needs.

An example of community participation is using community action to reduce knife crime and make a safer environment for young people. Decent housing is as important to health as getting a prescription from the doctor. An advantage of the social model of health and well-being is that it is broader than physical health. It considers mental health and well-being, and it focuses on community initiatives to prevent ill-health. It is focused on education, preventing ill-health, encouraging people to take responsibility for their own health, and it involves the community in a **grassroots approach** to health. A disadvantage of this model is that it is expensive, as it seeks to address all the underlying causes of ill-health. It also requires more time from professionals.

2.3 Factors which impact upon human growth and development

There are many positive and negative factors that influence how we grow and develop physically, socially, emotionally and cognitively.

Activity

Prepare a leaflet for young adults in which you outline both the medical model of health and well-being and the social model of health and well-being. Outline the advantages and the disadvantages of each model and include references.

🔑 Key terms

Grassroots approach refers to the people who form the main part of an organisation or movement, rather than its leaders, for example the community in health and social care.

Medical model of health and well-being is a scientific approach that sees the body as a set of systems, for example the respiratory system, the circulatory system, and it focuses on the biological/physical aspects of disease.

Social model of health and well-being is holistic and looks at the whole person and social, physical, emotional, cultural and economic influences on health and values individual experience.

Table 2.4 Factors which impact upon human growth and development

Factor	Positive impact	Negative impact
Biological, for example genetic inheritance	Inheriting certain genes for particular traits can give an individual an advantage in their environment, for example inheriting genes for being tall increases chances of growing tall.	Certain inherited genes may have a detrimental effect on the body and/or mind, for example inheriting the BRCA gene for breast cancer may reduce chances of living to old age.
Lifestyle	Having a healthy lifestyle helps the body and mind to function optimally, for example a non-smoker will have better lung function.	An unhealthy lifestyle can negatively affect the body and mind, for example a heavy smoker will have damaged lungs, may get breathless and develop lung cancer.
Health	A child who is active is more likely to be healthy and grow physically.	An inactive person is more likely to develop long-term health conditions such as heart disease or diabetes.

→

Factor	Positive impact	Negative impact
Education	Educational achievement opens doors, and gives opportunities for better jobs, higher income and a healthy diet. Children from higher-income families may have access to more opportunities.	Poor education limits opportunities. If a person cannot write or read, they will struggle to get a well-paid job, may not be able to afford a healthy diet for their children.
Employment	Having a job or career has a positive impact on self-esteem and mental health. We develop socially as we meet more people.	Being unemployed can lead to a lack of self-esteem and poor mental health. With no reason to go out, unemployed people can become socially isolated.
Socio-economic	Financial security may provide children with healthier food options and access to a wider choice of educational experiences. Being able to afford the necessities of life reduces this type of stress.	Being short of money increases stress. Parents in low paid jobs struggle to provide the basic requirements for their children's growth and development. They may not be able to afford fresh fruit and vegetables and the protein needed for growth. Those in higher social classes, such as professionals, may also have other work-related stresses.
Culture	Cultural influences may encourage people to work hard, and develop socially, emotionally and cognitively.	Some cultures discourage education, for example educational aspirations for females may be lower than for males. This restricts their social and cognitive development.
Environment	Green open spaces and safe parks encourage people to exercise and keep healthy.	An unsafe environment, for example a high prevalence of crime, might discourage people from exercising as they might stay indoors for safety.
Relationships	Supportive relationships encourage people to stay healthy, to value themselves and grow emotionally.	Abusive relationships can cause mental ill-health, restricting social and emotional growth.
Bullying	There are few positive aspects to bullying, except when a person has challenged the bully and developed emotional resilience.	Bullying causes stress and can cause severe mental ill-health. It restricts social development as the victim is afraid that others will be bullies too. Unless the victim challenges the bully, their emotional growth will be held back.
Aspirations	Having the motivation to achieve realistic hopes and dreams can contribute to a healthy body and mind.	Unrealistic aspirations, over which the person has no control, for example to win the lottery, can cause stress, depression and anxiety. It can restrict social, emotional and cognitive growth as the person relies on external forces to improve their life, rather than using their own resources.

Activity

Using your transcript for the vlog you developed in the activity for AC2.1, discuss at least three factors which impact upon human growth and development.

Include at least two relevant and traceable references and a reference list.

2.4 The importance of recognising and responding to concerns regarding an individual's growth and development

Health and social care practitioners have a professional duty set out in their code of conduct, as well as a moral duty, to recognise and respond to concerns about an individual's growth and development. Even before birth, babies are checked to ensure they are growing and developing as they should. For example, if an unborn baby stops growing, they may have to be delivered early by Caesarean section. At birth, the midwife checks the newborn. The community midwife visits for ten days then the health visitor is responsible for checking a baby's growth and development. During childhood and adolescence, community nurses and educational psychologists may be involved with monitoring growth and development if there are any concerns, along with social workers.

Intervention

Intervention is to take action to promote an individual's health and well-being. This is essential if there are concerns about a child's growth and development, because at this age, intervention may help to prevent harm. At birth, babies are screened to check their eyes, heart, hips and, in boys, the testicles (testes). Babies with hips that dislocate easily will be treated so they will be able to learn to walk. Children who are born deaf will be given the support they need to develop communication, whether a hearing aid so they can hear and learn to speak, or learning sign language.

A health visitor will check a child's height and weight. Children who fail to grow at the expected rate will be monitored closely. They may have genetic problems, such as sickle cell anaemia, a condition where red blood cells that carry oxygen around the body develop abnormally; or thalassaemia, a different blood condition which affects the red blood cells. Children with sickle cell anaemia will need specialist care throughout their lives.

Health and social care practitioners have a safeguarding duty towards children and vulnerable adults and must report any concerns. Sometimes, a child is brought to hospital with several broken bones and bruising. This may be due to a genetic condition, for example osteogenesis imperfecta (OI), or it may be due to child abuse. Health and social care practitioners must report any concerns so that intervention can take place. It may be that the child is investigated and found to have OI, then treatment can begin. If it is a case of child abuse, the needs of the child are of paramount importance. They may be placed in the care of the local authority in order to remove them from harm and to be kept safe.

Promote health and well-being

Health and social care practitioners have a duty set out in their code of practice to promote health and well-being. They do this by giving information and advice to individuals and to carers, encouraging them to take responsibility for their own health and well-being. They may advise about diet, exercise, and reducing risky behaviours such as smoking, drug taking or drinking too much alcohol. A midwife may provide a new mother with advice about breastfeeding. A practice nurse may advise about diet and exercise. A community psychiatric nurse will encourage a patient to take their medication. A social care worker may encourage an older person to remain active through music and movement sessions.

Meet individual needs

In **person-centred care**, individuals are always at the centre of health and social care services. Meeting individual needs means people get the right treatment and support at the right time so they can grow and develop, maintain healthier lives and remain independent for longer. The case study that follows is outlined to illustrate this.

Daisy was born with Down syndrome, a genetic condition which means she was born with an extra chromosome due to a one-off genetic change in the sperm or egg. Down syndrome is a genetic disorder but is not inherited. Down syndrome is characterised by floppiness (hypotonia), a small nose and flat nasal bridge, small mouth with a tongue that may stick out. The eyes slant upwards and outwards, the back of the head is flat, and the person has broad hands with short fingers with only one crease across the palm. They may also be below-average weight and length at birth (**www.nhs.uk/conditions/downs-syndrome**).

Daisy will be monitored closely by child health services, with different professionals involved in her care. She will be referred for an early intervention programme that aims to help a child with learning disabilities develop and support the family. It may include speech and language therapy to help with problems communicating or feeding. It may include physiotherapy to help with muscle weakness and it may include individual home-teaching programmes. A paediatrician gives regular health check-ups, tests hearing and vision, measures height and weight, takes blood to test for thyroid problems and checks for heart problems.

Daisy has mild learning difficulties which means she may take a bit longer to reach developmental milestones, such as walking and talking. She will be able to attend a nursery and then a mainstream school and have the support of a classroom assistant, or attend a specialist school with smaller classes and more individual care. Daisy will be under the care of child health and social care services until she is 18 when adult services will be responsible for her care. Between the ages of 16 and 18, she will start a 'transition' to adult services.

Daisy will be able to lead a fairly independent life, going on to college and gain qualifications if she wishes. When she is an adult, she may decide to leave home and live in supported housing with the support of care staff, according to her individual needs. Her social worker may help her find accommodation and an occupational therapist may offer practical advice on living independently. Daisy may need to learn to travel by herself on public transport, if she goes to college. This means managing to work out which bus to take and what fare to pay. Meeting her individual needs means this training will be included in her care plan. Daisy may decide to move in with a boyfriend, get married and have children. She may need extra support in the parenting role, especially if her partner has learning disabilities. Her needs will be assessed and met by health and social care professionals who see her as an individual with needs that differ not only from others, but from others with Down syndrome.

Meet the needs of others

Parents, carers, family, friends, and colleagues make up a network of informal care.

For example, parents of a baby with Down syndrome like Daisy might need support in understanding the condition and help when encouraging their child's learning and development. As part of the early intervention plan, a home visiting teacher or speech and language therapist may show new parents how to use toys and activities to encourage speech. Parents may need support to help their child be independent when completing everyday tasks, such as feeding and dressing or getting ready for bed. Family and friends may be uncertain

> ### Key term
>
> **Person-centred care** involves the health and social care practitioner placing the individual at the centre of their working practices. They must always act in the individual's best interests to ensure that the individual remains in control of their care and support.

how to interact with Daisy because she has Down syndrome. Health and care practitioners can help parents deal with this by providing information they can share with others. As Daisy grows, she will meet people who know nothing about Down syndrome or may be prejudiced. Health and social care practitioners can help parents to manage such situations.

Using the example of Daisy with Down syndrome shows the importance of recognising and responding to concerns regarding an individual's growth and development. It shows how health and social care practitioners can meet individual needs and the needs of others. In a similar way, health and social care practitioners meet the needs of individuals at all ages with different care needs.

Explain Activity

Prepare a presentation for health and social care students to explain the importance of recognising and responding to concerns regarding an individual's growth and development. Use a specific example, which you can create based on your knowledge so far. Look at what intervention might be needed, how to promote health and well-being, consider how to meet individual needs and meet the needs of others. Others may include parents or carers.

Check your understanding 2

1 What is the nature versus nurture debate about?
2 Explain the medical model of health and well-being.
3 Explain the social model of health and well-being.
4 Explain how three different factors can impact upon human growth and development.
5 Why is it important to recognise and respond to concerns regarding an individual's growth and development?

LO3 Understand significant life events across the lifespan

Significant life events are major changes in an individual's life. Some happen so early in our lives that we do not remember them, while others happen later and we do remember them.

3.1 Significant life events across the life stages

Although we are all individuals, certain life events will happen to us all. We are all born, go through various stages of growth and development, form social relationships and many reach old age. This section examines some of the main life events that happen to us through the life stages.

Infancy

As previously mentioned, infancy is generally defined as the first year of life but for the purposes of this section it refers to the first years of life up to starting school. During the first few months of life, babies form a close emotional bond with their primary care giver.

Separation is stressful for babies and children. Babies learn about the world through their senses, as Piaget first noted. If a baby can see, hear or smell their primary care giver, they feel secure. New babies like to be held close. As babies grow and begin exploring their world, they realise that things and people still exist when out of sight or sound. This starts at about the age of 4–7 months. Piaget calls this the stage of 'object permanence'. Until that stage, a baby may cry if they do not sense the primary care giver nearby.

Nursery usually starts at about 18 months to 2 years of age, although it is important to remember that not all children attend nursery as it is not compulsory. A family may live in a rural area, a long way away from a nursery or they may have family such as grandparents caring for their children. Nursery may be the first time a toddler has been separated from their primary care giver for any length of time. Nursery gives toddlers a chance to meet and play with other children, although at first they do not play together. Solitary play is usual until about the age of 2 or 3 years. After that, children play alongside others, perhaps watching them but still doing their own thing. This parallel play continues but pre-schoolers also develop associative play, working alongside others, occasionally sharing materials but producing their own story or picture. Later they develop co-operative play, sharing materials and working together towards one game, for example playing shop, where each person has a different role in the same game.

Weaning is the gradual introduction of solid foods, usually around six months of age. Up to that point a baby gets all it needs from breast milk or formula milk. Solid foods are gradually introduced so that any allergic reactions can be noted and the food omitted. The baby is ready for weaning when they can stay in a sitting position, swallow, hold their head steady and co-ordinate eyes, hands and mouth. This allows them to look at the food, pick it up and put it in their mouth. It is important never to add sugar or salt to food for babies. Babies should not have honey — it may contain bacteria. They should not have raw or lightly cooked shellfish, raw or lightly cooked eggs, or mould-ripened soft cheeses like brie or camembert. They should not be given hard food and should not have nuts as they can cause allergic reactions. Weaning should begin with soft pureed food and a variety of different tastes. Gradually, the range of foods can be increased. Babies must never be left alone while eating because they may choke (**www.nhs.uk/conditions/ pregnancy-and-baby/solid-foods-weaning**).

Toilet training refers to a child learning how to use a potty or toilet with a children's toilet seat. Readiness varies with each individual child. It is best to wait until these five signs are apparent before beginning toilet training:

1 Nappies are dry for at least an hour or two at a time.

2 They understand when they are having a wee and may say so.

3 When they have a wet or dirty nappy they may pull at it, take it off or ask you to change it.

4 The child may fidget when they need the toilet.

5 They know when they need to wee and may say so in advance.

(**Source: www.nct.org.uk**)

Accidents can happen and it is important not to make a fuss when they do. Just say 'never mind' and clean it up. Always praise a child for using the potty or toilet and they will then associate using the potty with something good. Remember to teach them to wipe from front to back — especially important for girls as this will reduce the chance of urinary tract infection. Teach them to wash their hands after using the potty or toilet. Children with older siblings may learn quicker than those without as they want to be like the older children. Some parents wait until summer for potty training when the weather is warmer and there are fewer clothes to remove.

Occasionally, a child who has learned to use the potty may regress and start to wet or soil themselves. This may be because they are not well or are going through a time of emotional upset. Perhaps there is a new baby taking their parent's attention or a parent is away from home and they miss them. Give the child reassurance if they do start wetting or soiling themselves and do not blame them. If it persists, a quick chat with the GP will check there is nothing else causing the problem. Regression like this usually sorts itself out.

Childhood

This refers to the period from about 5 years to puberty, which is a time of many growth and development changes.

School is a major life event, beginning at the age of four or five. Secure, confident children may enjoy meeting new friends. Other children with less social experience may take longer to settle in. This is the time when play becomes more focused and structured learning is introduced. It may also be the time when special educational needs and disabilities are noticed and a child may be referred for assessment to ensure they get the support they need.

Siblings refer to an individual's brothers and/or sisters, or half-brothers and/or half-sisters, who can in some cases help a child's social development. An older brother or sister may feel proud of helping with a new baby. A younger child may learn by watching their older siblings. When children are encouraged to be helpful and kind, having siblings can be a positive experience. When children are rivals for parental affection, or are compared negatively with one another, the sibling relationship can be less positive. Parents have a responsibility to foster good relationships between siblings.

Moving home can mean losing friends and familiar surroundings, moving to a new school, and getting used to a new way of life. It is even more traumatic when moving home means losing a parent figure, for example in the case of divorce. Children require a lot of emotional support at such times and may regress to an earlier stage of behaviour, for example asking for a bottle or wetting the bed, until they begin to feel secure in their new surroundings.

Adolescence

This period begins with the onset of puberty until the early twenties, when hormones cause physical changes in the body.

Puberty is a time of physical change, as described earlier in the unit. It is a major life event and can be difficult for young people. Hormones control their body. As they grow physically, they may go through a clumsy stage. Their appearance changes and their emotions are sometimes likened to a roller coaster. They may not understand what is happening to them.

Relationships outside the family become important. Maslow suggests that we all need to feel we are loved and belong. The esteem or respect of others becomes important. At this stage in life, adolescents may sometimes do things to earn the respect of others. They may work hard and study to gain good grades if that is valued in their group. As part of wishing to belong to a group, they may steal for a dare and if caught, get a criminal record which can limit their future career choices. Adolescents are vulnerable to being exploited because of their need to belong and gain respect. Some young people may be an easy target for organised gangs who lure them into criminal behaviour.

Leaving home is a natural part of growing up. Many people leave home to go to university or to take up a job. Growing up involves finding out your identity and gaining self-awareness. Most people who leave home go into rented and shared accommodation and learn to live with others who are not family, learning life lessons such as managing a budget, cooking a meal and keeping the house tidy. Inevitably, they will make mistakes but they learn independence, in readiness for the next life stage — adulthood.

Early, middle, late adulthood

Early adulthood

Adulthood is traditionally a time of independence, establishing a home of one's own and a family. The age at which this happens varies. In some cultures, adults stay in the parental home for longer. According to the Office for National Statistics, in the UK 26 per cent of 20–34-year-olds are living with their parents (**www.ons.gov.uk**). Increasingly, many young people move back to the parental home so that they can save up for a home of their own.

Employment is a key factor in whether young adults can be independent. Their career choice has an impact at this life stage. If they have a well-paid, permanent job, they might be able to afford to rent or get a mortgage to buy a home of their own and establish a family. However, sometimes people are employed on a zero-hours contract with no guarantee of work, or they may have a low paid full-time job making it difficult for them to afford rent. They may move back into their parental home or may move to a cheaper part of the country. Employment and earning capacity, i.e. the amount a person is likely to earn in their working life, are major factors in affecting life chances. Those in the low wage economy may be unlikely ever to buy their own home: however, just because a person is in a well-paid job does not necessarily mean their future is secure. Redundancy, for example when a company lays off workers, can happen at any time in adulthood. In 2008, when the global economy crashed, many well-paid people were made redundant. If they had saved, they were able to manage until they found another job. Some people who had no savings could not afford mortgage repayments and lost their homes.

Co-habitation or marriage occurs in adulthood. Marriage is the legal or formally recognised union of two people as partners in a personal relationship. Married couples have more legal rights and advantages than co-habiting couples. Co-habitation, when people live together as a couple without marrying, gives few rights. For example, according to Citizen's Advice Bureau, when two people co-habit and one partner dies without leaving a will, the surviving partner will not automatically inherit anything unless the couple owned property jointly (**www.citizensadvice.org.uk**). Co-habiting couples will have to pay tax on anything they inherit from their partner, while married couples have less tax to pay on what they inherit. Civil partnerships are legal relationships which can be registered by two people of the same sex, and provides same-sex couples with added legal rights and responsibilities. According to the ONS, there were 12.9 million married or civil partner couple families in the UK in 2017. This remains the most common type of family. The second largest family type was the co-habiting couple family at 3.3 million families, followed by 2.8 million lone parent families (**www.ons.gov.uk**).

Middle adulthood

This tends to refer to the period of **parenthood**, consolidating or breaking relationships, and sometimes forming new relationships.

When adults decide to have children, they are more likely to be in a stable relationship. In 2017, over two-thirds of births were to parents who lived together and just over a half of births were to parents who were married or in a civil partnership (**www.ons.gov.uk**).

Overall, the fertility rate is decreasing, with fewer children being born. According to government statistics, women are also delaying the age at which they have children. In 1975, the average age of mothers was 26 years. In 2017 it was 31 years. Reasons are varied — some women want to establish a career before having children, some women do not want more than one child while others do not want any children. There is no data on the age of fathers.

Divorce is the formal ending of a marriage. The rate of divorce is on the decline: in 2017, there were 8.4 divorces per 1,000 married men and women aged 16 years and over. This is the lowest divorce rate since 1973. It was highest for men aged 45 to 49 years and women aged 40 to 44 years. The average length of marriage was 12.2 years and the most common reason for divorce was unreasonable behaviour (**www.ons.gov.uk**). The impact on children is that they may for the first time be in a single parent family. They may have to move from the family home and friends. They may even have to move school. Most divorced families experience a financial change for the worse and this can affect parents and children. Such a life event is disruptive for parents and for children and may have an emotional impact on them. Sometimes children have to adapt to a new family as parents re-marry. This may have an emotional effect on them.

Late adulthood

This is characterised by a time of bereavement, retirement, age-related medical conditions and adapting to elderly care. However, it is important to remember that whilst these things are more common in late adulthood they can happen in earlier life stages, too. For instance, a young parent may die, leaving children to be cared for by their partner, and some people are able to retire in early or middle adulthood. Age-related medical conditions do not refer just to late adulthood. Juvenile arthritis affects children under 16, and dementia can occur in young adults too. Nevertheless, late adulthood is a time when people experience more of these life events.

Bereavement refers to the period of mourning after a loss, especially after the death of someone close. For those in long-term relationships, death of a partner is a time of grief. If a person has no family, they may have a pet cat or dog as a close companion and they grieve as they would for a family member when the animal dies. Grief is experienced in stages. The five stages described by the Kübler-Ross model are:

1 **Denial:** belief that the situation is somehow not real and refusal to accept reality.
2 **Anger:** once denial can no longer continue, the individual is angry with the person for dying and leaving the bereaved person behind, and also with others for not saving them.
3 **Bargaining:** involves the hope that an individual can avoid a cause of grief, i.e. 'If only it could have been me who died.'
4 **Depression:** a period of withdrawal, coming to terms with what has happened.
5 **Acceptance:** realising that the situation has happened and coming to terms with their emotions and their 'new' normal lives.

Retirement refers to giving up work, which may be gradual or quite sudden. They may be a company secretary on Friday, and retired with nothing to do on Saturday. Such an abrupt change may be hard to adjust to. Many people who can afford it and are nearing the age of retirement reduce the hours they work and increase their hobbies outside work, so the change is gradual and less of a shock to the system. Many replace full-time work with full- or part-time volunteering. For those with no interests outside work, retirement can be a time of stagnation and rapid physical and mental decline. Erikson described this stage as ego integrity v. despair, when people look back on their lives and are either thankful for the opportunities they have had or regret the opportunities they did not take.

Age-related medical conditions are, at this age, related to physical decline and tend to be degenerative disorders. For example:

- Osteoporosis refers to bones becoming more fragile as calcium is lost and fractures are common.
- Macular degeneration in the eye causes sight problems.
- Cardiovascular disease, high blood pressure, type 2 diabetes, cancer and dementia risks all increase with age.

Much can be done to delay their onset by leading an active and healthy life. The NHS promotes healthy diet and exercise for people of all ages so that they experience fewer of these age-related conditions.

Adapting to elderly care often means a loss of independence and, for many, this is the worst aspect of ageing. A person may need help with washing and dressing for a short period after coming out of hospital, or they may need support for longer. As far as possible, people are cared for in their own home with support from family and friends as well as care services. Most people find it frustrating that they can no longer care for themselves. Adapting to having others do things for you can be difficult when parents who have always seen themselves as carers now have to be cared for by their grown-up children. This adjustment may be equally difficult for the grown-up children. As people age, they may move to sheltered accommodation or a nursing or residential home.

Activity

Create a poster that outlines the significant life events across each life stage.

3.2 The impact that significant life events may have on an individual

The previous section examined some significant life events and touched on the emotions people may feel during these changes, including the impact on relationships and independence. The next section provides a little more detail on the impact these life events may have on the individual.

Emotion

Life events have a positive or negative emotional impact on individuals. In infancy, separation can have an emotional effect. In the 1970s, Bowlby and Ainsworth studied children in a hospital who were separated from their parents. They found three different attachment styles exhibited in these children:

1 Secure attachment — the infants showed distress on separation but eventually settled, knowing their care giver will return. When they did, the infant was easily comforted.

2 Ambivalent attachment — the infants showed distress on separation and couldn't settle as they didn't know if their care giver would return.

3 Avoidant attachment — the infants showed no emotion on separation or on being reunited with their care giver, treating their care giver the same way they treated a stranger.

Nursery provides an opportunity for happy experiences once the child feels secure. Weaning and toilet training offer opportunities for infants to feel proud of learning new skills.

Childhood events such as starting school can be an anxious time for children until they adjust. A new baby can cause jealousy.

Whether a child is the oldest, youngest or middle child can impact on their emotions. Moving home can be stressful. Childhood events can bring anxiety but can also provide opportunities for making new friends, growing in confidence and for developing pride in new achievements.

Adolescence brings emotional turmoil as hormonal changes in puberty affect the growing brain. An adolescent may become depressed, anxious about their appearance and what others think of them. Leaving home for the first time is stressful. They can be homesick but it can also be an opportunity to learn new skills, such as living with others, managing budgets and cooking meals.

Early, middle, and late adulthood involve a range of emotions. Employment, co-habitation or marriage and parenthood can bring happiness and a sense of fulfilment. Equally, if they do not go well, they can result in unhappiness. Divorce and bereavement bring sadness and regrets for some, but for others they can be an end to suffering. Retirement can bring regrets or happiness, and sometimes a mixture of both. A person may regret they did not save more for old age, or be glad if they did. Age-related medical conditions and adapting to elderly care can cause frustration and resentment but equally can be a chance to learn patience and acceptance.

Relationships

The first and most important relationship is that between a baby and its primary care giver, the person who is attentive and meets the baby's need for love. Bowlby suggested that babies who do not have a bond with a primary care giver in the first five years of life may find it difficult to form trusting relationships later on.

- Birth to 18 months is the time when a baby learns whether it can trust those around it.

- From 18 months to 3 years, a child with supportive relationships will gain confidence and independence.

- By 5 years, a child begins to use its initiative. A child who does not have supportive relationships will doubt themselves, may be reluctant to try new things in case they are wrong, and may feel guilt especially if told they are naughty.

Childhood relationships are primarily within the family although friendships begin to develop at school. Supportive relationships at home will encourage a child to gain new skills if praised for what they try as well as what they achieve. Children who are not supported by positive relationships may begin to feel inferior and become overly self-critical — seeing their mistakes rather than what they do right.

Adolescent relationships are still family focused, but increasingly, peer relationships become important. During this time, supportive relationships help the adolescent find out who they are, their strengths and their weaknesses. Supportive relationships at home and with peers help the adolescent gain a sense of self-worth. Unfortunately, at this age, relationships can have a negative impact. Vulnerable adolescents may be bullied face-to-face or by comments on social media from 'friends'.

Early adulthood is the main time for establishing relationships with a life partner. Some people establish intimacy and the relationship becomes a key source of support in their lives. Others might not find the right person they can trust, or the relationship they thought would last forever breaks down and they become isolated, with few or no supportive relationships.

Middle adulthood is time to build a career and create a family or a network of friends, supported by the positive relationships they have established. New relationships perhaps with children or grandchildren bring opportunities to support others. Sometimes people meet a new partner and build a new family at this stage in life. While it can be a time of fulfilment for adults, the effect on children of family splits and reformations can have a big impact socially and emotionally.

Late adulthood relationships focus on old friends, family and local community as retirement narrows the social circle. Some people continue to make new friends, establish positive relationships with people of all ages, and have a wider network of support. Some older adults use Skype and WhatsApp to keep in touch and maintain relationships with those not geographically nearby. Such supportive relationships help them pull through when ill-health and bereavement occur.

Independence

Infancy, childhood and adolescence are periods of increasing physical, social and emotional independence. Children learn to dress and feed themselves, and take care of their own personal hygiene needs. Early and mid-adulthood is the time of maximum physical, social and emotional independence and when financial independence is usually achieved. In later adulthood, independence may decrease due to age-related disorders. Physically, the person may not see or hear as well. They may have limited physical mobility and be reliant on others to do their shopping or help them have a shower. They may be financially dependent on the government or on family to help them with living costs as they may no longer work. However, not all older adults lose their independence. Many continue to live active lives well into their 90s.

Health

Health is not just the absence of disease but the sum total of physical and mental health, affecting every aspect of what we do in life. Genetic factors influence health. We cannot change the genes we have inherited, but we can try to keep healthy. Lifestyle factors such as diet and exercise affect physical and mental health. Keeping active and eating a healthy diet can do much to promote health throughout life and to slow the progress of age-related disorders (recommended activity levels were described earlier in the unit). Mental health is also very important and a person with good mental health adapts to change. A secure emotional bond with a primary care giver, and supportive relationships will help children, adolescents and adults develop good mental health.

Resilience

This refers to an individual's ability to recover quickly from difficulties. Physical resilience is measured by how quickly a person recovers from an illness. Babies and children can get sick quickly but also can recover quickly. The protection they get from mother's milk and from vaccinations gives them some protection, but in general, a physically healthy child will bounce back from an infection whereas an older person may take longer to recover.

Emotional resilience refers to the ability to recover mentally from situations. Babies and young children are emotionally resilient. A baby separated from its soother will yell furiously but the moment the soother is returned the baby is happy. Less resilient adolescents (and adults) faced with personal challenge may become increasingly anxious. Generally, those who adapt well to change are more emotionally resilient than those who do not. Emotional resilience increases self-esteem and can be learned.

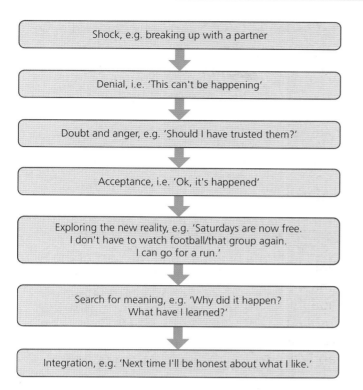

Shock, e.g. breaking up with a partner

Denial, i.e. 'This can't be happening'

Doubt and anger, e.g. 'Should I have trusted them?'

Acceptance, i.e. 'Ok, it's happened'

Exploring the new reality, e.g. 'Saturdays are now free. I don't have to watch football/that group again. I can go for a run.'

Search for meaning, e.g. 'Why did it happen? What have I learned?'

Integration, e.g. 'Next time I'll be honest about what I like.'

Figure 2.4 Transition model (adapted from **www.slideshare. net/Lucia_Merino/stages-of-change-15015562**)

Explain Activity

Write an article for a magazine to explain the impact that significant life events may have on an individual.

Either make up a fictitious person, or if it based on someone you know, ensure confidentiality by changing their name so they cannot be identified. Describe what the life events are and how they affect them.

 Check your understanding 3

1 Give an example of a life event for each of these stages of life:
  ● Infancy ● Adolescence
  ● Childhood ● Adulthood.
2 For each of the examples you gave for Question 1, describe how the life event might affect the person's emotions and relationships.
3 How might the life events impact on an individual's independence and health?
4 Explain, using examples, what is meant by 'emotional resilience'.

LO4 Understand how health and social care services meet the care needs of individuals through the lifespan

When the National Health Service (NHS) was introduced in 1947, it was proudly declared that the government provided care from 'cradle to grave', i.e. from birth right through to the end of life. Health services were provided nationally so it did not matter where you lived in the country, you were still entitled to access to health care. Social care is provided by local councils and planned according to local need, so if there are a lot of children in an area, the local council provides more children's services. If a local authority has a lot of older people, they will provide more services for older people.

4.1 Care needs of individuals through the life stages

Our need for care changes. Infants and children require more care because they are unable to care for themselves. Most adults can care for themselves but as they get older, they may need help.

Infancy

This is a period of total dependency on adults. Infants cannot buy and cook food, turn on the heating or run a bath. They need someone to feed them, wash them, change their nappy and love them. They need physical, social and emotional support to grow and become independent.

Childhood

This is a time of increasing independence. Young children learn to dress themselves, clean their teeth, and go to the toilet. Although they can do many things for themselves, they still need help, for example at around six or seven years old, they may learn to make toast, but they cannot plan and cook meals. They can feed themselves but may not, if left to their own devices, choose a healthy diet. They may need someone to show them how to share and take turns. They need encouragement to try new things and keep going, for example when learning to read and write. They still need physical, social and emotional support to grow and become independent.

Adolescence

This is a time of physical independence. While many adolescents can cook a basic meal and shop for the ingredients, they need help at this stage to understand and cope with physical changes in their bodies, as well as the social and emotional changes puberty brings. Adolescents may need help to develop social confidence and emotional resilience if they do not have this already.

Looking at the cause of death at different ages can help us decide what health care is needed. If people are dying from infectious diseases we can plan to control those diseases through vaccinations. If they are dying from mental health issues such as suicide, we can put more resources into preventing deaths from mental ill-health. Support for mental health is particularly important in adolescence. Research into adolescent mental health can be found on the National Institute of Mental Health website (**www.nimh.nih.gov/about/ advisory-boards-and-groups/namhc/ reports/blueprint-for-change-research- on-child-and-adolescent-mental-health. shtml**).

Early, middle, late adulthood

Adults often feel they should be able to look after themselves and ignore their own needs, either because they are too busy caring for others, or are too busy building a career.

By looking at the reasons why adults die, we can work out where care is needed.

According to the Office for National Statistics, from 2001 to 2017, the most frequent cause of death for 20- to 34-year-olds was suicide followed by traffic accidents, liver disease and homicide (**www.ons.gov.uk**). These are related to unhealthy lifestyle choices as young adults establish themselves and either die trying to live up to their ideal of being tough or feel rejected by their peers and commit suicide. It is now thought that adolescence lasts until the twenties and the part of the brain responsible for judgement matures less quickly. Poor judgement may be a factor in death from road traffic accidents and alcohol intake. Improved mental health services are needed however, as statistics show that many are not getting the support they need. In the age group 20–40, women attended a GP twice as often as men, yet the suicide rate shows that young men need mental health support (**www.menshealthforum.org.uk**).

Mental health support is needed for middle-aged men. In 2017, suicide remained the leading cause of death for males aged 35 to 49 years, followed by heart disease which is linked to lifestyle factors. For females of this age, breast cancer followed by cirrhosis and other diseases of the liver were the main causes of death. There is a need for effective health education and effective health promotion in this age group as many of these are preventable deaths.

For older adults, aged 50 to 64 and 65 to 79 years heart disease, lung cancer and for females aged 50 to 64 years, breast cancer, are the main causes of death. These are largely preventable. Heart disease and lung cancer are related to smoking. These individuals require help to give up smoking and make healthier lifestyle choices. Health promotion and disease prevention services are needed. Poor air quality also contributes to lung disease.

For adults aged 80 years and over, dementia and Alzheimer disease remained the leading cause of death followed by heart diseases, influenza and pneumonia, cerebrovascular diseases (strokes) and respiratory diseases (**www.ons.gov.uk**). People over 80 years of age have the cumulative effects of multiple health problems and are less able to fight off infections. They need services to enable them to remain active, to reduce heart disease and strokes. Flu vaccinations reduce the number of deaths from influenza and respiratory infections. The causes of dementia are not yet understood but it is thought that remaining active and independent for as long as possible may delay the onset. Therefore health promotion for this age uses a holistic model and is targeted at keeping people healthy and active, with day centres for activities, and free travel passes to encourage older people to get out and stay active.

Description Activity

Write an account which describes the care needs of individuals through each life stage.

A minimum of two relevant and traceable references must be used, referenced briefly within the text and in full in a reference list at the end.

4.2 How health and social care services meet the care needs of individuals through the life stages

Health and social care services are there to meet the needs of all ages. The government allocates money gathered from taxes to pay for these services but demand is increasing. Improving technology means we can save premature babies who are so small they can fit into the palm of an adult's hand. They need months of intensive care. Older people live longer and need hip replacements. Funding is scarce for services and this can impact availability and accessibility.

Local authorities

Local authorities have a broad public health role, ensuring waste is not left rotting in the street, controlling rats and other vermin that spread disease, and checking the food hygiene standards of eating places. They have a social role too, providing housing and schools (**www.local.gov.uk**). In addition to these broad public health roles, they have specific functions to provide information about how the care and support system works and the services available, such as to:

- promote a range of high-quality providers so people can choose what they need
- co-operate with other local organisations
- integrate services
- provide early interventions to reduce dependency on services.

Some services are available at any time of life, for example everyone is entitled to an assessment of their needs and a care plan for identified needs. Carers too are entitled to an assessment and if needs are identified, they are given information about services. If eligible for help, a personal budget may be given to them to purchase required services, or the money may be used on their behalf to organise the services they need. The social worker will review the care plan with them periodically to make sure there have been no changes. If a person is not entitled to financial help, they must still be told what services are available so they can purchase the services for themselves with their own money.

Local authorities have special responsibilities for children and vulnerable adults, for example those with learning difficulties or complex needs. Children's services include:

- Children's Advice and Support Service — a single point of contact for professionals and members of the public who want support or are concerned about a child.

- Emergency duty teams — social workers respond to any concerns about children reported by the public or professionals.

- Early help — for children and their families. A Family Plan is drawn up to identify what is needed to help the family. Services come from a range of organisations working together.

- Family support is offered at Children's centres (see below).

- Youth Offending — for 10- to 17-year-olds. Local authority children's services, probation, police, education, health and voluntary agencies work together to deliver projects that reduce youth offending and look at the underlying causes of crime.

- Children in care — children and young people may be cared for by the local authority for a short while, for example if their parents are unwell, or for longer if a court has ordered it is in their best interests to be in the care of the local authority. Children stay with foster parents who have been screened for suitability. Occasionally, children will live in residential care (a children's home). Where possible they are placed in their local areas so they can go to the same school. They would have a social worker, a care plan and regular reviews to ensure the care suits their needs.

- Care leavers — all young people leave care when they turn 18 years old, but can stay with their foster carers after this if both the young person and their carers agree. If they are in care for at least 13 weeks after they turn 16 years old, they are entitled to leaving care support until the age of 21 (or 25 if still in full-time education). Leaving care support helps with accommodation, further education and employment.

- Adoption and fostering — adoption is permanent. It means becoming the legal parent(s) to a child who is no longer able to live with their birth family. Where possible, children who are to be adopted are placed early with their adoptive parents rather than going to a temporary foster parent. Local authorities are responsible for vetting prospective parents and ensuring the suitability of the placement.

- Fostering is a temporary arrangement and may be short or long term. Foster parents offer the child a family, but do not take on the legal responsibility of a parent. They are trained over a period of six months and supported in their role by the local authority. Sometimes a child returns to their own family or they go on to be adopted. At other times they are fostered until they leave care (adapted from **www.birminghamchildrenstrust.co.uk**).

A similar assessment and care planning process takes place for adults with care and support needs aged 18 and over who may have:

- a learning disability
- a mental health need or dementia or a personality disorder
- a long- or short-term illness
- an addiction to a substance or alcohol
- age-related ill-health

Elderly people and people with disabilities can also have an assessment by an occupational therapist in their home to establish their needs and give advice. They may suggest hand rails, lever taps or a downstairs bathroom. After a financial assessment, some people are able to get financial help for changes through the Disabled Facilities Grant.

Supported living is an alternative for adults with learning/physical disabilities, sensory problems, or mental health problems. Older people, those who are moving out of hospital, and adults and young people with a disability who are moving towards independent living may also live in supported housing. It allows them to have their own tenancy where they are supported by care workers for between a few hours a day to 24-hour care.

Safeguarding children and vulnerable adults is part of the role of local authorities. The Safeguarding Adults Board works together with police, the NHS and the fire service, to protect adults with care and support needs from abuse and neglect. They review serious cases to draw lessons for how to improve care. The Safeguarding Children Board does a similar thing to protect children to the age of 18.

Hospitals

Hospitals offer secondary care for all ages. People are referred there by the general practitioner (GP). Some hospitals, but not all, offer accident and emergency (A&E) services, where you can just turn up (self-referral) or be taken by ambulance following a 999 call. Some hospitals, but not all, offer maternity services. Some regional hospitals offer specialist services, for example mental health services or children's services.

General Practitioner services

General Practitioner services provide primary care in the community for all ages. As well as GP services from a general doctor, the local clinic may offer diabetic screening, flu vaccinations, counselling, baby clinics and other services such as family planning.

Day centres

These provide services for adults and offer a variety of activities to help people stay well and socially engaged. Activities include arts and crafts, IT workshops and health and well-being classes. Day centres can be organised in purpose-built centres alongside health clinic and chiropody services or they can be in community centres or places of worship.

Some day centres offer specialist dementia services with gentle music-based activities for adults and their carers.

Children's centres

These are run by local authorities and offer a range of support services to all children aged 0–5 years old and their families. These universal services include:

- Early education and childcare
- Sessional care, for example playgroups
- Health services, for example midwives and health visits
- Parenting support
- Family support
- Support for parents looking for training or job opportunities.

Residential homes

Residential homes offer accommodation and care for older people who can no longer manage at home but are not ill. They are usually privately owned but have a contract with a local authority to provide places for those funded by the local authority. Some also take private clients. Residential homes have staff on duty 24 hours a day but care homes with nursing have a registered nurse on duty at all times. Some offer specialist dementia care.

Residential homes for children under the care of the local authority are decreasing as fostering services increase.

Community

Home support or domiciliary care is often preferred by adults who want to stay in their own home as long as they can. Carers come in and help with basic needs, such as washing and dressing, and may call again later in the day to help the person get ready for bed. Most domiciliary care agencies are privately owned, get contracts from the local authority and also take private clients.

Community health services cover 'cradle-to-grave' services mostly in people's homes. Teams of nurses and therapists co-ordinate care, working with professions including GPs and social care workers. Community health provides preventative and health improvement services, often with partners from local government and the third or voluntary sector. Community midwives, health visitors and school nurses look after the needs of children. Physiotherapists, occupational therapists, speech and language therapists and podiatrists help people to recover from a major health event such as a stroke. Community nurses care for people with long-term conditions and provide care for those at the end of life (**www.nhsconfed.org**).

Rapid response teams assess people who have either suddenly become unwell or have a long-term condition that has suddenly worsened. They provide care at home to avoid unnecessary hospital admissions. A rapid response team will include nurses, mental health nurses, therapists, rehabilitation assistants and social workers.

Rehabilitation

This is the process of restoring someone to health or normal life through training and therapy after addiction or illness.

Older people take longer to recover from illnesses and accidents than younger people. They lose muscle strength when they are not active, and so it is important to rehabilitate them as quickly as possible. Physiotherapy may be needed, for example for exercise after a knee replacement. Occupational therapy may be needed to ensure people can cope with activities of daily living such as washing and dressing. While younger

people may have family to support them after discharge from hospital, this is not always the case for older people. Sometimes, older people are fit for discharge but need a period of rehabilitation before they are ready to live alone. They may be transferred to a step-down bed in a care home as they recover while a care package is set up for when they are at home.

For those with addictions needing rehabilitation, for example drugs or alcohol, it can be expensive. It may be provided by the NHS or by one of many charities as a residential course. It may also be offered as a private fee-paying service.

Mental health rehabilitation aims to help people suffering from long-term mental health issues cope with daily life without long stays in hospital. Mental health rehabilitation may begin in hospital, with support from counselling and medication, to help the person develop effective ways of coping. They may then move to live in the community with continuing support from the team.

Counselling

This is an effective form of therapy. It is a talking therapy that involves a trained therapist listening and helping you find ways to deal with emotional issues. It is effective for treating depression, anxiety and eating disorders, after bereavement, and for anger management. Counsellors do not judge; they listen and help the person gain a better understanding of their thoughts and feelings so they can find their own solutions to problems.

Counselling can be face-to-face, in a group, over the phone, by email or online through live chat services. A person can be referred by their GP or refer themselves for therapy (self-referral). Their GP does not have to be informed unless they are a risk to themselves or others. They must be over 16, 17 or 18 years old depending on the area, but children and young people who are not eligible for psychological therapies can get support with mental and emotional problems from their local child and adolescent mental health service (CAMHS).

Cognitive behavioural therapy (CBT) is particularly effective as it helps the person understand how their thoughts affect their behaviour, and how changing their thoughts can change the way they interact with others. CBT deals with current problems the person has, and helps them manage overwhelming problems by tackling them in smaller, more manageable portions (**www.nhs.uk/ conditions/cognitive-behavioural-therapy-cbt**). Other types of counselling are used in mental health services but CBT is the most frequently used.

Charities

Sometimes called the voluntary or third sector, charities provide a lot of care that perhaps might be expected from the NHS or social services. Some provide services for a specific age group, for example:

- The National Society for the Prevention of Cruelty to Children (NSPCC) works to prevent child abuse. It has statutory powers and can take action to safeguard children at risk of abuse. It also runs ChildLine, a support and advice service for children online or by phoning 0800 1111, where trained counsellors can respond and help them.

- Age UK is the largest charity for older people. It provides advice and support on health, well-being and care issues (**www.ageuk.org.uk**).

Some charities fill the gap in mental health services. For example:

- Samaritans is a free, one-to-one helpline on 116 123 for people going through a difficult time and at risk of suicide. It is open 24 hours a day (**www.samaritans.org**).

- MIND provides advice and support for those experiencing a mental health problem (**www.mind.org.uk**).

- The Alzheimer's Society provides information and support in the community for people with dementia (**www.alzheimers.org.uk**).

Some charities provide a service that is not usually offered in the NHS. Hospice care for the terminally ill is mostly provided by charities. Hospices work in local communities and offer holistic care tailored to individual needs. For example:

- Acorns, a Midlands charity, provides specialist palliative nursing care and support for those aged 0–18 years with life-limiting or life-threatening conditions. It supports their families, including the bereaved. It is funded by charitable donations (**www.acorns.org.uk**).

- The Marie Curie organisation supports adults with terminal illness, providing Marie Curie nurses in the person's own home, and hospice services as well as advice and information (**www.mariecurie.org.uk**).

Explain Activity

Prepare a presentation for young people interested in health and social care services in which you explain how services meet the care needs of individuals through the life stages. Use examples to support the explanation.

A minimum of two relevant and traceable references must be used, referenced briefly within the text and in full in a reference list at the end.

Note: The activity for AC4.1 focuses on the needs, but activity AC4.2 focuses on how the needs are met. You may wish to build on the AC4.1 activity by saying how each need is met by health and care services, thus meeting AC4.2. Use an example to show each need and how it is met by health and care services.

Check your understanding 4

1 How do physical needs vary across life stages?
2 How do health and social care services meet these needs?
3 How do the emotional needs of infants, adolescents and those in late adulthood differ?
4 How do health and social care services meet these needs?
5 How do social needs vary across life stages?
6 How do health and social care services meet these needs?

 Classroom Discussion

Some young people carry knives. How much does peer pressure contribute to this? How far do you think gang culture influences this behaviour? What need or needs does this fulfil? How else could these needs be met? From your knowledge of young people, what reasons do they give for carrying knives? Do these reasons seem valid to you? What problems might there be with carrying a knife? Does anyone else have a responsibility in this situation, for example the school or police?

 Case scenario

N ran away from home when she was 15 years old after being abused by her mum and step-dad. She ended up sleeping on the streets where she was groomed to pack and carry drugs. She was taken to out-of-town trap houses for weeks at a time, given a mobile phone and told she had to sell the drugs. Having lost contact with her family, friends and school, and needing a place to eat and sleep, she became completely dependent on those exploiting her.

1 What are N's physical, emotional, social and cognitive needs at this point in her life?
2 How could health and social care services, including charities, meet those needs?
3 What needs might she have in the next ten years?
4 How could health and social care services meet those needs?

Read about it

Ahern, N., 2008, 'Resilience and coping strategies in adolescents', *Paediatric Nursing*, vol. 20, no 10 www.nursingacademy. com/uploads/6/4/8/8/6488931/ adolescentresiliency.pdf

Segal, N. L., *Born together, Reared apart* – a study of twins http://drnancysegaltwins.org/ index.php/born-together-reared-apart

Bowlby's theory of maternal deprivation www. simplypsychology.org/bowlby.html

ChildLine service for children and young people at risk of harm www.childline.org.uk

Citizen's Advice – Living together and marriage: legal differences www.citizensadvice.org.uk

Cognitive behavioural therapy www.nhs.uk/ conditions/cognitive-behavioural-therapy-cbt

Erikson's theory of psychosocial development www.learning-theories.com/eriksons-stages-of-development

Female menopause www.nhs.uk/conditions/ menopause

Genie: Feral Child www.youtube.com/ watch?v=YQNBSPY4QUc

Information about counselling services www. nhs.uk/conditions/Counselling

Information about dementia www.alzheimers. org.uk

Male menopause www.nhs.uk/conditions/ male-menopause

Mental health rehabilitation services www. rcpsych.ac.uk

Minnesota centre for twin and family research http://mctfr.psych.umn.edu/

New rapid response teams will 'dissolve boundary' between GPs and community nurses, 21 November 2018 www.nursingtimes.net

Osteoporosis www.nhs.uk/conditions/ osteoporosis

Piaget's theory of cognitive development www. simplypsychology.org/piaget.html

Puberty – what happens www.nhs.uk/live-well/sexual-health/stages-of-puberty-what-happens-to-boys-and-girls

Restricted growth or achondroplasia www.nhs. uk/conditions/restricted-growth

Types of households 2017 – Office for National Statistics www.ons.gov.uk/ peoplepopulationandcommunity/ birthsdeathsandmarriages/families/bulletins/ familiesandhouseholds/2017#multi-family-households-have-grown-the-fastest-but-which-household-type-is-the-most-common-in-the-uk

What are community health services? www. nhsconfed.org

How will I be graded?

The table below shows what learners must do to achieve each grading criterion. Learners must achieve all the criteria for a grade to be awarded. A higher grade may not be awarded before a lower grade has been achieved, although component criteria of a higher grade may have been achieved.

Grade	Assessment Criteria number	Assessment Criteria/What you need to show
D1	1.1	Outline the life stages of human growth and development.
D2	1.2	Outline social, emotional, cognitive and physical development within one (1) life stage.
D3	1.3	Describe holistic development. Examples may be used to support the description.
D4		A minimum of one (1) relevant and traceable reference must be included.
C1	2.1	Outline the nature versus nurture debate in relation to human growth and development.
C2	2.3	Discuss factors which impact upon human growth and development. A minimum of three (3) factors which impact upon human growth and development must be discussed.
C3	3.1	Outline significant life events across each life stage.
C4	4.1	Describe care needs of individuals through each life stage.
B1	2.2	Outline the: ● medical model of health and well-being ● social model of health and well-being.
B2	2.4	Explain the importance of recognising and responding to concerns regarding an individual's growth and development.
B3		A minimum of two (2) relevant and traceable references must be included. A reference list must be included.
A1	3.2	Explain the impact that significant life events may have on an individual.
A*1	4.2	Explain how health and social care services meet the care needs of individuals through the life stages. Examples must be used to support the explanation.
A*2		References must be present throughout to show evidence of knowledge and understanding gained from wider reading. References must be relevant and traceable.

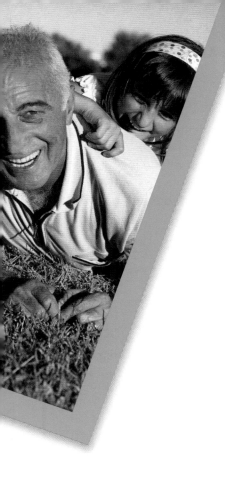

Safeguarding and protection in health and social care

About this unit

Safeguarding individuals and protecting them from harm and abuse is one of the most important responsibilities of a health and social care practitioner. This unit will provide you with the knowledge about the relevant safeguarding legislation, policies and procedures that exist. You will also develop your understanding of the responsibilities the health and social care practitioner has, including understanding the different types of abuse and what makes an individual more vulnerable to being abused or harmed.

You will explore the actions to take in response to evidence or concerns that an individual is at risk or has been harmed or abused, including the boundaries of confidentiality. Finally, you will consider the many benefits that exist for the health and social care practitioner working in partnership with others to safeguard and protect individuals.

Learning Outcomes

LO1: Understand legislation, policies, procedures and codes of practice in relation to safeguarding and protection.

1.1 Safeguarding:

- central to high quality health and social care provision
- protection of health, well-being and human rights
- freedom from harm and abuse.

Protection:

- detecting and preventing harm and abuse.

1.2 Legislation, policies, procedures and codes of practice in relation to the safeguarding and protection of:

- children and young people
- adults.

Children and young people:

- Equality Act 2010
- Children Acts 1989, 2004
- Children and Social Work Act 2017
- Human Rights Act 1998
- General Data Protection Regulation (GDPR) 2018
- Public Interest Disclosure Act 1998
- United Nations Convention on the Rights of the Child 1992
- Working Together to Safeguard Children 2013, 2015, 2018
- the role of the Local Safeguarding Children Board
- related policies and procedures
- codes of practice relevant to the sector
- current legislation as relevant to Home Nation.

→

Adults:

- Care Act 2014
- Health and Social Care Act 2012
- Equality Act 2010
- Mental Capacity Act 2005
- No Secrets 2000
- Human Rights Act 1998
- General Data Protection Regulation (GDPR) 2018
- Public Interest Disclosure Act 1998
- The Modern Slavery Act 2015
- Female Genital Mutilation Act 2003
- local multi-agency Safeguarding Adults policy and procedures, the role of the Local Safeguarding Adults Boards
- related policies and procedures
- codes of practice relevant to the sector
- current legislation as relevant to Home Nation.

LO2: Understand the role and responsibilities of the health and social care practitioner in relation to safeguarding.

2.1 How the health and social care practitioner safeguards individuals:

- work within policies and procedures
- duty of care
- person-centred practice
- monitoring, observation, reporting, recording
- partnership working
- confidentiality
- whistleblowing.

2.2 How the health and social care practitioner safeguards themselves:

- working within policies and procedures
- duty of care
- personal care
- physical contact
- technology
- confidentiality
- record keeping
- whistleblowing.

LO3: Understand types of abuse.

3.1. Types of abuse:

- self-neglect
- physical
- emotional
- sexual
- domestic
- financial

- institutional
- bullying.

3.2 Signs, symptoms, indicators and behaviours which may cause concern:

- as related to the types of abuse in 3.1.

3.3 Factors which contribute to an individual being vulnerable to harm or abuse:

- age
- health
- substance abuse
- disability
- isolation
- social media
- environment.

LO4: Understand action to be taken by the health and social care practitioner in response to evidence or concerns that an individual is at risk or has been harmed or abused.

4.1 Actions to take if harm or abuse is suspected or disclosed:

- work within policies and procedures
- lines of reporting and responsibility
- maintain safety
- preservation of evidence
- confidentiality
- listening, reassurance, non-judgement.

4.2 The responsibilities of the health and social care practitioner in relation to whistleblowing:

- reporting concerns of practice
- reporting to external body in response to no action being taken.

4.3 The boundaries of confidentiality in relation to the safeguarding, protection and well-being of individuals:

- duty of care
- consent
- need-to-know
- policy and procedures.

LO5: Understand the benefits of working in partnership in relation to safeguarding and protection.

5.1 The benefits of working in partnership in relation to safeguarding and protection:

- expertise
- working together towards shared goals
- defined roles and responsibilities
- intervention
- referrals.

LO1 Understand legislation, policies, procedures and codes of practice in relation to safeguarding and protection

1.1 Safeguarding and protection

What is safeguarding?

Safeguarding children and adults is central to high quality health and social care provision because it involves providing individuals with:

- safe care that stops abuse or neglect wherever possible
- effective care that supports them in making choices and being in control so they can decide how they want to live
- effective care so they know the course of action to take should they or someone else have a concern about their safety or well-being
- care that gives them the best outcomes in life, focusing on improving their lives.

Safeguarding children and adults includes the protection of health, well-being and human rights because it involves:

- promoting individuals' health, development and well-being
- preventing the impairment of individuals' health, development and well-being
- promoting individuals' human rights to live safely, free from **abuse** and **neglect** (you will learn more about individuals' human rights in 1.2).

Safeguarding children and adults includes freedom from **harm** and abuse because it involves:

- protecting individuals from maltreatment
- preventing individuals from being placed in danger

- preventing individuals from experiencing harm, abuse and neglect.

Everyone who works with children and adults has a responsibility to keep them safe. For example, health and social care practitioners can do this by recognising when an individual is being harmed or abused and knowing the actions to take. When safeguarding individuals, it is their needs, interests and views that must come first. For example, health and social care practitioners can do this by listening to what an individual would like to happen as a result of the safeguarding process. They should be working closely with them to find the best outcome.

 Key terms

Abuse is when a person is mistreated in a way that causes them pain and harm.

Harm is when someone is at risk either physically or emotionally; this may be intentional (i.e. abuse) or unintentional (i.e. an accident).

Neglect is when a person's needs are not met through failure to care.

What is protection?

Protection of children and adults is closely linked to safeguarding because it involves detecting and preventing harm and abuse. It is important that all those who work with children and adults, such as individuals' families, health and social care practitioners, advocates and professionals, such as GPs, nurses and social workers:

- understand their own and each other's responsibilities in the safeguarding process
- work together to understand the different types of abuse, recognising what signs to look for out for that may indicate that an individual is in danger of being harmed and abused

- respond to abuse and neglect when it occurs
- work together to prevent individuals from being harmed and abused by raising awareness of and promoting well-being.

Everyone who works with children and adults has a responsibility to protect them from being harmed and abused. For example, health and social care practitioners can do this by attending regular training sessions on safeguarding. When protecting individuals, it is their safety and well-being that must come first. Health and social care practitioners can do this by, for example, ensuring that individuals have a representative when they need it during the safeguarding process.

Description Activity

Discuss with someone you know what the terms 'safeguarding' and 'protection' mean. Describe why safeguarding and protection are relevant when providing care and support to children and adults.

1.2 Legislation, policies, procedures and codes of practice in relation to the safeguarding and protection of:

- **children and young people**
- **adults**

Health and social care practitioners can safeguard and protect children and young people by being aware of the current **legislation** that exists in both the UK and internationally. They can do this by ensuring that their ways of working comply with their employer's safeguarding **policies** and **procedures** and the **codes of practice** that exist across the health and social care sector. Some of the main pieces of legislation, policies, procedures and codes of practice that are relevant to safeguarding are outlined in this section.

Equality Act 2010

The **Equality Act** safeguards and protects individuals, including children and young people, by making it unlawful to discriminate and treat individuals unfairly. Children and young people are protected from discrimination by, for example:

- organisations, such as retail shops that provide services
- health and care providers, such as hospitals
- education providers, such as schools.

Under the Equality Act, there are nine protected characteristics and if discrimination happens because of one or more of these then it is considered unlawful. The nine characteristics that are relevant to everyone, including children and young people, are:

- age
- disability
- gender reassignment
- marriage or civil partnership (in employment only)
- pregnancy and maternity
- race
- religion or belief
- sex
- sexual orientation.

Children Acts 1989, 2004

The **Children Act 1989** safeguards children (up to the age of 18) and promotes their welfare by:

- ensuring that safeguarding is everyone's responsibility (e.g. local authorities, courts, parents, health and social care practitioners)
- establishing the paramountcy principle. This means that a child's welfare is the most important factor when making any decisions about a child's upbringing

- avoiding (or at least reducing) delays when making decisions about a child's welfare. This is because delays are likely to prejudice the welfare of the child

- establishing the 'no order principle'. This means that the court will not make an order in relation to the welfare of the child, unless doing so is better for the child than making no order at all.

The Children Act 2004 safeguards and protects children (up to the age of 18) at risk from harm and abuse by:

- promoting the child's welfare. For example, when a local authority applies for an **emergency protection order** to remove a child from the family they live with because there is a serious concern that the child is likely to be harmed.

- promoting the child's right to be consulted. A child's wishes must be listened to and taken into consideration when making decisions concerning them.

- promoting the child's right to be represented. A child has a right to have an independent person such as an **advocate** act on their behalf during the safeguarding process.

- establishing the aims for services for children. Under the *Every Child Matters* document, the five aims include supporting children to:
  1 be healthy
  2 stay safe
  3 enjoy and achieve
  4 make a positive contribution
  5 achieve economic well-being.

- promoting services working in partnership. This is when different services involved in protecting children work together by sharing information to avoid any misunderstandings.

- establishing the role of the Children's Commissioner. This person champions the views and interests of children and reports to Parliament.

- establishing Children Safeguarding Boards. These boards represent the best interests of children and develop safeguarding policies and procedures for local areas.

Key terms

Advocate refers to an independent person who represents the views, needs and interests of individuals who are unable or unwilling to do so themselves, and supports them to express their views, i.e. during a safeguarding inquiry.

Codes of practice set out the standards or values that health and social care practitioners must follow to provide high-quality, safe, compassionate and effective care and support.

Emergency protection order is an order issued by the court in an emergency that enables the child to be removed from where they are living because they are at risk of physical, mental or emotional harm.

Legislation are the laws that must be followed, for example Acts of Parliament, as well as regulations, such as the General Data Protection Regulations (GDPR).

Policies are statements of how an organisation works based on legislation, such as a safeguarding policy.

Procedures are step-by-step guides of how to put a policy into practice.

Children and Social Work Act 2017

The **Children and Social Work Act 2017** has amended the **Children Act 2004** and made changes to safeguarding arrangements for children and young people by:

- establishing a new national Child Safeguarding Practice Review Panel. The panel's role is to identify and review local safeguarding cases that are complex or of national significance. This is so that improvements can be made to safeguard and promote the welfare of children.

- abolishing Local Safeguarding Children Boards and instead placing duties on three 'safeguarding partners':

  1 the local authority

  2 any **Clinical Commissioning Groups (CCGs)** operating in the area

  3 the Chief Officer of Police.

  These safeguarding partners will be responsible for safeguarding children in their area.

- establishing new Child Death Review Partners who will consist of local authorities and any clinical commissioning groups for the local area. They will undertake a review of every death of a child usually resident in their area, and of children not usually resident in their area (if appropriate).

- extending the protection of whistleblowers (i.e. against employment discrimination) to include those who work in children's social care roles, local authorities and other providers of statutory social care services.

Human Rights Act 1998

The **Human Rights Act** protects the human rights of every person living in the UK. This includes safeguarding the human rights of children and young people by:

- promoting the child's human rights. For example, to live with dignity and free from abuse; to develop and fulfil their potential.

- promoting the child's right to not be at risk from harm. For example, local authorities have a duty to protect the human rights of

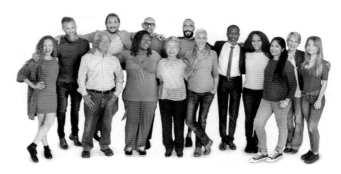

Figure 3.1 How are people's human rights protected in the UK?

children that are in care, making sure they are not subjected to degrading or cruel treatment.

General Data Protection Regulation (GDPR) 2018

The **General Data Protection Regulation (GDPR)** came into effect in May 2018. It protects the rights of everyone who has personal information or data recorded, used, stored and shared by organisations. Personal data applies to both paper-based and electronic records. It includes information such as:

- email addresses

- telephone numbers

- health records or social information held about individuals.

The GDPR is a law that replaced the Data Protection Act 1998. It gives people more rights over their personal information and how it is processed. In relation to children and young people, the GDPR does this by claiming that data protection is everyone's responsibility and must be child-centred.

Under the GDPR, all organisations must obtain individuals' consent to collect, store and use their personal data. Individuals also have the right under the GDPR to withdraw their consent for use of their personal data or ask for it to be deleted or erased. The

GDPR also allows parents and guardians to give consent for their children's data to be used. The GDPR states that consent must be given freely and be specific, informed and unambiguous.

Public Interest Disclosure Act 1998

The **Public Interest Disclosure Act** safeguards individuals, including children and young people, who have care and support needs from abuse or harm by:

- requiring that organisations have **whistleblowing** procedures in place

- ensuring that any suspicions and allegations of abuse can be reported by health and social care practitioners, free from fear of repercussions from their employers.

 Key terms

Clinical Commissioning Groups (CCGs) are local public bodies made up of doctors, nurse specialists, lay people and others such as service users. They commission (buy) care services from private and NHS providers to meet the needs of their local community.

Whistleblowing is when a person discloses or reports any information or activity that is deemed illegal or unethical, such as unsafe practices or abuse.

United Nations Convention on the Rights of the Child 1992

The **United Nations Convention on the Rights of the Child** is an international set of human rights for all children and young people (aged 17 and under) irrespective of their gender, religion or abilities. It safeguards and protects children by:

- establishing the rights that all children and young people have, for example the right to think and believe what they choose; the right to privacy; the right to education; the right to play; the right to be safe from violence.

- promoting working in partnership by setting out how everyone, including people and governments, must work together to ensure children's rights are upheld.

Working Together to Safeguard Children 2013, 2015, 2018

Working Together to Safeguard Children 2013 provides guidance to adults working with children and families in England, replacing the previous guidance of 2010. It safeguards and protects children by:

- confirming that safeguarding is everyone's responsibility.

- promoting a child-centred approach to safeguarding children (i.e. one that is based on the needs and views of children).

- confirming that everyone who works with children must share safeguarding information in a timely manner.

- ensuring that **Local Safeguarding Children Boards** co-ordinate their work to safeguard children locally, monitoring and challenging the effectiveness of local systems in place.

- publishing **serious case reviews (SCRs)** if the safeguarding process goes wrong, being transparent about any mistakes that were made so lessons can be learnt.

Working Together to Safeguard Children 2015 provides guidance to adults working with children and families in England. It replaces the previous guidance of 2013 by introducing three key changes.

These changes safeguard and protect children and young people by:

- providing guidance on how to refer allegations of abuse against those who work with children. It requires local authorities to have a designated officer or team of officers for managing allegations of abuse against people who work with children.

- clarifying the requirements on local authorities to notify serious incidents. It clarifies a notifiable incident as one involving the care of a child, which meets any of the following criteria:

1 a child has died (including cases of suspected suicide), and abuse or neglect is known or suspected

2 a child has been seriously harmed and abuse or neglect is known or suspected

3 a looked-after child has died (including cases where abuse or neglect is not known or suspected)

4 a child in a regulated setting or service has died (including cases where abuse or neglect is not known or suspected).

- clarifying the definition of serious harm for the purposes of serious case reviews. For example, a child being seriously harmed includes, but is not limited to, cases where the child has sustained, as a result of abuse or neglect, any or all of the following:

1 a potentially life-threatening injury

2 a serious and/or likely long-term impairment of physical or mental health

3 a serious and/or likely long-term impairment of physical, intellectual, emotional, social or behavioural development.

In addition, it states that if a child recovers, this does not mean that they have not sustained serious harm.

Working Together to Safeguard Children 2018 has been published and replaces the previous guidance of 2015 in light of the Children and Social Work Act 2017. The guidance applies to all children up to the age of 18 years whether living with their families, in state care, or living independently, and to all schools. The key changes that have taken place and that safeguard and protect children and young people include the following:

- The replacement of the Local Safeguarding Children's Boards with Safeguarding Partners (see the section that follows for more information about the new system).

- The replacement of Serious Case Reviews (SCRs) by a new system of national and local child safeguarding practice reviews.

- The transfer of responsibility for child death reviews to new Child Death Review Partners who will consist of local authorities and any clinical commissioning groups for the local area.

- A new section has been added requiring organisations to have clear policies in place regarding allegations against people who work with children.

- A new section has been added requiring employees and volunteers in sports clubs and organisations to be aware of their safeguarding responsibilities.

- Other new sections included are in relation to: referrals; assessments of disabled children and their carers, young carers and children in secure youth establishments; designated healthcare professionals; Multi-Agency Public Protection Arrangements (MAPPA), and children's homes.

The role of the Local Safeguarding Children Board

In 2016, the function of the Local Safeguarding Children Boards was reviewed. They are responsible for co-ordinating the work to safeguard children locally, monitoring and challenging the effectiveness of local systems in place. As a result of this review, it was agreed that:

- The boards will be replaced with three safeguarding partners per local authority area: the local authority, a chief officer of police and a clinical commissioning group.

- It will be the responsibility of the **safeguarding partners** to make arrangements to work with relevant agencies (i.e. organisations and agencies whose involvement is considered essential to safeguarding) in order to protect the welfare of children in their area.

- The safeguarding partners must decide how they will best work together and which local safeguarding agencies they would like to work with in their locality.

- Their main responsibilities are:
  1 to involve relevant agencies in their area
  2 to identify and supervise the review of serious safeguarding cases in their area
  3 to publish and review their local safeguarding arrangements, in order to determine how effective the arrangements have been.

Key terms

Local Safeguarding Children Boards are responsible for overseeing different organisations in each local authority. They ensure that these organisations work together to develop effective systems for safeguarding and protecting children and young people from harm and abuse.

Safeguarding partners are those agencies who work together to safeguard individuals such as the police, the local authority, the NHS, health and social care organisations and education providers.

Serious case reviews (SCRs) refer (in this section) to an enquiry into the death or serious injury of a child where abuse or neglect is known or thought to be a factor. SCRs provide lessons that can be learned to prevent similar incidents occurring again.

Related policies and procedures

A range of local and national policies and procedures are in place to safeguard and protect children and young people.

- **Organisations' policies and procedures.** At a local level, all organisations providing care and support to children and young people will need to have agreed ways of working in place to safeguard and protect them. Although these may vary between different organisations, they will typically define the meaning of safeguarding and protection and outline how to:
  - identify when a child is being abused or harmed
  - safeguard children from abuse and harm
  - report concerns and explain the arrangements in place for whistleblowing.

- **People in Positions of Trust.** The Working Together 2018 national guidance emphasises the importance of organisations' responsibility to have clear policies in place regarding allegations against people who work with children. This includes all educational organisations, Early Years settings, healthcare professionals, child carers, children's homes, charities, voluntary organisations, social enterprises, faith-based organisations, and private sectors.

- **Safeguarding needs in sports clubs.** The Children and Social Work Act 2017 legislation states that staff (either paid or voluntary) at sports clubs and organisations need to be aware of their safeguarding responsibilities. They will need to work effectively with safeguarding partners to uphold the safeguarding arrangements that are in place.

- **Serious Case Reviews 2018.** This is a new system put in place to learn from national and local safeguarding case reviews. At a national level, the Child Safeguarding Practice Review Panel is responsible for how we learn from the serious safeguarding reviews. At a local level, the safeguarding partners will have this responsibility. They will then send copies of the reviews that they carry out to the Child Safeguarding Practice Review Panel, who will then decide if any of the reviews need to be made on a national level.

- **Child Death Review Partners.** The Children and Social Work Act 2017 (the Act) replaces Local Safeguarding Children Boards (LSCBs) with new local safeguarding arrangements that will be led by three safeguarding partners, i.e. local authorities, chief officers of police, and clinical commissioning groups. The responsibility for the child death reviews is being transferred to the new Child Death Review Partners. They will be responsible for the reviews of all child deaths of those who are normally residents in the local area, as well as non-resident children who have died in their local area (if deemed appropriate).

Codes of practice relevant to the sector

The main code of practice relevant to the sector is Working Together to Safeguard Children 2018. In addition, there are another two pieces of guidance that are relevant in England:

- **'What to do if you're worried a child is being abused: Advice for practitioners' (Department for Education, 2015).** This guidance outlines the indicators of abuse and neglect, including the actions to take if you think a child is being abused or neglected. It is relevant for anyone who comes into contact with children and families while working and applies to the statutory, voluntary and independent sectors.

- **'Mandatory reporting of female genital mutilation (FGM) – procedural information' (Home Office, 2015).** This guidance provides health and social care practitioners, teachers and the police with information on their responsibilities on how to report FGM.

Current legislation as relevant to Home Nation

Each of the UK's four nations England, Northern Ireland, Scotland and Wales have their own safeguarding laws to help protect children from abuse and neglect. You have learned about the safeguarding legislation relevant to England, but here is some more information about other legislation that is relevant to Northern Ireland, Scotland and Wales:

Safeguarding legislation for Northern Ireland

- **The Children (Northern Ireland) Order 1995** sets out the rights and responsibilities of parents, as well as the duties and powers of public authorities, to safeguard and promote children's safety and welfare.

- **The Safeguarding Board Act (Northern Ireland) 2011** established the Safeguarding Board for Northern Ireland.

- **The Children Services Co-operation Act (Northern Ireland) 2015** sets out the requirements for public authorities to promote the well-being of children and young people. This is in relation to their physical and mental health; their enjoyment of play and leisure; their learning and achievement; and their living conditions, rights, and economic well-being.

Safeguarding legislation for Scotland

- **The Children (Scotland) Act 1995** sets out the rights and responsibilities of parents, as well as the duties and powers of public authorities, to safeguard and promote children's safety and welfare. Under this Act, local authorities have a duty to assess the needs of care leavers up to the age of 26.

- **The Children and Young People (Scotland) Act 2014** promotes the rights of children and young people in planning services. Under this Act, a **Named Person** must advise and support the child or young person in accessing a service or support.

Safeguarding legislation for Wales

- **The Children Acts 1989, 2004** apply to both England and Wales. Some aspects of this Act have been amended or replaced by the Welsh pieces of legislation (see the following legislation).

- **The Social Services and Well-being (Wales) Act 2014** established a National Adoption Service and gave children and young people more control over the care and support they receive. It introduced a National Outcomes Framework for setting out what children and families can expect from social services.

- **The Well-being of Future Generations (Wales) Act 2015** established Local Safeguarding Children Boards in Wales; these are being replaced with Safeguarding Children Boards.

Outline Activity

Create a poster that outlines how a piece of legislation, policy, procedure or code of practice relates to the safeguarding and protection of children and young people.

1.2 Legislation, policies, procedures and codes of practice in relation to the safeguarding and protection of adults

Legislation, policies, procedures and codes of practice are also in place for the safeguarding and protection of adults with care and support needs, relevant to the practices of health and social care practitioners.

Care Act 2014

The **Care Act** replaced the No Secrets guidance (you will learn about this later on in the unit). It sets out how local authorities and other organisations must work together to protect adults at risk of abuse or neglect. It promotes their safety and well-being by ensuring that:

- Local authorities work in partnership with other organisations, such as the NHS and the police, to prevent abuse and neglect from happening. Abuse and neglect must be identified as early on as possible and stopped immediately when it does occur.

- Local authorities carry out Safeguarding Adults Reviews when an adult with care and support needs dies as a result of neglect or abuse. They will investigate any concerns that more could have been done to prevent their death.

- Safeguarding Adults Boards are responsible for developing effective systems for safeguarding and protecting adults from abuse. They promote the importance of sharing information between agencies, such as adults who may be at risk from abuse.

- Adults with care and support needs have access to an independent advocate during the safeguarding process.

Health and Social Care Act 2012

This Act promotes the safeguarding and well-being of adults by:

- improving the quality of the care and support provided to adults through the working partnership of adult social care services and other organisations.

- establishing Clinical Commissioning Groups (CCGs) responsible for safeguarding adults who access health and social care services, i.e. by identifying or undertaking an inquiry when abuse has taken place in a service.

- establishing **Health and Well-being Boards** responsible for overseeing the provision of health and social care services in each local area.

> ### Key terms
>
> **Health and Well-being Boards** refer to health and social care organisations who work together to improve the health and well-being of all those who live in the local area.
>
> **Named Person** refers to a person who works with children, young people and their families to protect the interests of the child or young person.

Equality Act 2010

As you will have learned in AC1.1, the Equality Act promotes the rights of individuals to not be treated unfairly because of their differences in relation to their age, disability, sex, sexual orientation, gender reassignment, marriage or civil partnership, pregnancy and maternity, race, religion or belief.

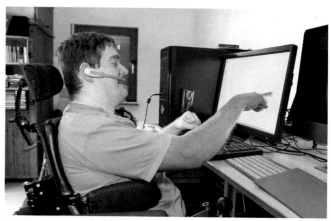

Figure 3.2 How do you support an individual's right to participate in their local community?

It also establishes the four main types of discrimination that are unlawful: direct, indirect, harassment and victimisation. Adults may, for example, experience discrimination when seeking employment (i.e. refused a job because of their age); accessing education (i.e. refused access to a course because of a disability); or using public transport (i.e. not provided with wheelchair access when boarding a train).

Mental Capacity Act 2005

The **Mental Capacity Act** promotes the rights of individuals who are unable to make choices and decisions for themselves because they lack the capacity to do so. This may be because, for example, they have an illness or a disability. It is based on the following five key principles:

1 Always assume that individuals are able to make their own decisions; never assume that they don't have the capacity to do so because they have an illness or disability.

2 Support individuals so that they can make their own choices and decisions.

3 Respect individuals' rights to make decisions that others may not agree with.

4 All decisions made on an individual's behalf, i.e. when they lack capacity, must always be in their best interests.

5 All decisions made on an individual's behalf must be the least restrictive option, i.e. the option that respects the individual's right to as much freedom as possible.

No Secrets 2000

The **No Secrets** guidance was published by the government to develop and implement multi-agency policies and procedures that protect **vulnerable adults** from abuse. The guidance reinforced that there can be no secrets or hiding places when it comes to exposing the abuse of vulnerable adults. It includes information on the:

- Different types of abuse, how and why abuse might occur, and why a vulnerable adult is at risk.

- Roles and responsibilities of different agencies working to safeguard vulnerable adults.
- Principles and policies to safeguard vulnerable adults.
- Procedures for responding to allegations and suspicions of abuse.

Human Rights Act 1998

As you will already know, the **Human Rights Act** promotes the human rights of everyone who lives in the UK. In relation to adults this includes, for example, promoting individuals' rights to privacy, dignity, equality, respect, freedom and to not be treated cruelly.

General Data Protection Regulation (GDPR) 2018

The **General Data Protection Regulation (GDPR)** replaced the Data Protection Act 1998. It protects the rights of everyone who has personal information or data recorded, used, stored and shared by organisations. You may find it useful to refer to your previous learning in AC1.1.

For example, an organisation providing care and support services to an adult needs to make sure that the safeguarding data they have aligns with the GDPR. They will need to review the safeguarding data and consider:

- Where and when they got it.
- Where they keep it and how it's kept secure.
- Who it's shared with and why.
- Who has access to it and why.
- Why it is needed and for how long.
- What the individual and/or their representative was told about the purpose for collecting the data.

Key term

Vulnerable adult, in the context of No Secrets, is defined as a person aged 18 years and over who is (or may be) in need of community care services, by reason of mental or other disability, age or illness. They are not (or may not be) able to take care of themselves, or cannot protect themselves against significant harm or abuse.

Public Interest Disclosure Act 1998

As you will have learned in AC1.1, the **Public Interest Disclosure Act** protects workers who disclose information about malpractice in their organisation by putting whistleblowing procedures in place. This includes abuse of adults at their current or former workplace.

The Modern Slavery Act 2015

The **Modern Slavery Act** safeguards adults by making slavery, servitude and forced or compulsory labour and human trafficking unlawful. The UK government estimates there are tens of thousands of people in slavery in Britain today. In 2017, over 5,000 people were referred to British authorities as potential victims of slavery, up one-third from 2016 (Anti-slavery organisation, 2019).

Female Genital Mutilation Act 2003

The **Female Genital Mutilation Act** safeguards and promotes the well-being of women by making it unlawful to perform **Female Genital Mutilation** (FGM). This includes UK nationals performing FGM outside of the UK.

Local multi-agency Safeguarding Adults policy and procedures, the role of the Local Safeguarding Adults Boards

Every local area has local multi-agency Safeguarding Adults' policy and procedures in place that set out the approach to be taken by agencies and practitioners working together to safeguard individuals from abuse. They represent good practice in safeguarding adults. They include information about the key safeguarding principles on which they're based, and how to:

- prevent harm and abuse and promote well-being
- recognise and report abuse and neglect
- respond to safeguarding concerns
- support individuals during the safeguarding process
- work in partnership when sharing information about individuals during the safeguarding process.

Under the Care Act 2014, every local area will also have a **Safeguarding Adults Board (SAB)**. The role of the SAB is to:

- ensure the effective safeguarding of adults with care and support needs
- undertake **Safeguarding Adults Reviews (SARs)**
- make information available to the public, health and social care practitioners, adults with care and support needs and their families, i.e. by publishing a report every year of its work and findings of any Safeguarding Adults Reviews
- take into account the views of the local community including the adults with care and support needs, their families and health and social care practitioners when planning safeguarding.

> ## 🔑 Key terms
>
> **Female Genital Mutilation (FGM)** refers to a range of procedures which involve the partial or total removal of the external female genitals for non-medical reasons.
>
> **Safeguarding Adults Reviews (SARs)** refers to, in this section, an enquiry into the death or serious injury of an adult with care and support needs, where abuse or neglect is known or thought to be a factor. They aim to provide lessons that can be learned to prevent similar incidents occurring again.

Related policies and procedures

Every organisation will have safeguarding policies and procedures that detail the agreed ways of working that employees must follow. They should include information on the:

- organisation's aims and principles relating to safeguarding, for example preventing the abuse and neglect of adults with care and support needs and promoting their well-being.
- roles and responsibilities of everyone involved in safeguarding, for example individuals, health and social care practitioners and/or other agencies.
- arrangements that are in place when there are safeguarding concerns, including who to contact and how to record concerns.
- useful sources of information and advice relating to safeguarding, including lessons learned from previous safeguarding incidents (either locally or nationally).
- arrangements in place for the use of advocacy.

There are also national safeguarding policies and procedures formed by the UK government and other organisations. These can be a useful source for information and guidance, such as the:

- **Safeguarding Adults Protocol – Pressure Ulcers and the Interface with Safeguarding Enquiries (Department of Health and Social Care, 2018).** This guidance aims to help practitioners and managers in health and social care services to provide appropriate responses to individuals who are at risk of developing pressure ulcers and therefore are at risk of harm.
- **Revised Prevent Duty Guidance for England and Wales (HM Government, 2016).** The Prevent Strategy is part of the government's response to counter-terrorism. Its aim is to reduce the UK

threat of terrorism by stopping people from becoming terrorists or supporting terrorism.

- **NHS Accountability and Assurance Framework (Department of Health, 2015).** This document provides information about the safeguarding roles, duties and responsibilities of all organisations in the NHS.

- **Safeguarding: Roles and Responsibilities in Health and Care Services (Department of Health, Local Government Association, ADASS, Association of Chief Police Officers, 2013).** This guidance details the roles and responsibilities of the key agencies involved in adult safeguarding. The aim is to ensure that the correct steps are taken by the appropriate people at the right time, working within their own agency and with partners.

- **Prevention in Adult Safeguarding (Social Care Institute of Excellence, 2011).** This report shares findings from research, policy and practice on prevention in adult safeguarding. It presents a wide range of approaches that can help prevent abuse and neglect.

Codes of practice relevant to the sector

There are codes of practice in relation to safeguarding that are relevant to the health and social care sector.

Deprivation of Liberty Safeguards (DOLS) Code of Practice (Ministry of Justice, 2008)

The Deprivation of Liberty Safeguards Code of Practice outlines how to identify when a person is, or is at risk of, being deprived of their liberty and how a deprivation of liberty may be avoided. It also explains how the safeguards ensure that a deprivation of liberty, where it does occur, is lawful.

The Deprivation of Liberty Safeguards apply to:

- People living in England and Wales.
- Adults who are 18 years or older.
- People who have a condition, such as dementia, a mental illness, learning disability or brain injury.
- People who live in a care home or are staying in hospital, who are lacking capacity to agree to be there.
- For whom deprivation of liberty is considered to be necessary in their best interests, in order to protect them from harm.

Mental Capacity Act 2005 Code of Practice (Department of Constitutional Affairs, 2007)

This code of practice provides guidance and information about how the Act works in practice. It is aimed at those who work with, or care for, adults who may lack capacity to make decisions for themselves. It provides guidance in relation to the following:

- How the Mental Capacity Act links to the code of practice.
- The principles on which the Mental Capacity Act is based and how they should be applied.
- How people should be helped to make their own decisions.
- How the Mental Capacity Act defines a person's capacity to make a decision and how capacity should be assessed.
- How the Mental Capacity Act protects people caring for individuals who lack capacity to consent.
- What the Act says about **Lasting Power of Attorney (LPA)**; the role of the **Court of Protection**; and of the **Independent Mental Capacity Advocate (IMCA) service.**

Current legislation as relevant to Home Nation

You will have learned about the safeguarding legislation that applies to adults in England, but here is some more information about other legislation that is relevant to Northern Ireland, Scotland and Wales:

Safeguarding legislation for Northern Ireland

- **Mental Capacity Act (Northern Ireland) 2016** protects the rights of individuals who lack capacity to make decisions.

- **Human Trafficking and Exploitation (Criminal Justice and Support for Victims) Act (Northern Ireland) 2015** prevents the abuse and **exploitation** of individuals and promotes their rights to safety and well-being.

- **The Public Interest Disclosure (Northern Ireland) Order 1998** promotes the rights of whistleblowers to report safeguarding concerns.

Safeguarding legislation for Scotland

- **Adults with Incapacity (Scotland) Act 2000** protects and safeguards the welfare and finances of adults who lack capacity.

- **Human Trafficking and Exploitation (Scotland) Act 2015** prevents the abuse and exploitation of individuals, promoting their rights to safety and well-being.

Safeguarding legislation for Wales

- **The Social Services and Well-being (Wales) Act 2014** gives individuals more control over the care and support they receive and safeguards adults at risk or experiencing abuse or neglect.

- **Violence against Women, Domestic Abuse and Sexual Violence (Wales) 2015 Act** requires local authorities and their partners to develop consistent services and support when safeguarding individuals against domestic abuse and sexual violence.

 Key terms

Court of Protection refers to the specialist court for all issues relating to people who lack the capacity to make decisions.

Exploitation refers to taking advantage of someone unfairly for your own benefit.

Independent Mental Capacity Advocate (IMCA) service is a service available in England to support individuals and their carers who wish to make a complaint about their NHS treatment or care. It is a not for profit organisation that represents a person where there is no one independent of services, such as a family member or friend, who can represent them.

Lasting Power of Attorney (LPA) refers to when a person (or persons) are appointed to make decisions about an individual's personal welfare, including healthcare, property and affairs. A way of giving someone else power to decide what is in the best interests of the person. There are two types: financial and health and welfare.

Outline Activity

Outline how adults can be safeguarded and protected by one piece of legislation, policy, procedure or code of practice you've learned about.

 Check your understanding 1

1 Give two differences between the terms 'safeguarding' and 'protection'.
2 Name two ways how the Children Acts 1989 and 2004 safeguard and protect children from abuse and harm.
3 Give two examples of codes of practice that provide guidance on safeguarding adults.
4 Outline how the Public Interest Disclosure Act 1998 safeguards and protects children, young people and adults.

LO2 Understand the role and responsibilities of the health and social care practitioner in relation to safeguarding

2.1 How the health and social care practitioner safeguards individuals

All health and social care practitioners must work within the requirements of current legislation to safeguard individuals. They must also follow their employer's requirements and good practice as relevant to the sector.

Work within policies and procedures

Health and social care practitioners can work effectively within relevant policies and procedures, such as those in relation to safeguarding, confidentiality and whistleblowing. They should:

- read them, i.e. as part of their **induction** to their job role or during safeguarding training
- understand them, i.e. understand how they are related to their job role and responsibilities to safeguard individuals
- follow them, i.e. know the process to follow if they suspect an individual is at risk of abuse
- seek advice, i.e. seek guidance from their manager if they are unsure about their responsibilities.

There may be cases were the health and social care practitioner provides care and support to an individual that is also their employer. In these instances, safeguarding practices will be developed and agreed with the individual and/or their representative. It may also be included in an employment contract or explained verbally.

Duty of care

All health and social care practitioners are legally required to have a **duty of care** towards the individuals that they provide care and support to, as well as others who they work with, such as colleagues, other professionals and individuals' families. In relation to individuals, health and social care practitioners can fulfil their duty of care towards them by:

- always acting in the best interests of individuals when carrying out their responsibilities, i.e. by ensuring all decisions that are made in relation to safeguarding individuals take into consideration first and foremost what will be best for the individuals in terms of keeping them safe and promoting their well-being.
- always taking action to prevent harm to individuals, for example if a health and social care practitioner has concerns that an individual may be in danger of harm, then they must report their concerns immediately to protect the individual.
- always working within the responsibilities of their job role, i.e. health and social care practitioners will have a **job description** that describes their job role and responsibilities. They will have agreed to carry out these responsibilities of the role with their employer, including safeguarding practices. For example, they must promote individuals' well-being at all times when providing them with care and support; they might also have to attend safeguarding training.
- always promoting individuals' well-being, for example by promoting individuals' human rights to privacy, dignity, choice and respect.

Key terms

Duty of care refers to the health and social care practitioner's legal obligation to ensure the safety and well-being of individuals and others, such as their colleagues and visitors, while providing care and support.

Induction is an introduction to an organisation, work setting or job role by an employer.

Job description is a document that details the purpose and responsibilities to be carried out as part of a job role.

Person-centred practice

Working in person-centred ways is essential for safeguarding individuals. This is because it involves health and social care practitioners:

- placing individuals at the centre of their care and support. If a health and social care practitioner knows and understands an individual, they will be more likely to meet their needs and preferences. They will also be able to recognise any changes in behaviour that may be a cause for concern.

- supporting individuals' rights to make their own choices and decisions, enabling them to be in control of their care and support. If an individual feels respected, valued and confident in their abilities, then they will be less likely to be abused or harmed because they will understand that it is their right to live free from harm and abuse and will therefore be more likely to report this should it occur.

- supporting individuals' rights to take risks and manage them safely. If an individual is aware of the benefits and consequences that their choices can have, then they are more likely to be protected from harm.

Not following person-centred practice must be avoided, otherwise health and social care

practitioners will be failing in their duty of care to promote individuals' rights and to provide high-quality care and support.

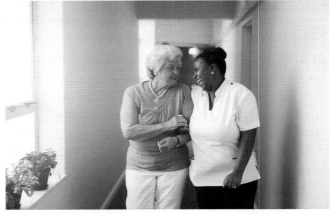

Figure 3.3 How do you contribute to person-centred practice?

Monitoring, observation, reporting, recording

As you will have already learned, safeguarding individuals is a very important responsibility of health and social care practitioners. It is part of the duty of care they have towards individuals and involves:

- **Monitoring**: Getting to know the individuals they support and care for so that they can promote their wishes, preferences and needs. Health and social care practitioners must also be vigilant about any unusual changes in an individual. For example, if an individual appears withdrawn and refuses to eat after every visit from a family member, it is important to check immediately why this might be happening. The change in the individual's behaviour might be a sign that they are being abused: this is why this must not be ignored. You will learn more about the signs and behaviours that may give cause for concern later in AC3.2.

- **Observation**: Observing individuals and noting any unusual changes in behaviour can help to safeguard against abuse. For example, if an individual has a bruised arm and seems reluctant to explain how it happened, then it may be possible that they have been harmed. This must be acted on immediately by working within set policies and procedures. You will learn more about the actions to take if harm or abuse is suspected in AC4.1.

- **Reporting**: Ensuring that all concerns are reported immediately will mean that senior colleagues, such as your manager, will be able to take the necessary actions to maintain the individual's safety. You will learn more about the lines of reporting and responsibility in AC4.1.

- **Recording:** Noting any incidences accurately and as soon as possible will ensure that there is a written, permanent record with the full details of the incident, and will allow for the individual to be removed from the risk of any further abuse and harm. You will learn more about the importance of accurate recording in the safeguarding process in AC4.1.

Partnership working

Health and social care practitioners can only safeguard individuals effectively if they work together with other people, such as their manager, colleagues, individuals, individuals' families, advocates and other professionals, such as the GP or social worker.

Health and social care practitioners can use partnership working to safeguard individuals. This is because it involves:

- working with different practitioners and agencies to provide person-centred care and support. This promotes the individuals' rights and safety with the aim to protect them from abuse or harm. You will learn more about the factors which contribute to an individual being vulnerable to harm or abuse in AC3.3.

- opportunities to get to know individuals well as others may have worked with

individuals for longer periods of time. Working in this way means that it will be easier to recognise any unusual changes in individuals' behaviour.

- sharing information and ideas for effective approaches when safeguarding individuals. Everyone involved will be working together in line with best practice, therefore safeguarding and protecting individuals from harm or abuse.

Description Activity

Identify an individual that you've seen in the media that was harmed or abused. Reflect on what happened. Describe how this individual should have been safeguarded from harm or abuse, using examples.

Confidentiality

Health and social care practitioners have a responsibility to maintain individuals' confidentiality during the safeguarding process. How to do so will be detailed in their agreed ways of working in relation to safeguarding. Therefore, it is important that health and social care practitioners understand the basic rules regarding confidentiality and how they relate to their practices:

- Knowing what **confidential information** means in the safeguarding process.

- Knowing what information can and can't be shared.

- Knowing when an individual's confidentiality may not be able to be maintained, i.e. if the individual discloses that they have been harmed.

All information sharing in the sector, including when maintaining confidentiality in relation to safeguarding, is guided by legislation such as the General Data Protection Regulation 2018 and by standards such as the **Caldicott Principles**. **Figure 3.4** describes what these are.

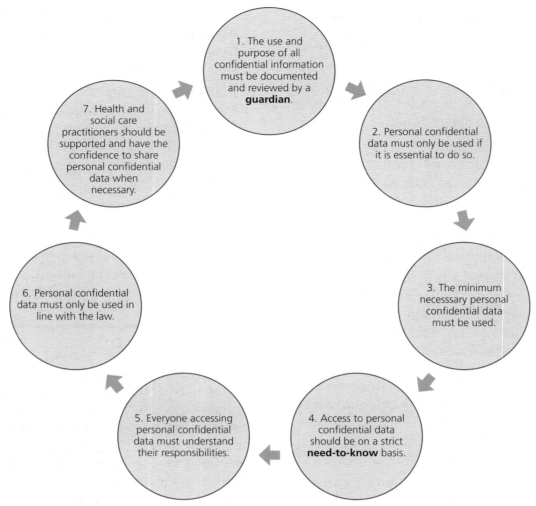

Figure 3.4 The Caldicott Principles

1. The use and purpose of all confidential information must be documented and reviewed by a **guardian**.

2. Personal confidential data must only be used if it is essential to do so.

3. The minimum necesssary personal confidential data must be used.

4. Access to personal confidential data should be on a strict **need-to-know** basis.

5. Everyone accessing personal confidential data must understand their responsibilities.

6. Personal confidential data must only be used in line with the law.

7. Health and social care practitioners should be supported and have the confidence to share personal confidential data when necessary.

Whistleblowing

All health and social care practitioners have a duty of care to report all unsafe or illegal working practices. This is referred to as whistleblowing. As you will have learned, the Public Disclosure Act 1998 and organisations' whistleblowing policy and procedures protect whistleblowers from having their career prospects or employment affected as a result of them reporting unsafe or illegal practices. You will learn more about whistleblowing responsibilities in AC4.2.

Key terms

Caldicott Principles are a set of standards aimed at improving information handling in health and social care.

Confidential information refers to all information that is personal or sensitive, and that is not available in the public domain.

Guardian is the lead person for safeguarding an individual's confidential information.

Need-to-know refers to when confidential information is shared with others who need it, i.e. when an individual discloses that they are being harmed.

2.2 How the health and social care practitioner safeguards themselves

Supporting individuals who have been harmed and abused can be upsetting and stressful. This means that the health and social care practitioner also has a responsibility to not only safeguard individuals, but also know how to safeguard and take care of themselves.

Working within policies and procedures

Working within policies and procedures relating to safeguarding means that the health and social care practitioner will safeguard themselves. They will be working in ways that comply with the law and their employer's policies and procedures, reflecting best practice.

Duty of care

Health and social care practitioners must maintain their duty of care to safeguard individuals as well as themselves. Not doing so can have serious consequences for individuals because it could lead to the risk of abuse or harm. For example, if a health and social care practitioner does not report their concerns about an individual being at risk of abuse, then this could result in them being held responsible for prolonging the individual's suffering. It may result in the practitioner losing their job; their work setting being declared unsafe and closed down; or even being prosecuted.

Personal care

Supporting individuals with personal care activities, such as dressing and undressing, eating and drinking, and daily hygiene (e.g. skin care) requires the health and social care practitioner to be sensitive and empathetic. This is because these tasks involve making physical contact with the individual.

The health and social care practitioner can safeguard themselves when carrying out personal care by:

- respecting the individual's rights to:
  - personal privacy, for example closing the door when an individual is getting dressed
  - being safe
  - independence, i.e. supporting the individual to do as much for themselves as possible
  - being valued by being treated with dignity and respect.

  Not doing so will mean that the individual's welfare and well-being are not being promoted.

- complying with agreed ways of working, i.e. only provide support with personal care tasks that they are trained to carry out and that have been agreed and documented in the individual's care or support plan. Similarly, if the care plan states that two practitioners must be present when providing personal care, then ensure best practice is followed. Not doing so may place the health and social care practitioner at risk of having allegations made against them.

- record and report all concerns, i.e. any unusual changes in an individual's behaviour when carrying out a personal care task must be recorded and reported in line with the employer's safeguarding policy and procedures. Not doing so will result in the health and social care practitioner failing in their duty of care.

Physical contact

Never making physical contact with individuals as a health and social care practitioner is unrealistic. The health and social care practitioner can safeguard themselves by following their employer's agreed ways of working. They should also consider whether it is:

- part of the individual's care and support, for example helping an individual to hold a fork when eating or supporting them when getting dressed

- appropriate, for example placing an arm around an individual who is upset (but only if the individual feels comfortable with this contact: if not, kind words could be used instead)

- necessary, for example when an individual requires first aid treatment

- preventative, for example if an individual self-harms by biting their arms or banging their head against a wall, then physical contact may be necessary to keep them safe. This is referred to as **restrictive practice**. It must only be used legally and as the last resort by practitioners who have had the relevant training.

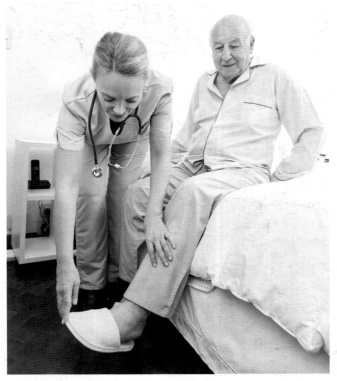

Figure 3.5 Safeguarding when making physical contact – what do you need to think about?

Technology

The use of technology such as the internet, social networking sites (e.g. Facebook, Twitter) and electronic devices (e.g. mobile phones, tablets) can present potential risks to health and social care practitioners. It is important that they are aware of what these risks are and develop their knowledge about online safety so that they can safeguard themselves.

- **The internet** may be a good source of information but it is also a means of sharing personal information with others who may then abuse or use this information dishonestly. All personal information, including names and addresses, must be kept safe. It is also important to only use official sites when searching for information; if not, there is a risk of finding information that is offensive or sexually explicit in nature. Similarly, when receiving emails from someone unknown, it is best to confirm their identity before any information is shared with them.

- **Social networking sites** are a good way of keeping in touch with family and friends. But it is important that health and social care practitioners do not share any personal information or photographs that they do not want to be shared publicly, i.e. that may be read and seen by the individuals they provide care and support to, their families or other professionals.

- **Electronic devices** such as mobile phones and tablets are used by many people on a daily basis. These devices often hold personal information including the names and contact numbers of family members and friends, photographs and apps for things such as bank accounts. Health and social care practitioners must keep these devices secure using passwords and switching on the appropriate privacy settings. This will restrict the information that can be accessed by others.

Confidentiality

Confidentiality is essential for ensuring that health and social care practitioners respect individuals' personal information and privacy. They must be aware that they can only share individuals' personal information with others when there is a reason to do so. In the safeguarding process, this is very important because the information being shared may be sensitive in nature. However, the information has to be shared securely and with the relevant persons in order to safeguard the individual from further abuse or harm. Avoid situations that may involve unintentionally sharing information with the person who abused the individual.

Maintaining an individual's confidentiality may not always be possible. For example, when an individual discloses that they have been abused to a health and social care practitioner but do not want anyone else to know. In this situation, to safeguard themselves, the health and social care practitioner must:

- always tell the individual who has disclosed abuse that it is their duty of care to share the information with a named person. They

should explain how this will be done in the strictest of confidence.

- only share the information with a named person, i.e. as outlined in their employer's policy and procedures.

If the individual does not agree with this information being shared, then apart from explaining the health and social practitioner's responsibilities, there is not much more than can be done. The information and individual's wishes must be recorded and reported in line with the agreed ways of working.

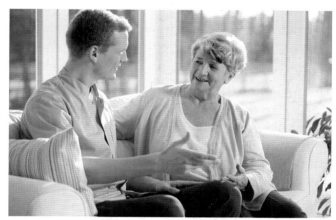

Figure 3.6 Keeping it confidential when it matters

Record keeping

Recording all concerns and allegations that an individual may be being abused or harmed will safeguard the health and social care practitioner. This is because a true and accurate record of what has happened is maintained. The health and social care practitioner will be responsible for ensuring that:

- only factual information is recorded. They must only include the details that they have seen and/or been told, using the words the individual (or another person) has used when documenting what has happened.

- full details are recorded. This includes their concerns or suspicions being documented clearly and accurately, including the reasons for their concerns. This must be based on facts, evidence and observations, not on opinions.

- following their agreed ways of working. All record keeping should be completed in private and made secure so that confidential information cannot be accessed by others who are not authorised. They should also use the agreed methods of recording, for example incident forms or concerns reports, in a timely manner, i.e. the earliest opportunity so the details are not forgotten.

Whistleblowing

The health and social care practitioner can safeguard themselves when whistleblowing by ensuring that they have a reasonable belief that disclosing their concerns is in the interest of the public. This is the key principle of whistleblowing.

Health and social care practitioners should follow their employer's policy and procedures to access the relevant information and advice about whistleblowing. They can also attend training sessions provided at their workplace, which can be provided by external organisations such as the Care Quality Commission. You will learn more about whistleblowing procedures in AC4.2.

> **Key term**
>
> **Restrictive practice** refers to actions that deliberately limit an individual's movement or freedom. They might be used legally in, for example, an emergency, when an individual requires life-saving treatment or when escaping violent behaviour.

> **Check your understanding 2**
>
> 1 Give two examples of how working within policies and procedures can safeguard individuals.
> 2 Describe how effective partnership working can safeguard individuals from abuse or harm.
> 3 Give two examples of how the health and social care practitioner can safeguard themselves when using technology.
> 4 Describe two ways in which the health and social care practitioner can safeguard themselves when record keeping in relation to the safeguarding process.

LO3 Understand types of abuse

Health and social care practitioners can only carry out their role and responsibilities to safeguard individuals from abuse, harm and neglect if they are aware of and can recognise the **signs**, **symptoms**, **indicators** and **behaviours** that may give cause for concern.

Table 3.1 outlines the main types of abuse and provides you with examples of the most common associated signs, symptoms, indicators and behaviours. It is important to remember that because all individuals are unique, the way they may experience abuse or harm will also be unique. Therefore, this means that may not all show the same signs, symptoms, indicators and behaviours associated with each type of abuse.

As you have learned so far, getting to know individuals and working in partnership with others are two of the most effective ways that the health and social care practitioner can safeguard individuals from being abused or harmed.

Key terms

Behaviours are the ways in which an individual acts physically and emotionally, for example self-harming or not eating, including when interacting with others.

Indicators are the changes in an individual that are shown and might give cause for concern.

Signs are symptoms that are outwardly visible to others, for example bruises, swelling and cuts.

Symptoms can be emotional and are experienced and felt by individuals, for example emotions such as feeling distressed, upset and/or angry; physical symptoms include feeling unwell, lack of sleep or poor appetite.

3.1, 3.2 Types of abuse and the signs, symptoms, indicators and behaviours which may cause concern

Outline Activity

Produce an information handout that outlines four different types of abuse. For each type of abuse, describe one sign, one symptom, one indicator and one behaviour that could be associated with each of these.

Table 3.1 Signs, symptoms, indicators and behaviours of abuse

Types of abuse	Signs and symptoms	Indicators and behaviours
Self-neglect – a failure of an individual to meet their own needs, for example poor personal hygiene, not eating or drinking, not taking prescribed medication.	malnutrition dehydration weight loss not wearing clean clothes feeling confused being low in mood	listlessness being withdrawn being isolated from others
Physical abuse – unwanted contact leading to injuries or pain, for example hitting, pushing, biting, restraining an individual incorrectly, such as by tying them to a chair.	bruises cuts pressure marks broken bones burns being in pain and discomfort being anxious being tearful	flinching in the presence of the abuser showing fear getting angry getting upset wearing long-sleeved clothing/jackets in hot weather to cover up bruises/cuts
Emotional abuse – actions that make an individual feel worthless and humiliated, for example threats, controlling, harassment, isolation, withdrawal of services.	anxiety disturbed sleep inability to eat feeling unwell	very under confident low self-esteem feeling anxious
Sexual abuse – unwanted sexual contact and involvement in sexual activities and relationships, for example rape, sexual harassment, subjection to pornography.	pain and bruises around the thighs, breasts and genital area unexplained bleeding stained or torn underclothing feeling angry	sexually transmitted infections (STIs) inability to take part in physical activities due to pain or discomfort difficulty in walking or sitting being withdrawn

Types of abuse	Signs and symptoms	Indicators and behaviours
Domestic abuse – threatening behaviour, violence or abuse between individuals who are related, for example honour-based violence (this may also include emotional abuse and/or physical abuse).	the signs and symptoms associated with the other types of abuse included in this table could be signs of domestic abuse	the indicators and behaviours associated with the other types of abuse included in this table could be signs of domestic abuse
Financial abuse – the unauthorised use of a person's property, money or possessions, for example theft, fraud in relation to financial transactions, wills, property.	lack of money large withdrawals of money not being able to pay bills feeling anxious	not wishing to spend money on day-to-day essentials such as food valuable items disappearing being fearful of not having enough money
Institutional abuse – the focus of the service is on the needs of the organisation and its staff, rather than on the needs of the individuals who access the service, for example no provision made available to meet individuals' needs, rigid routines and systems.	poor care standards lack of choice lack of individuality low self-esteem	inadequate staffing a lack of positive responses to individuals' needs getting frustrated and angry
Bullying – repeated behaviour which is intended to hurt someone, either emotionally or physically. It is often aimed at certain people because of their race, religion, gender or sexual orientation or any other aspect such as appearance or disability. Types of bullying can include physical assaults, verbal abuse, threatening behaviour and cyber bullying (i.e. via a mobile phone or online).	being upset being anxious being tearful feeling under-confident	self-harming suicidal thoughts being withdrawn being isolated

3.3 Factors which contribute to an individual being vulnerable to harm or abuse

Being aware of the factors that can make an individual more vulnerable to harm or abuse is useful. It can enable the health and social care practitioner to monitor and observe the individual, taking action at the earliest opportunity to prevent any abuse or harm from taking place.

Age

A young individual such as a child who is unable to defend themselves, or an older adult who may be physically frail, may be more vulnerable to abuse. This is because their vulnerability can be exploited by others since it is unlikely that they will be able to defend themselves from any abuse or harm they experience.

Health

Poor physical and/or mental health may mean that the individual depends on others, such as family members and health and social care practitioners, for their care and support. This includes all of their personal care. Because of this close relationship, the individual might be reluctant to report any abuse because they fear that their abuser will get into trouble, or that they will lose their care or have to be moved from where they are living.

Substance abuse

An individual with a history of substance abuse, such as alcohol and/or drugs, may experience memory difficulties, hallucinations and periods of unconsciousness. This may make them more vulnerable to abuse because they may not be able to recall what has happened. An individual with substance abuse may also have been involved in crime and be known to the police for making false allegations. Therefore, they might be more at risk of not being believed when they make an allegation that they have been harmed or abused.

Disability

An individual who has a disability is more likely to be vulnerable to abuse. For example, if an individual has a physical disability and uses a wheelchair, they may be unable to defend themselves from a physical assault. Or if an individual has a learning disability, they might not be able to understand and/or be able to express clearly that they have been abused.

Isolation

An individual who lives on their own and away from the people who know them well, such as their family or friends, may be more vulnerable to abuse. This is because they might have very few (if any) visitors who might recognise that they are being abused. An individual who is isolated might also be taken advantage of by an abuser: they might see the abuser as a friend because they visit them regularly and/or do activities together.

Social media

Social media can be used to abuse individuals by, for example, posting comments, photographs and videos that intimidate, bully and/or humiliate the individual. Some individuals who have care and support needs might know how to use the internet, but may not understand the dangers of social media. Educating individuals about online safety and speaking to them about the dangers and risks can reduce their vulnerability to abuse.

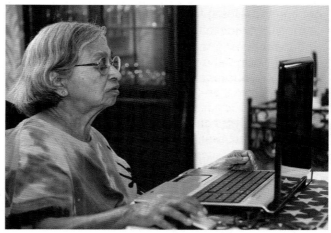

Figure 3.7 Do you know how to promote online safety?

Environment

The environment that an individual lives in can also influence whether or not they are vulnerable to abuse. For example, if an individual lives in a care setting where health and social care practitioners are not being supported or trained effectively, then the individual might be at risk. Similarly, in environments where family members or health and social care practitioners feel stressed, then this may result in inadequate care or support to the individual. If left unmonitored and unsupported, this stress could potentially lead to the individual being vulnerable to abuse.

Classroom Discussion

Discuss what makes individuals more vulnerable to harm or abuse. Include in your discussion what can be done to reduce the likelihood of individuals being harmed or abused.

Description Activity

Go back to the activity that you completed for AC2.1, where you identified an individual you have seen in the media that was harmed or abused. Using this example, describe the factors that increased the likelihood of that individual being made more vulnerable to harm or abuse.

Check your understanding 3

1 Give two examples of different types of abuse.
2 Name the signs, symptoms, indicators and behaviours associated with the two different types of abuse you identified in Question 1.
3 Describe how isolation can contribute to an individual being vulnerable to harm or abuse.
4 Describe the reasons why an individual with a disability may be more vulnerable to harm or abuse.

LO4 Understand action to be taken by the health and social care practitioner in response to evidence or concerns that an individual is at risk or has been harmed or abused

If a health and social care practitioner has evidence or concerns that an individual is at risk or has been harmed or abused, the appropriate action must always be taken. This is their legal duty of care to safeguard and protect the individual.

4.1 Actions to take if harm or abuse is suspected or disclosed

Work within policies and procedures

Employers' policies and procedures will outline the actions that a health and social care practitioner should take if there is evidence or any suspicion that an individual is at risk or has been harmed or abused. This will be in line with their job role and responsibilities. When a health and social care practitioner is employed directly by the individual with care or support needs, then they will need to follow their responsibilities as set out in their contract of employment, as well as the local authority's policies and procedures.

Not working within policies and procedures may mean that essential evidence of harm or abuse is jeopardised and individuals cannot be safeguarded. It can also mean that the health and social care practitioner may lose their job as a result of failing in their duty of care.

Lines of reporting and responsibility

Safeguarding policies and procedures will also outline how evidence or concerns of harm or abuse must be reported, including how to escalate to the appropriate lines of responsibility. The health and social care practitioner must always comply with these so that the individual can be safeguarded from any further danger, harm or abuse. Although each work setting will have their own safeguarding procedures and lines of reporting, there are some actions that must be taken. These include:

- Reporting all evidence and concerns immediately, so that the individual can be safeguarded.
- Reporting all evidence and concerns to a named person, i.e. manager or team leader.
- The named person ensuring that the individual at risk of harm or abuse is safeguarded.
- The named person informing the individual and relevant authorities about the action that has been taken, i.e. the police, Care Quality Commission.

Other responsibilities that must also be carried out include:

- Ensuring that no one else is placed in danger, for example other individuals, visitors.
- Getting help – for example, if medical care is required then an ambulance and/or the police will be called.
- Preserving all evidence (you will learn more about what this involves later on in this unit).
- Recording all actions that have been taken, by whom and when.

Description Activity

Identify an employer's safeguarding policy and procedure. Discuss with someone you know the actions that must be taken when abuse is suspected, or has happened, and the reasons why.

Maintain safety

Maintaining the individual's safety is very important when there is evidence or concerns that they have been harmed or abused. This may involve removing the individual from the environment where they have been harmed or abused or moving them to a place of safety. The health and social care practitioner, as you will have already learned, must also safeguard themselves and others by not placing themselves or others in any danger of being harmed or abused. This might involve calling for help, such as from the police; leaving an unsafe environment and waiting for help to arrive; or supporting others to move to a place of safety.

Preservation of evidence

The health and social care practitioner must also ensure that any evidence of an individual being at risk or being harmed or abused, is preserved. This is so that:

- an investigation into what happened can take place
- the abuse of harm caused can be proved
- the person carrying out the abuse can be prosecuted and brought to justice.

Figure 3.8 describes how evidence of abuse or harm can be preserved.

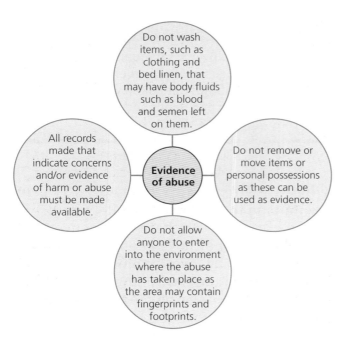

Figure 3.8 Preserving evidence of abuse

Confidentiality

Ensuring confidentiality is maintained when reporting and recording evidence or concerns regarding incidences of potential harm or abuse is essential. This is to make sure that the individual is safeguarded and evidence is preserved. You will learn more about the boundaries of confidentiality in AC4.3.

Listening, reassurance, non-judgement

As you will have learned in AC3.2, individuals can experience a range of emotions when they have been abused or harmed. How the health and social care practitioner responds to abuse or harm being disclosed is therefore very important. They need to listen carefully and make the individual feel as comfortable as possible, especially since they have had the courage to admit they are suffering. It is also important that the individual is reassured that they are being taken seriously and are believed. The health and social care practitioner must not show any shock or disbelief so that the individual does not feel that they are being judged about what has happened.

4.2 The responsibilities of the health and social care practitioner in relation to whistleblowing

Reporting concerns of practice

The health and social care practitioner has a legal duty to follow their employer's policies and procedures when reporting any concerns that they have regarding illegal or unsafe practices. For example, witnessing a colleague verbally abuse an individual or administering medication without the proper training. Not reporting concerns of practice may result in the individual being placed in prolonged danger. The health and social care practitioner might even be prosecuted for enabling the abuse or harm to continue.

In the first instance, any concerns of practice must be reported to the practitioner's senior, such as a manager or team leader. If the concerns are about the practitioner's senior, then these must be reported to someone even more senior in the organisation they work in, such as the Director, Chief-Executive or Safeguarding Lead.

Reporting to external body in response to no action being taken

When the health and social care practitioner has reported concerns of abuse or harm, but no action has been taken by the employer or organisation, then they must report directly to the Care Quality Commission. This can be done anonymously by telephoning or emailing them their concerns. When the concerns raised are of an illegal nature, and therefore a criminal offence, the police must be contacted.

> ### Description Activity
>
> Talk to someone you know about the responsibilities that health and social care practitioners have in relation to whistleblowing. Describe the process for reporting concerns and, if they are not followed up, what actions must be taken.

4.3 The boundaries of confidentiality in relation to the safeguarding, protection and well-being of individuals

Maintaining confidentiality when safeguarding and protecting individuals from abuse or harm is essential, especially when complying with legislation, policies and procedures.

Duty of care

As you will have learned, the health and social care practitioner has a legal duty of care to maintain individuals' confidentiality. They must work in ways that safeguard and protect individuals, promoting their overall well-being. To fulfil their duty of care, the health and social care practitioner must follow their work setting's policies and procedures. They must also ensure that individuals understand what this duty of care means and why it is important.

Consent

Individuals who have been abused or harmed might refuse to allow the health and social care practitioner to share the information they have disclosed to them. This might be because they are fearful of what could happen next.

In the first instance, the health and social care practitioner must reassure the individual that what happened to them is not their fault. They should also explain that it is their duty of care to maintain the individual's safety. In these situations, the individual's safety is paramount and, therefore, the information disclosed must be reported in the strictest of confidence.

Need-to-know

One of the ways that the health and social care practitioner can maintain confidentiality when safeguarding individuals is by sharing information on a need-to-know basis. This refers to information being shared only with those who need to know about it, in order to carry out their job role and responsibilities. For example, a health and social care practitioner might report a concern about an individual becoming withdrawn. They must share this information with their manager or the safeguarding officer at their workplace. However, it would not be appropriate to share this information with the individual's family, who do not necessarily need to know this particular information.

Policy and procedures

All policies and procedures in relation to confidentiality when safeguarding, protecting and promoting individuals' well-being are guided by the Caldicott Principles. You may find it useful to review your previous learning about these standards in AC2.1.

Description Activity

Describe to someone you know the limits of maintaining confidentiality in relation to the safeguarding, protection and well-being of individuals.

 Check your understanding 4

1 Describe best practice when supporting an individual who has disclosed that they have been abused or harmed.
2 Name the responsibilities the health and social care practitioner has when following whistleblowing procedures.
3 Describe what is meant by sharing information on a 'need-to-know' basis.

LO5 Understand the benefits of working in partnership in relation to safeguarding and protection

5.1 The benefits of working in partnership in relation to safeguarding and protection

Working in partnership when safeguarding and protecting individuals will include working with individuals and their families, friends, advocates, colleagues, managers and others, such as individuals' GPs, social workers and the police. Working in partnership effectively involves:

- being clear about each other's roles and responsibilities to encourage mutual trust and respect
- good communication by ensuring that all partners are aware of the information that they need to know so that individuals can be safeguarded
- showing positive behaviours, such as respectful communications, **active listening** and a genuine commitment to safeguarding individuals and promoting their well-being.

Table 3.2 includes some of the benefits of working in partnership in relation to safeguarding and protection.

Table 3.2 Benefits of working in partnership in relation to safeguarding and protection

Benefits of working in partnership	Reasons why
Expertise	Working with different professionals and agencies means that everyone can draw on each other's varying levels of knowledge, skills and expertise about the individual and the safeguarding process. Good practices can also be shared among the team.
Working together towards shared goals	Agreeing to work together as one team and towards agreed goals means that the individual will be provided with safe, consistent and effective care. Working in this way means that the individual will be placed at the centre of all working practices.
Defined roles and responsibilities	Having defined roles and responsibilities promotes an understanding of each other's roles and responsibilities. It encourages mutual respect and trust in each other's level of expertise, views and contributions when safeguarding individuals.
Intervention	Working in partnership will mean that early intervention will be more likely when there are concerns about an individual's safety or well-being. Responses to safeguarding concerns will also more likely be quicker and more effective.
Referrals	Working in partnership will mean that working relationships will have been developed with different partners and therefore referrals to, for example, agencies that provide support or assistance with housing can be made to support the individual.

Key term

Active listening is a communication technique that involves understanding and interpreting what is being expressed through verbal and non-verbal communication.

Case scenario

Pete is a young person with a learning disability and lives on his own in a flat. His friend, George, is worried that there is something wrong with Pete because he refuses to come out with him as he used to on a Friday night. Pete attends college twice a week and his teacher has noticed that Pete appears to be finding it difficult to concentrate, which is very unlike him. Last week, Pete asked his sister to go with him to the GP, as he thinks he might be depressed because he is feeling low in himself.

1 What could be wrong with Pete? Why?
2 How could George, Pete's teacher and his sister work in partnership to safeguard Pete and promote his well-being?
3 Describe the benefits of George, Pete's teacher and his sister working in partnership to help Pete.

Read about it

Care Quality Commission, 2018, 'Equally outstanding Equality and human rights – good practice resource', Care Quality Commission

Department for Education, 2018, 'Working together to safeguard children 2018', Department for Education

Department of Health, 2014, 'Positive and Proactive Care: reducing the need for restrictive interventions', Social Care, Local Government and Care Partnership Directorate

Information Commissioner's Office, 2018, 'Guide to the General Data Protection Regulation', Information Commissioner's Office

Action on Elder Abuse – (information about abuse that happens to older people) www.elderabuse.org.uk

Care Quality Commission (CQC) – (information about the Mental Capacity Code of Practice) www.cqc.org.uk/sites/default/files/Mental%20Capacity%20Act%20Code%20of%20Practice.pdf

Care Quality Commission (CQC) – (information about whistleblowing) www.cqc.org.uk/contact-us/report-concern/report-concern-if-you-are-member-staff

Department of Health and Social Care – (factsheets about the Care Act 2014) www.gov.uk/government/publications/care-act-2014-part-1-factsheets/care-act-factsheets

Equality and Human Rights Commission – (information about the European Convention on Human Rights) www.equalityhumanrights.com/en/what-european-convention-human-rights and

Government Equalities Office – (information about equality legislation and policy) www.gov.uk/government/organisations/government-equalities-office

Skills for Care – (information about the Care Act 2014) www.skillsforcare.org.uk

The British Institute of Human Rights – (information about the Human Rights Act 1998) www.bihr.org.uk/thehumanrightsact

UNICEF – (information about the United Nations Convention on the Rights of the Child 1989) www.unicef.org.uk/what-we-do/un-convention-child-rights/

How will I be graded?

The table below shows what learners must do to achieve each grading criterion. Learners must achieve all the criteria for a grade to be awarded. A higher grade may not be awarded before a lower grade has been achieved, although component criteria of a higher grade may have been achieved.

Grade	Assessment Criteria number	Assessment of learning/What you need to show
D1	1.1	Describe what is meant by: ● safeguarding ● protection.
D2	1.2	Outline: ● one (1) piece of legislation, policy, procedure or code of practice in relation to the safeguarding and protection of children and young people ● one (1) piece of legislation, policy, procedure or code of practice in relation to the safeguarding and protection of adults.
D3	3.1	Outline types of abuse. A minimum of four (4) types of abuse must be outlined.
D4		A minimum of one (1) relevant and traceable reference must be included.
C1	3.2	Outline signs, symptoms, indicators and behaviours which may cause concern.
C2	4.1	Describe actions to take if harm or abuse is suspected or disclosed.
B1	4.2	Describe the responsibilities of the health and social care practitioner in relation to whistleblowing.
B2	2.1	Describe how the health and social care practitioner safeguards individuals. Examples may be used to support the description.
B3		A minimum of two (2) relevant and traceable references must be included. A reference list must be included.
A1	2.2	Describe how the health and social care practitioner safeguards themselves. Examples may be used to support the description.
A2	4.3	Describe the boundaries of confidentiality in relation to the safeguarding, protection and well-being of individuals.
A*1	3.3	Describe factors which contribute to an individual being vulnerable to harm or abuse. A minimum of four (4) factors must be described.
A*2	5.1	Explain the benefits of working in partnership in relation to safeguarding and protection.
A*3		References must be present throughout to show evidence of knowledge and understanding gained from wider reading. References must be relevant and traceable.

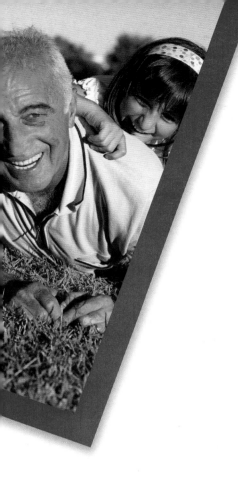

HSC M4
Communication in health and social care

About this unit

Communication is an essential skill, not only for health and social care, but for general life. This unit will provide you with the knowledge and understanding required for communication in health and social care. You will learn about the different types of communication, how to use communication effectively and the communication and language needs of different individuals. Communication also helps to establish and maintain professional relationships in health and social care, and it is important that you are able to distinguish between a professional and a personal relationship. Managing information that may be confidential is an important responsibility of professionals. In this unit, you will learn about the legislation, policies, procedures and codes of practice that relate to managing information and maintaining the security of data. You will also gain an understanding of the tension between maintaining confidentiality and the need to disclose information when carrying out the duty of care.

Learning Outcomes

LO1: Understand effective communication.

1.1 Types of communication:

- verbal
- non-verbal: body language, written, electronic, specialist.

1.2 Communication and language needs and preferences of individuals and others:

- aids, adaptations, augmentative approaches
- Makaton
- objects of reference
- picture exchange communication system (PECS)
- speech and language services
- interpreting and translation services
- advocacy services.

1.3 The skills of an effective communicator:

- active listening
- clarifying/checking understanding
- proximity
- pace
- intonation
- language
- body language
- cultural awareness.

LO2: Understand professional relationships in health and social care.

2.1 The difference between a professional relationship and a personal relationship:

- working within policies and procedures
- limits and boundaries of professional relationships

→

- underpinned by health and social care values
- confidentiality.

2.2 Working relationships that a health and social care practitioner will have:

- individuals
- health and social care practitioners
- parents/carers
- colleagues
- external partners.

2.3 The role of communication in building and maintaining professional relationships in health and social care:

- listening
- empathising
- decision-making
- informing care
- concern
- reassuring
- building trust
- confidence
- confidentiality
- positive personal regard.

LO3: Understand legislation, policies, procedures and codes of practice relating to the management of information.

3.1 The term confidentiality.

3.2 Legislation, policies and procedures relating to the management of information:

- Care Act 2014
- Health and Social Care Act 2012
- General Data Protection Regulation (GDPR) 2018
- Human Rights Act 1998
- Common Law Duty of Confidentiality
- related policies and procedures
- codes of practice relevant to sector
- current legislation as relevant to Home Nation.

3.3 How the health and social care practitioner maintains security of data:

- work within policies and procedures aligned with current legislative practices
- verify identification
- passwords
- consider method of transmission
- environment
- need-to-know
- accessing, storing and sharing information including online and paper-based records.

3.4 The tension between maintaining confidentiality and the need to disclose information:

- duty of care
- consent
- need-to-know.

LO1 Understand effective communication

Effective communication is a two-way process. The intended message is composed, sent, received and understood as intended. Then, a response is composed, sent, received and understood. This process is often shown as a cycle, which is illustrated in **Figure 4.1**.

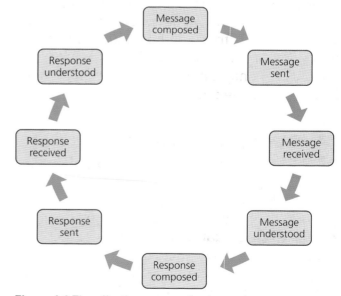

Figure 4.1 The effective communication cycle

Communication requires a:

- sender
- receiver
- message
- **medium** or way of transmission.

The medium or way of transmission may be verbal, for example talking to someone face-to-face or on the phone. Or, it may be visual, for example a welcoming smile, a written letter or a diagram. Here is an example of effective communication:

A person arrives at the hospital and asks the receptionist for directions to the outpatient department. The person has verbally composed the message in a face-to-face situation, i.e. 'Where is the outpatient department please?' The receptionist receives the message, understands it and composes a response, explaining verbally which route to follow.

Sometimes, the communication cycle can be broken, leading to ineffective communication. For example, if the person had asked for directions in Welsh and the receptionist spoke only English, the message would not have been understood. As another example, an individual with a visual impairment might be sent a letter from the hospital that is not in Braille, or an individual with a hearing impairment might not hear when their turn is called out by the doctor.

1.1 Types of communication

There are two main types of communication: verbal and non-verbal. **Verbal communication** works if people speak the same language and dialect. **Non-verbal communication** manifests itself in many different ways, including through body language, written, electronic and specialist forms. For example, individuals

may read another person's body language and sense whether or not they are welcome or perceived as a nuisance. They may read written communication in a letter or leaflet or an email. There are specialist types of communication developed for specific individual's needs. Each type of communication uses the communication cycle, and each can lead to miscommunication.

Verbal

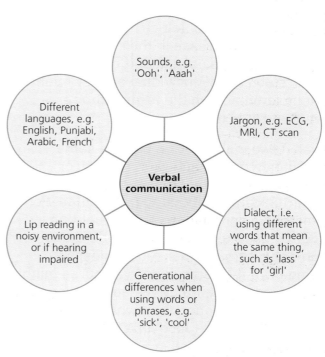

Figure 4.2 Types of verbal communication

Verbal communication usually refers to speech or spoken words, but it may also refer to using sounds to convey meaning. For example, a teenager may grunt a response in answer to a parent's question; an unconscious person may groan if they are in pain; and a baby will coo, cry or babble long before they learn words, but we can still gain an insight into whether they are happy or uncomfortable. A health and social care practitioner needs to be sensitive to sounds, as well as words, as part of understanding verbal communication.

Sometimes, the same language uses different **jargon**. Verbal communication is more likely to be effective if both the sender and receiver speak the same language; but, if the health and social care practitioner uses jargon that a person does not understand, this can make communication ineffective. Jargon is often used because it is quicker to convey what is meant rather than using the official term in full. However, this can lead to miscommunication. For example, a nervous individual with chest pain may not understand a paramedic when they say they are going to perform an 'ECG' (electrocardiograph), leading to an increase in their anxiety. Even if the full term is used, it still might not be understood by the individual as they might not be familiar with the term and/or a medical context.

Even if two individuals speak the same language, there might be variations or differences in dialect that can make communication difficult to understand. For example, a person born and brought up in one region might not always understand someone from another region, despite being from the same country. A nurse might ask an individual if they've had anything to eat, and not understand when they say they've had 'fittle' ('food' in a Black Country dialect) or 'snap' (food in a Yorkshire dialect). Generational differences in language may also cause confusion. For example, 'sick' might mean 'unwell' to an older person, but to an adolescent, it can also mean 'impressive'.

Sometimes, the physical environment or a disability might hinder communication. An individual might have partial hearing or be temporarily or permanently deaf. They might be able to lip read another person speaking if the area is well-lit with light directed towards speaker's face, but in a dim environment, this task might be more difficult. Someone using a hearing aid might find all noise is louder, even background noise, which can make it difficult for them to follow a conversation.

Different languages also influence verbal communication. Health and social care practitioners may well care for people who do not speak English for various reasons. This might be because they work with minority ethnic groups, so it can be helpful to learn a few key words in the spoken language to ensure that the individuals feel comfortable. This is also the case for health and social care practitioners working with the deaf community, where learning sign language would be beneficial to meet the needs of the individuals they care for and support.

Non-verbal: body language, written, electronic, specialist

Non-verbal communication refers to the behaviour and elements of speech (aside from words) that convey meaning. These can be split into categories, which are outlined in this section.

Body language

Body language in an important way of communicating. Professor Albert Mehrabian studied communication and found that over 55 per cent of our communication pertaining to feelings and attitudes is in facial expression, 38 per cent of communication pertaining to feelings and attitudes is in the way words are said. Body language involves physical movements that send subtle messages, such as:

- the position of a person's arms, hands, legs and feet, for example arms crossed, hands clasped together, feet tapping
- eye movements and where the individual is looking
- body posture.

One of the key skills for health and care practitioners to develop involves how to observe and understand body language effectively. For example, an observant practitioner will know that the person pacing around a waiting room might be anxious without having to ask them how they feel. Crossed arms and legs might indicate that an individual is feeling defensive. Looking down or over someone's shoulder implies that an individual is not really interested or listening to what the person is saying.

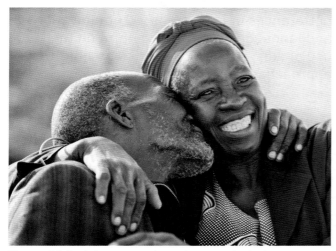

Figure 4.3 Body language shows how people feel

Written language

Written language is a representation of non-verbal communication by means of a writing system. Some examples might include:

- a personal hand-written letter
- a birthday card
- an informative leaflet
- a newspaper or online article.

However, written language is only an effective means of communication if the individual can read and understand the language. For example, if the individual only understands English and Punjabi, but a message is written in French, then they won't understand the intended meaning of the message. Sometimes, written language can cause miscommunication, for example jargon may not be understood or taken to mean something else, or a message written as a joke might be misunderstood and offend the individual.

Electronic communication

Electronic communication is increasingly becoming a part of daily life. Emails, social media, texts, WhatsApp and Facebook messenger are just a few examples of how we use electronic communication to communicate. Some people believe that electronic messaging is replacing a lot of face-to-face communication, leading to a loss of vital communicative skills such as reading body language, making eye contact and interacting face-to-face with others.

In 2010, US adolescents spent an average of 8.5 hours per day interacting with digital devices, up from 6.5 hours in 2006 (Rideout *et al.*, 2010).

Research by Twenge *et al.* (2019) found that adolescents with less face-to-face social interaction and high social media use reported the most loneliness.

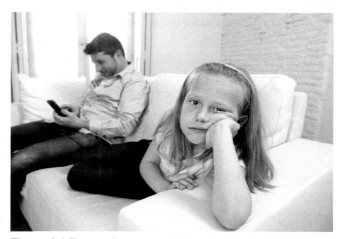

Figure 4.4 Electronic communication can replace face-to-face communication

Specialist communication

Sometimes, it is necessary to use specialist communication to convey intended messages to an individual who has specific needs. For example, an individual who has had a stroke that affected their speech might require a communication board to indicate their needs and wishes, or someone who was born deaf might need to learn sign language as their first language. These forms of communication are non-verbal, as they require alternative ways of conveying meaning other than just speaking.

Key terms

Jargon refers to technical language or terms and abbreviations that are difficult for those not in the group or profession to understand.

Medium is the method of transmitting the message. This may be verbal, spoken or visual.

Non-verbal communication refers to the behaviour and elements of speech (aside from words) that convey meaning. Examples include pitch, tone, speed, volume, gestures, body language, posture, eye movements, proximity to the listener and even dress or appearance.

Verbal communication refers to the use of sounds and words to express yourself and convey meaning.

Activity

Design a poster for a school open day that outlines at least two types of communication.

1.2 Communication and language needs and preferences of individuals and others

Each individual is unique with their own set of personal needs and preferences. This means that the way we communicate with others is also individual and will change over time. For example, the communication we use for a baby will not necessarily suit a seven-year-old child. It is also important to consider different communication requirements throughout the life stages: for example, at 70 years old, an individual might develop hearing loss and will need to adjust to life by communicating in a different way to how they have in the past.

Aids, adaptations, augmentative approaches

It is possible to meet the needs and preferences of individuals' communication and language requirements through the use of aids, adaptations and augmentative approaches. These are detailed below.

Aids

People with profound hearing loss may require the use of aids, such as hearing aids or **cochlear implants**, to help them to receive verbal messages clearly. Some hearing aids can be linked via Bluetooth to an Apple, Android, or Amazon Fire device, delivering sound to the individual's hearing aid.

Adaptations

Smartphones are becoming increasingly useful in our daily lives, for those with and without disabilities. Some smartphones have increased amplification or hearing aid compatibility. For those with visual impairments, messages can be enlarged to help those with a visual impairment read the text clearly. Some smartphones have large buttons while others have Bluetooth-enabled braille displays (**www.rnib.org.uk**).

Some electronic devices have built-in screen readers that are operated by gestures. Individuals with visual impairments can move their finger over the screen to hear information. Gestures can magnify the screen, change the font and screen colours too, making reading easier. Apple products (e.g. iPhones, iPads) have a screen reader called 'Voiceover', while Android products have 'TalkBack' and Amazon's Fire tablets have 'Screen reader' (**www.sense.org.uk**). Voice recognition software, such as speech-to-text, enables people to dictate emails and other documents. For example, Microsoft Windows 10 has its own in-built software for this that enables those with a visual impairment to hear their messages. This software works on computers, smartphones or tablets and is also used by those who have no communication issues but may be short of time and want to dictate or hear a message while performing another task.

Amazon's Alexa and Echo technology (and other similar devices) enable people to search the internet, play music, create lists, and control smart home devices, such as adjustable heating and lighting, using only their voice. Technology that once was specialised for people with disabilities is increasingly being refined and used by others, which helps to break down the barriers between those with and without communication disabilities.

Augmentative approaches
Alternative and Augmentative Communication (AAC) refers to methods that aid communication for people with speech difficulties. Many AAC methods use technology, such as the text-to-speech or speech-to-text facility mentioned earlier. Some devices turn symbols into speech and can be operated by switch or eye gaze. AAC devices must be tailored to the individual and their needs.

An example that illustrates the effectiveness of augmentative communication is Professor Stephen Hawking, a famous theoretical physicist who had Motor Neurone Disease (MND). This disease affects the cells that control muscle activity and affects the individual's ability to speak. Professor

Hawking used a voice synthesiser to communicate when he lost the ability to do so himself: however, it spoke in an American dialect, not British! Individuals with MND in Yorkshire and the Black Country have been given voice synthesisers that reflect their own regional accents. Eventually, more regional accents will be available to meet individuals' communication and language needs (**www.bbc.co.uk/news/av/uk-38871649/synthetic-yorkshire-voice-for-mnd-sufferer-jason-liversidge**). Developers at the Anne Rowling Clinic and University of Edinburgh are collecting samples of regional voices to provide communication aids that sound more like the individual's own voice (**www.annerowlingclinic.org**).

Another example is comedian Lee Ridley who performs under the stage name 'Lost Voice Guy'. He is unable to speak due to **cerebral palsy** and uses the voice app Proloquo2Go. He won *Britain's Got Talent* and performed at the Royal Variety Show. His humour helps people laugh with him about disability and ridicule those who are patronising or prejudiced (**lostvoiceguy.com**).

Other types of alternative and augmentative communication systems include signing, gestures, written words, symbols and picture books. Symbol charts, large pictures or objects of reference are increasingly being produced in electronic format.

Makaton
Makaton is a language programme to support spoken language. It uses signs and symbols with speech, following the order of spoken words. It is used with children who might have limited speech. In time, some children drop the use of signs and symbols as they develop speech, although others may continue to use Makaton. Signs have associated symbols and reinforce the word used (**www.makaton.org**).

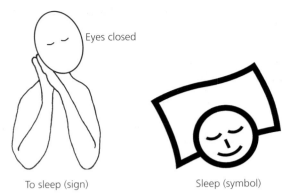

Eyes closed

To sleep (sign)

Sleep (symbol)

Figure 4.5 Makaton uses signs and symbols to support speech

Objects of reference

Objects of reference are items used to represent something, for example a cup could represent having a cup of tea or coffee, a leaf might represent going to the park. Objects of reference are useful to help people who have Profound and Multiple Learning Disabilities or visual impairment to communicate. As they associate the object with the activity, for example, a leaf with going outside, more objects can be added to the vocabulary. Each person might have their own set of objects that have a specific meaning to them. The objects should be kept together in a bag or box near the person, so that they can use them often. They can then express choice, for example indicate the paint brush or the leaf for their choice of activity. More objects of reference are introduced as the individual requires. Oxfordshire Inclusive Communication, which is part of Oxford NHS Foundation Trust, has useful suggestions online for suitable objects of reference: **www.oxfordhealth.nhs.uk/oxtc/good-advice/objects-of-reference**.

Picture Exchange Communication System (PECS)

The **Picture Exchange Communication System (PECS)** is a commercially produced, augmentative training package for children and adults with autism and other communication difficulties, such as problems with cognition or physical movement. A key advantage of the system is that it allows the individual with communication difficulties to start communication by showing a picture of what they want, for example a glass of water. The teacher or carer gives the water immediately. The individual associates the picture with receiving that item. This means the individual with communication difficulties does not have to wait to be asked what they want: they can start the conversation. The system is based on B.F. Skinner's work in behavioural psychology, building in stages so the individual learns to discriminate between different pictures, learns to build sentences and comment and respond to questions. Although speech is not used in PECS, some children and young people have developed speech as a result of using the system (**https://pecs-unitedkingdom.com/pecs**).

Speech and language services

Speech and language services are offered through the National Health Service (NHS), usually in the community, but are also offered privately on a fee-paying basis. They can help those with communication difficulties, such as babies who were born with issues such as a cleft lip or palate that make it difficult for them to develop speech. Communication difficulties can also occur later in life, perhaps as a result of brain injury or a stroke. Speech and language therapists also help with individuals who have:

- difficulty swallowing, for example families with premature babies when the baby has to learn how to swallow or older people who have difficulty swallowing after a stroke
- stammers
- problems producing and in understanding communication.

Look back to the start of the section at **Figure 4.1** and remind yourself where problems can arise and disrupt the communication cycle.

Interpreting and translation services

Interpreting and translation services are offered through the NHS, although they are commissioned or purchased from private companies who make a contract with the local NHS. Interpreting is hearing someone speaking, and saying those same things in another language. It also refers to saying what someone may have signed using sign language, such as British Sign Language (BSL). Interpreting may be done face-to-face, through telephone or video interpreting, or visual relay interpreting. **Translation** refers to written material, including Braille. Translation is reading a text and then writing it in another language that means the same thing, for example from Bengali to English, or from English to Braille.

Communication is essential for good quality care. When people do not understand what the health and social care practitioner is saying, or if the practitioner cannot understand the individual, mistakes can be made, appointments missed and treatment not followed. It is very important that we have interpreters in the health and social care sector. For example, without an interpreter, a diabetic person who speaks only Arabic may not understand the importance of diet, which could severely affect their health. As a result of ineffective communication, the person might go into a diabetic coma resulting in death.

Advocacy services

Advocacy services help people have their voice heard. An advocate speaks for an individual who may not be able to speak for themselves. They are independent of the NHS and social services. Local councils must provide an advocate for those who experience difficulty:

- understanding and remembering information
- communicating their views
- understanding the benefits and drawbacks of different options
- finding a family member or friend to represent them.

Paid carers cannot act as a person's advocate because they will have a conflict of interest. Someone employed by the NHS or local social services might be influenced by the needs of the service, rather than the needs of the individual needing advocacy. For example, an older person may be ready to be discharged from hospital but is unable to go home until arrangements have been made. However, the hospital may need the bed for an emergency and the nurse might be influenced by the fact that a casualty needs a bed, so could not act as advocate for the individual to ensure they go home to a safe environment.

Advocates help people to:

- understand the care and support process
- express their views about their care
- make decisions
- challenge decisions made about the person's care and support.

Advocates can also write letters for the individual and attend meetings with them, providing support during assessments, care planning meetings, safeguarding and reviews. Those with mental health issues and/or who lack capacity to make their own decisions are entitled to the services of an **Independent Mental Capacity Advocate (IMCA)**. In England, IMCAs are appointed by a local authority. You can read more about this in *Unit HSC 09: Mental health and well-being.*

Key terms

Alternative and Augmentative Communication (AAC) is the term used to describe various methods of communication, such as 'text-to-speech' technology, that can be used to assist people with speech difficulties.

Cerebral palsy is a group of lifelong conditions that affect movement and co-ordination, caused by a problem with the brain that occurs before, during or soon after birth.

Cochlear implants are surgically implanted hearing devices.

Independent Mental Capacity Advocate (IMCA) refers to a person who can represent those in need when there are no family members or friends able to help.

Makaton is a language programme to support spoken language. It uses signs and symbols with speech, following the order of spoken words, and is used by individuals who have learning difficulties.

Picture Exchange Communication System (PECS) is a non-verbal method of communication using symbols and pictures.

Translation refers to the process of translating words or text from one language into another.

Description Activity

In preparation for your school or college open day, you have been asked to design a leaflet describing the communication and language needs and preferences of both the individuals accessing services at the school, and of those supporting them, such as family members and carers. Use examples to support the descriptions and give at least one reference.

You may find it easier to base this on a fictional person you have made up, who has specific communication or language needs and preferences.

1.3 The skills of an effective communicator

Effective communicators know that **communication** is a two-way process. It involves listening as much as it involves sending out a message. The skills for effective **communication** can be learned and are essential in any health or social care-related work.

Active listening

Active listening is when the listener fully concentrates, understands, responds and remembers what is being said. An active listener's body language is open, leaning forward slightly, sitting at an angle to the speaker rather than directly opposite, which can be confrontational. Active listening involves focusing on what is said and how it is said. For example, an individual might say they are fine but their body language and tone of voice could indicate otherwise. Active listening includes listening with eyes and ears. The words 'I'm fine' may be belied by a downcast expression, drooping stance and sad tone of voice.

Active listening also involves asking an individual open questions to encourage them to keep talking. Instead of asking a closed question, such as 'Are you OK?' which requires a simple yes or no answer, asking an open question such as 'How are things?' will provide the individual with an opportunity to talk further and convey more information.

Clarifying/checking understanding

Effective communicators check and clarify they have understood what the individual intended to say, for example 'So, do you mean you enjoy your job but you feel stressed at the moment?' They encourage the individual to talk by using phrases such as, 'Tell me a bit more about that.' This helps an individual to clarify their thoughts.

Sometimes, just saying 'Yes, I see', while they are talking will encourage them to open up. The Samaritans, a charity that provides a confidential listening service for those who need to talk, has useful tips on effective communication: **www.samaritans. org/active-listening**.

Proximity

Proximity, or 'nearness', affects communication. Different people from different cultures require varying amounts of personal space when they communicate. For example, if someone is standing too far away, the individual might interpret this as them not being interested in their conversation. If they are too near, the individual might feel uncomfortable as their personal space is violated. It is always better to check that the position and proximity is acceptable for the other person before getting into a listening situation. Sitting directly opposite someone or standing over them can be threatening. A desk can also be a barrier to communication. For effective communication, it is better to sit at about 90 degrees with no barrier between the two people.

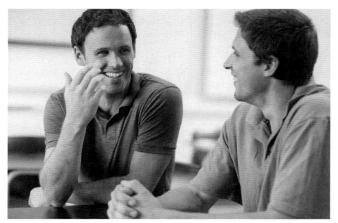

Figure 4.6 Body language and proximity in active listening

Pace

The pace of communication can influence whether or not it is effective. For example, an individual who speaks too quickly may not get their message across to the other person. Speaking too slowly may irritate the listener, causing them to switch off and stop listening. Effective communicators should match their pace to that of the individual they are communicating with.

Intonation

Intonation refers to the sound changes produced by the rise and fall of the voice when speaking. It adds a different layer of meaning to a message; for example, 'Come here!' can be either a command or an invitation to something nice, depending on the speaker's intonation. Sometimes, people with communication issues or who are communicating in a language which is not their first language, may miss the message conveyed by the tone of voice. For those using assistive technology, intonation could also be limited. Effective communicators should be aware of the limitations of technology when it comes to communicating through intonation.

Language

Language can be verbal or written, and even includes body language. In **Figure 4.2**, you will have seen the different types and variations of verbal communication. Effective communication involves both people using not just the same language, but the same **register**. Health and social care practitioners must be prepared to learn different registers; for example, a hospital consultant may formally refer to a psychoactive substance by its medical name, whereas a young patient might use **slang** to refer to it. The health and social care practitioner must be able to communicate effectively with both the hospital consultant and the patient in the appropriate register. If the health and social care practitioner does not know the formal language of an individual, they may need to use an interpreter to help them to communicate.

Body language

Body language conveys information to others about an individual's mood and feelings. It is non-verbal but one of the most powerful ways to communicate. Most people are unaware of their body language, but an effective communicator can pick up clues that indicate how they are feeling. For example, crossed legs and arms are a sign that the individual might feel vulnerable and defensive. A power stance, taking up lots of room by spreading legs or arms, or sitting with legs spread, denotes confidence and can be seen as arrogant or ignoring the needs of others. A slumped posture, downcast eyes and low energy levels may indicate the person is depressed.

Cultural awareness

Cultural awareness is extremely important for effective communication. As a health and social care practitioner, it is likely that you will encounter individuals from various cultural backgrounds who might speak or behave differently to you. It is therefore critical that you are able to communicate effectively with them in order to improve relationships, experiences and avoid any incidences of miscommunication. For example, in some cultures:

● men and women do not shake hands when being introduced

● individuals call older people 'uncle' or 'aunty' as a term of respect, rather than denoting that they are their blood relative

● maintaining close family ties is extremely important, whereas in other cultures this is regarded as less important, for example brothers and sisters may only meet at family events such as weddings or funerals

● individuals from close-knit communities might be reluctant to seek help externally, feeling that 'outsiders' do not understand their way of doing things and worry about what their community will think.

Body language varies in different cultures too. For example, in China it is considered impolite to make too much eye contact, but in the UK too little eye contact is seen as rude or denotes uncertainty or a lack of confidence. Effective communicators in health and social care need to be ensure that they are culturally sensitive in their practices so that they can understand those they care for.

Key terms

Active listening is a communication technique that involves understanding and interpreting what is being expressed through verbal and non-verbal communication.

Communication refers to a two-way process between individuals, involving a sender and a receiver who are composing, sending, understanding and responding to a message.

Register refers to the degree of formality of language, or the language used by a group of people who share similar work or interests, for example doctors or lawyers.

Slang is a type of language that is regarded as very informal. It is more common in speech than in writing and is often restricted to a particular context or group of people.

Explain Activity

Write an article for the school magazine. The article should explain the skills and techniques needed for effective communication.

Check your understanding 1

1 Describe the difference between communication and effective communication.
2 What different types of communication are there?
3 Give three examples of language needs and preferences.
4 Name three skills of an effective communicator and explain how they use these skills.

 Classroom Discussion

Discuss the possible benefits if health and social care practitioners learn to be effective communicators.

● How might it benefit individuals using the service?
● How might it benefit others, such as carers?
● How might it benefit colleagues?
● How might it benefit the health and social care practitioner themselves?
● How might it benefit employers?

 Case scenario

Maggie is three years old and has Down's syndrome (trisomy 21), an extra chromosome which causes some health problems. Like many children with Down's syndrome, Maggie has delayed development in speech and language, but she can understand very well. It just takes her a bit more time to answer if she is asked a question. She attends the clinic for a check-up with her mother.

The practitioner who sees her speaks slowly and clearly, looking at Maggie while asking her 'How are you feeling?' She then shows Maggie two pictures, one with a smiley face, and one with a sad face. Maggie points to the sad face. The practitioner looks at Maggie, makes a sad face herself and says with concern, 'I am sorry you feel like that. Why are you sad?' Maggie then turns to her mother and opens her bag, taking

out a picture of a rabbit and says 'Snuffles'. The practitioner looks interested and says 'Tell me more …'

Using signs, pictures and gestures to help her words, Maggie explains that her rabbit is sick. Having established effective communication with Maggie, the practitioner then goes on to explain what the check-up involves and what will happen. She speaks slowly, clearly and maintains eye contact.

1 Is this an effective method of communication? Give reasons for your answer.
2 How are Maggie's communication needs catered for in her check-up?
3 What changes might the practitioner make to her communication methods when communicating with Maggie's mother, who does not have Down's syndrome?

LO2 Understand professional relationships in health and social care

Relationships and interactions are important. Humans do not survive and thrive in total isolation and they live longer healthier lives when they help each other.

2.1 The difference between a professional relationship and a personal relationship

There are many different types of relationships. Some are personal, for example the relationship between parents and children or between life partners. Some relationships are professional and are those that we form with people we work with, whether colleagues or people who use a service. While personal relationships may have few boundaries or restrictions, professional relationships are limited by **policies** and **procedures** in organisations. There are limits and boundaries imposed by the nature of the professional relationship and they are regulated by health and social care values, such as confidentiality.

Professional relationships are limited by time. A social worker or health care professional is on duty for a specific amount of time but, during their time away from work, another professional may take over the care of the person they have been working with. Professionals do not spend their spare time with those who they care for professionally.

Professional relationships have a specific role and purpose. For example, to find a person suitable accommodation on discharge from hospital, or to support a person in a mental health crisis until they are admitted to a crisis house or hospital. The professional relationship requires practitioners to hand over care to other professionals when appropriate. A social worker planning the discharge of a patient into the community will not continue to visit them once the person is back in the care of the community team. A midwife will not continue to visit a new mother and her baby for longer than ten days as the health visitor is then responsible for their care. It is unprofessional for a health and social care worker to overstep these requirements because it undermines other professionals and the service user may be confused about who is responsible for their care.

Professional relationships tend to follow a structure. This will involve:

- A beginning, for example assessing needs
- A middle, for example planning to meet those needs and implementing the plan
- A review of care to assess how effective the planned care has been.

Once the professional relationship has reached the review stage, it may end and another professional may then take over the person's care.

Professionals have a depth and breadth of knowledge that a person using the service may lack. Professionals also have authority, for example a GP can refer a patient to hospital; or a community psychiatric nurse can decide that a patient in the community needs to be referred again to hospital. Such knowledge and authority places a professional in a powerful position. In order to empower the individual using the service, professionals must follow policies, procedures and codes of conduct that regulate their professional relationship with those using the service. They must explain what course of action they suggest and why, the risks and advantages, and must ensure the individual is aware of their rights and aware of the complaints procedure.

Working within policies and procedures

Codes of professional conduct, such as the Nursing and Midwifery Code published by the Nursing and Midwifery Council, and the Code of Conduct for Healthcare Support Workers and Adult Social Care Workers published by Skills for Health, set out the rules for professional relationships.

Code of Conduct for Healthcare Support Workers and Adult Social Care Workers in England

1 Be accountable by making sure you can answer for your actions or omissions.

2 Promote and uphold the privacy, dignity, rights, health and well-being of people who use health and care services and their carers at all times.

3 Work in collaboration with your colleagues to ensure the delivery of high quality, safe and compassionate healthcare, care and support.

4 Communicate in an open, and effective way to promote the health, safety and well-being

of people who use health and care services and their carers.

5 Respect a person's right to confidentiality.

6 Strive to improve the quality of healthcare, care and support through Continuing Professional Development.

7 Uphold and promote equality, diversity and inclusion.

(**Source:** www.skillsforhealth.org.uk/standards/item/217-code-of-conduct)

The Social Care Institute for Excellence suggests that relationships should be based on openness, transparency and empathy, whether with individuals, their families, carers or fellow professionals and colleagues.

Each organisation has policies and procedures for sharing and storing information and for maintaining confidentiality, including when it is appropriate to break confidentiality, for example if a person's life is in danger.

Professional relationships may involve multi-agency working in order to meet the range of needs of individuals. A GP may work with a social worker and drugs support worker to help a person who is addicted. Sometimes, multi-agency protocols must be followed, for example when sharing information or for keeping information confidential, such as the location of a refuge for abused families.

The underlying principle is to remain person-centred, not organisation-centred. The needs of the person are more important than the needs of the organisation. An understanding of an individual's cultural and ethnic background is essential for person-centred care. It is important that the professional recognises their own limitations and involves advocates and/or interpreters where needed in order to ensure a full understanding of people's needs.

Limits and boundaries of professional relationships

Professional relationships should be client-focused and person-centred. Health and social care practitioners are expected to put the needs of individuals using their services at the centre of care. They must avoid giving information about themselves and their personal life to those in their care.

Professionals must never have more than one relationship with an individual. For example, if a social worker is working with an individual, they cannot start a personal relationship with them or employ them. A doctor or nurse should never treat a member of their own family. A counsellor may not be employed to give therapy to a person and then start dating them. Professionals who ignore these guidelines risk being struck off from the professional register and losing their qualification.

Professionals must always acknowledge the limits of what they can do and they must refer the individual on when further help or treatment is needed. For example, a domiciliary care worker must report if a person's mobility gets worse and they need two care workers to help them get out of bed, rather than the one already allocated. A nurse is not a counsellor and must refer a person to the counsellor if they need such help. It is equally important that professionals recognise when they are unable to fulfil their role properly, for example due to stress or burnout, and refer themselves for help.

Underpinned by health and social care values

Values are the principles or beliefs that individuals and groups hold. Values can relate to work, to how people treat others to how different sections of society treat each other. Values guide what we do and influence our judgements about right or wrong, helping us with decision-making.

Health and social care values underpin how those who work in the sector treat others. A lot of documentation has been produced around care values and at times it can be confusing for professionals to know which documentation to follow.

In 2012, Skills for Care summarised care values as:

- Support people in maximising their potential.
- Support people in having a voice and being heard.
- Respect people's beliefs and preferences.
- Support people's rights to appropriate services.
- Respect people's privacy and right to confidentiality.

(**Source:** Skills for Care, 2012, cited in The Open University (2018) 'Section 1.3 Principles of care practice,' *K101 An introduction to health and social care, Learning Guide 4: Developing Care relationships*)

There is also the 2018 Code of Conduct for nurses and midwives – you can find out more information in AC3.2. The common principle in health and social care values is to work collaboratively with others for the benefit of the individual under their care. This may be working with other professionals, for example a psychiatric nurse working with a social worker, or a GP working with a practice nurse. It may also mean working with advocates who represent the views of the person being cared for.

It includes working directly with the individual themselves in a professional way, ensuring that they are at the centre of the care process, supporting them in having a voice

and being heard. It also includes maximising the individual's potential, supporting their rights to appropriate services and respecting their beliefs, preferences and needs. The case study that follows illustrates how this principle works.

Zara has just started at college but is struggling to cope. She feels permanently low, as though she is under a dark cloud that is weighing her down. She decides to see her GP, who listens to how she feels, then suggests she may have depression. By listening, the GP has shown respect for her views. The GP offers her a choice of options and explains the advantages and drawbacks of each option. The options are:

- *To wait and see how she feels in a couple of weeks. She may get better, stay the same or get worse.*
- *To make some lifestyle changes, such as doing the Couch to 5K NHS health programme. The advantages are that she may get fitter doing more exercise, feel healthier and recover from depression. There are few disadvantages if she is otherwise healthy.*
- *To have details and self-refer to psychological well-being services or a community mental health team (CMHT). The advantages are that she will have access to specialists who have allocated time to help her recover. The disadvantages are that there may be a waiting list for services such as counselling in her area.*

By giving her choices, the GP is supporting Zara in maximising her potential, having a voice and being heard, and supporting her rights to appropriate services, while also respecting her beliefs and preferences. Zara decides to make some lifestyle changes. She finds out about the Couch to 5K programme but also takes up the offer to refer herself to psychological well-being services. She is given an appointment for counselling. Both the counsellor and the GP keep Zara's information confidential.

Confidentiality

One of the underpinning values in health and social care is to respect people's privacy and their right to confidentiality. According to NHS guidance, which also covers social care, 'A duty of confidence arises when one person discloses information to another (for example, patient to clinician) in circumstances where it is reasonable to expect that the information will be held in confidence' (Confidentiality; NHS Code of Practice). An example of this might be that a person is about to leave their life partner, or that 20 years earlier, they had an abortion. Such information is personal and confidential.

Professionals are entrusted with many types of information. Identifiable information includes:

- Name
- Address and full postcode
- Date of birth
- Any pictures, photographs, videos, audio-tapes or other images of the individual
- NHS number and local patient identifiable codes
- Anything else that could identify a patient directly or indirectly.

Such identifiable information must be kept confidential to protect the person. It might be that an abusive ex-partner is trying to find out where they live. A professional who gives this information is breaching confidentiality and may be endangering the individual.

Record holders are those who obtain and record information, for example when completing a care assessment or admitting a person to hospital. Record holders must tell people what the information will be used for, give them the choice to give or withhold their consent, and must protect identifiable information from accidental disclosure. People can object to the use and disclosure of their confidential information to other health professionals. If this means that care options are limited because other health professionals are involved in their care, or do not have the information they need, patients must be informed of this.

Disclosure, i.e. sharing information, can only happen when the person gives consent, when required by law, when the person lacks capacity, when they have an advocate and it is in their best interests, or when it is in the public interest to prevent harm to the person or to others. When information is disclosed it is on a need-to-know basis, and the information is limited to only what is needed. You can read more about this in *Unit HSC M1: Equality, diversity and rights in health and social care.*

The Health and Care Professions Council, which regulates 16 health and care professions, publishes guidance on confidentiality. The key principles are:

- Take all reasonable steps to keep information about service users safe.
- Make sure you have the service user's consent if you are passing on their information (unless there are good reasons not to, for example it is necessary to protect public safety or prevent harm to other people).
- Get express consent, in writing, if you are using identifiable information for reasons which are not related to providing care, treatment or other services for them.

- Only disclose identifiable information if it is necessary, and, when it is, only disclose the minimum amount necessary.
- Tell service users when you have disclosed their information (if this is practical and possible).
- Keep appropriate records of disclosure.
- Keep up to date with relevant law and good practice.
- If appropriate, ask for advice from colleagues, professional bodies, unions, legal professionals or us.
- Make your own informed decisions about disclosure and be able to justify them.

(**Source: www.hcpc-uk.org/registration/ meeting-our-standards/guidance-on-confidentiality**)

Explain Activity

Write an article for your school journal to explain the difference between a professional relationship and a personal relationship. Use examples to support what you say and use one reference.

2.2 Working relationships that a health and social care practitioner will have

Health and social care practitioners do not work in isolation. They work as part of a team and have working relationships with many others, which is illustrated in **Figure 4.7**.

Individuals

Individuals refer to many different people, such as patients in a hospital or in the community, residents in a care home, or service users living in their own homes.

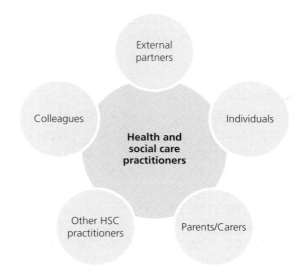

Figure 4.7 Working relationships

Health and social care practitioners

Health and social care practitioners include professionals such as social workers, social work assistants, nurses, nursing assistants, occupational therapists, psychologists, and counsellors as well as many others.

Parents/carers

Parents or carers might be the parents of babies, children, or of young people with disabilities. Carers might be elderly themselves, for example a 70-year-old caring for a 90-year-old parent.

Colleagues

Colleagues are individuals who work with health and social care practitioners. They might be in the same department or establishment, for example nurses on a ward, or social workers working for the same local authority.

External partners

External partners may be statutory bodies, for example, health and social care practitioners work with schools, the police and the probation service. A mental health practitioner may work with social workers and teachers to support a young person still in education.

Description Activity

Prepare an article for a careers fair and describe a minimum of three working relationships that a health and social care practitioner will have. Use at least two relevant and traceable references and include a reference list.

2.3 The role of communication in building and maintaining professional relationships in health and social care

Effective communication, as outlined earlier, encourages positive professional relationships. It refers to a set of skills that can be learned with practice, and these are listed in this section.

Listening

Listening and hearing are not the same. It is possible to hear someone but not listen, so that whatever they say washes over the person who is supposed to be listening. Active listening, as mentioned earlier in the unit, is truly listening and requires focus. Body language must be open, non-threatening and non-judgmental, with friendly eye contact and comfortable proximity. When a person is really listening, they may mirror the other person's body language unconsciously. If one person leans their chin on their hand, the other may do so. This shows they are in tune with one another.

Empathising

Empathising means understanding, which is different to sympathising. When you empathise with someone, you try to understand what they are feeling and experiencing. Empathising is described as walking in the other person's shoes. When you sympathise, you feel sorry for them. A social worker listening to the needs of a carer may feel sorry for them, but sympathy is not what is needed in a professional working relationship. Empathy is understanding what it is like to care for someone 24 hours a day, getting up in the night because their elderly partner with dementia has wandered downstairs and may turn the gas on. Empathy is about understanding the needs of others.

Decision-making

Decision-making is a delicate balance between empowering individuals to make informed choices for their care and knowing what is feasible. A carer may be worn out and would like to have a weekend of respite care as a break from caring, but they may be reluctant to leave their partner with dementia or their child with multiple needs in a strange place, knowing it will confuse and upset them. The social worker assessing the carer's needs must allow carers to decide for themselves whether they want the respite care. The social worker must give full information but allow the person to make their own decisions.

Informing care

Communication builds and maintains professional relationships and has a role in informing care and sharing information to improve the care given. For example, an elderly man falls downstairs and his wife calls 999. When the paramedics arrive, she tells them her husband is allergic to penicillin. The paramedic who was told that information then relays it to the emergency team in the A&E department. This is noted on the patient's notes and he is given a different antibiotic. Communication such as this can inform care and save lives.

Concern

Concern relates to feelings of worry or anxiety. It can be expressed through body language. For example, simple eye contact can show a person they are not being overlooked and that the professional cares about what happens to them. In a busy outpatient department, the clinic is running over an hour late because the surgeon is still in theatre operating on a difficult case. A health care assistant can avoid looking at the waiting queue while he goes to the clinical room, or he can express concern for those waiting, and explain that the doctor is still in theatre.

Reassuring

Reassuring is not about telling lies. It is not reassuring to tell a patient that everything will be fine if the outcome of treatment is uncertain, because if things go wrong, the person will lose faith in professionals. It is far better to be honest and communicate in a gentle way, saying statements such as 'We will do all we can' rather than offer false reassurance. Expressing concern for others, empathising, really listening and keeping others informed is all reassuring for the individual. Other professionals also value being kept informed. Service users and patients appreciate that someone understands how they feel. Using effective communication skills like these reassures people they are in capable hands.

Building trust

When people feel reassured, they develop trust in the professional who is caring for

them. They are more likely to open up about any concerns they have and this gives the professional a greater understanding of their problems, which can result in better care. For example, a person who is being abused by their partner may only disclose that information when they can trust the professional.

Confidence

Effective communicators inspire confidence. They give clear messages, respect others and actively listen to them, and do not avoid unpleasant realities. A domiciliary care worker may have only 30 mins to help Mr X get up, have a wash and have breakfast, but if the care worker has built up a relationship of trust and shown her concern, Mr X is more likely to have confidence in the care he receives.

Confidentiality

As discussed earlier, confidentiality is a key skill of working relationships. Knowing what information to keep confidential and when to break that confidentiality is essential to professionalism.

Positive personal regard

Positive personal regard means not judging others but accepting them for what they are, however much they differ from yourself. Health and social care professionals are not there to judge others. They are there to care for all, regardless of gender, ethnicity, religion and race. Carl Rogers, the humanistic psychologist, suggested that for a person to develop emotionally, they need an environment that accepts them positively without judgement, and with empathy which means being listened to and understood (**www.simplypsychology.org**).

Key terms

Empathising refers to the ability to understand or feel what another person is experiencing from their point of view, i.e. putting oneself in another's position.

Positive personal regard refers to not judging another person but accepting them as they are. It is about respect for others and belief in their genuineness, even if we disagree with them.

Activity

You have been invited to contribute to a newsletter for people interested in care work. Write an account in which you discuss the role of communication in building and maintaining professional relationships in health and social care. Use examples and cover at least three different professional relationships. Use at least two relevant and traceable references and include a reference list.

Check your understanding 2

1. Give at least three ways that personal relationships differ from professional relationships.
2. Explain at least three working relationships that a health and social care practitioner will have, using examples.
3. How can effective communication build and maintain professional relationships in health and social care?

LO3 Understand legislation, policies, procedures and codes of practice relating to the management of information

3.1 The term confidentiality

In *Unit HSC M1: Equality, diversity and rights in health and social care*, it explains that confidentiality means to keep something private. It refers to protecting an individual's personal, sensitive or restricted information and only disclosing it to those who need to know it, for example others in the care team in relation to an individual's health condition. All health and social care organisations have a confidentiality policy and a procedure to guide their employees in how to maintain confidentiality and when and how confidentiality may be broken. These policies and procedures are the agreed ways of working in an organisation.

Activity

Define the term 'confidentiality', using examples to support the definition.

3.2 Legislation, policies and procedures relating to the management of information

Legislation refers to the laws which, if broken, can lead to prosecution and could result in a professional person losing their registration. Policies set out an organisation's commitment, for example how to manage information safely. Procedures set out how this will be done. Managing information includes obtaining, using, sharing, storing and disposing of information, as well as giving information.

Care Act 2014

The Care Act 2014 deals with aspects of social care. As part of this Act, local authorities must make sure that people who live in their areas receive services that prevent their care needs from becoming more serious. Local authorities must ensure people can get the information and advice they need to make good decisions about care and support. Local authorities must have a range of high-quality, appropriate services to choose from.

According to the Care Act 2014, the local authority must provide information and advice on these matters in particular:

- How the system operates in the authority's area.
- The choice of types of care and support, and the choice of providers, available to those who are in the authority's area.
- How to access the care and support that is available.
- How to access independent financial advice on matters relevant to the meeting of needs for care and support.
- How to raise concerns about the safety or well-being of an adult who has needs for care and support.

Many local authorities provide this information on their websites and also in printed form in various languages.

Local authorities are allowed to share information with those carrying out a needs assessment for carers, or an adult to whom the assessment relates, for assessment purposes. For example, a person might be applying for funding to have their home adapted with grab rails and a walk-in shower following a stroke. If the person or their carer is not eligible for help, local authorities must give them information about what can be done to meet or reduce the needs, or prevent or delay the development of needs for care and support in the future. They may give a list of approved workpeople who carry out the work required, along with an estimate of the cost. The example that follows outlines this.

Bob is caring for his wife Janet. She has multiple sclerosis and needs the kitchen and bathroom adapted if she is to be able to stay in her own home. A social worker assesses their needs and Bob provides them with details of his and his wife's income. They are eligible for funding and the adaptations are done. Janet is provided with a power-assisted wheelchair, which enables her to get out and do the shopping. Bob can then go back to work part-time. By providing this support, the local authority are prolonging the time Janet can be independent and Bob can work.

The Act provides individuals with a legal entitlement to a personal budget. The personal budget must be included in every care plan, unless the person is only receiving intermediate care. It is an agreed amount of money allocated to the individual by their local council after an assessment of needs. They can receive it directly as a Personal Independence Payment (PIP). The individual controls the money and makes decisions how it is used in relation to their care and support. For example, an individual has cerebral palsy might buy a car adapted to their needs so that they can get to work.

Safeguarding Adults Boards (SAB) help and protect adults in cases where a local authority suspects that an adult in its area (whether or not ordinarily resident there):

- has needs for care and support (whether or not the authority is meeting any of those needs)
- is experiencing, or is at risk of, abuse or neglect
- as a result of those needs, is unable to protect him- or herself against the abuse or neglect (or the risk of it).

Examples of abuse include forced marriage, psychological (mental), physical, sexual, financial, emotional abuse or honour-based violence.

Safeguarding Adults Boards can request a person to supply information to assist the SAB to exercise its functions, if the information relates to the person to whom the request is made, or is a function of that person, for example a social worker managing the person's case.

Health and Social Care Act 2012

The Health and Social Care Act is covered in detail in *Unit HSC M1: Equality, diversity and rights in health and social care* and *Unit HSC 09: Mental health and well-being.* Information held under this Act relates to purchasing or commissioning services and may be confidential, for example the cost of services from different competing private providers bidding to get a contract with the NHS or Social Services.

General Data Protection Regulation (GDPR) 2018

The General Data Protection Regulation (GDPR) 2018 links with the Data Protection Act 2018. These are key pieces of legislation about how to manage information.

The Information Commissioner's Office (ICO) is the UK's independent authority set up to uphold information rights in the public interest, promoting openness by public bodies and data privacy for individuals. This office publishes guidance about data management and data protection.

GDPR applies to 'controllers' and 'processors'. Controllers decide the purposes and means of processing personal data. Processors are responsible for processing personal data on behalf of a controller. The GDPR places specific legal obligations on processors; for example, they must maintain records of personal data and processing activities. They have legal liability if they are responsible for a breach. Processors might be social workers or health professionals completing an assessment or care plan.

The GDPR sets out seven key principles:

1 Lawfulness, fairness and transparency

2 Purpose limitation

3 Data minimisation

4 Accuracy

5 Storage limitation data

6 Integrity and confidentiality (security) measures

7 Accountability.

The GDPR provides individuals with:

1 The right to be informed of the purposes for processing their personal data, retention periods for that personal data, and who it will be shared with.

2 The right of access to their personal data.

3 The right to have inaccurate personal data corrected, or completed if it is incomplete.

4 The right to have their personal data erased.

5 The right to restrict or suppress processing of their personal data.

6 The right to obtain and reuse their personal data for their own purposes across different services. An example of this is where a GP and hospital have access to a patient's medical records.

7 The right to object to the processing of their personal data in certain circumstances.

8 Rights in relation to automated decision-making and profiling. For example, a GP inputs the height, weight, blood pressure and blood test results of a person into an automated programme to decide whether that person should start medication to reduce cholesterol levels. The individual's consent must be obtained (adapted from 'Guide to the General Data Protection Regulation (GDPR)' **www.ico.org.uk**).

Under GDPR, measures must ensure the 'confidentiality, integrity and availability' of the system, services and personal data. In 2018, the NHS was criticised for relying on fax machines and outdated data technology. This put the security of data at risk, and so doctors have called for a secure system for communicating patient data between different parts of the NHS.

Human Rights Act 1998

The Human Rights Act is covered in detail in *Unit HSC M1: Equality, diversity and rights in health and social care* and *Unit HSC O9: Mental health and well-being*. Important articles relating to the management of information include:

- **Article 8** which protects the right to respect for private life, family life, home and correspondence, for example letters, telephone calls and emails.

- **Article 10** which protects a person's right to hold their own opinions and express them freely without government interference, including the right to express views openly, for example public protest and demonstrations; or through published articles, books, leaflets, television or radio broadcasting, works of art, the internet and/or social media. It also protects an individual's freedom to receive information by being part of an audience or reading a magazine.

Restrictions do apply as everyone has a duty to behave responsibly and respect other people's rights. Public authorities may restrict the right to freedom of expression if they can show that their action is lawful, necessary and proportionate in order to protect national security; territorial integrity (the borders of the state) or public safety. Authorities may restrict freedom of expression if someone expresses views encouraging racial or religious hatred (**www.equalityhumanrights.com**).

Common Law Duty of Confidentiality

Common law is law based on previous court cases decided by judges and is also called 'judge-made' or case law. Common law is based on a precedent, or examples of similar cases. Generally, if information is given in situations where a duty of confidence is expected, that information cannot normally be disclosed without the information provider's consent. All patient/client information, however it is held, i.e. whether on paper, computer, visually or audio recorded, or even held in the memory of the professional, must not normally be disclosed without the consent of the patient/client.

Disclosure of confidential information is only lawful:

- where the individual to whom the information relates has consented

- where disclosure is necessary to safeguard the individual, or others, or is in the public interest

- where there is a legal duty to do so, for example a court order.

Under common law, health or social care providers wishing to disclose a patient/client's personal information to anyone outside the team providing care, should first seek the consent of that patient/client. If it is not possible to get consent, legal advice should be sought before the information is disclosed. If a disclosure is made which is illegal under common law, the patient/client could bring a legal action against the organisation and the individual responsible for breaching confidentiality.

Any decision to disclose should be fully documented. Disclosures required by court order should be referred to the organisation's legal advisers immediately.

Related policies and procedures

Each organisation will have its own policies and procedures derived from the laws and regulations. Professionals must be made aware of these as part of their induction when joining the organisation and they must update themselves as part of their Continuing Professional Development.

Codes of practice relevant to sector

The Nursing and Midwifery Council updated the Code of Practice for nurses and midwives in 2018 to include nursing associates, a role that exists in England. The Code sets out the professional standards that registered nurses, midwives and nursing associates must uphold. These are:

- Prioritise people.
- Practise effectively.
- Preserve safety.
- Promote professionalism and trust.

The following standards relate to information management:

- **Standard 3.3:** professionals must act in partnership with those receiving care, helping them to access relevant health and social care, information and support when they need it.
- **Standard 5:** respect a person's right to privacy in all aspects of their care.
- **Standard 6.1:** any information or advice given is evidence-based, including information relating to using any health and care products or services.
- **Standard 7:** communicate clearly.
- **Standard 8:** work co-operatively.
- **Standard 10:** keep clear and accurate records relevant to practice.
- **Standard 17.2:** share information if you believe someone may be at risk of harm, in line with the laws relating to the disclosure of information.

(**Source:** www.nmc.org.uk)

In England, the social care Code of Conduct says that health care support workers or adult social care workers must respect people's right to confidentiality, including:

- Treat all information about people who use health and care services and their carers as confidential.
- Only discuss or disclose information about people who use health and care services and their carers in accordance with legislation and agreed ways of working.
- Always seek guidance from a senior member of staff regarding any information or issues that you are concerned about.
- Always discuss issues of disclosure with a senior member of staff.

(**Source:** www.skillsforhealth.org.uk)

Current legislation as relevant to Home Nation

Legislation in England, Wales, Northern Ireland and Scotland is very similar, laying out similar responsibilities that professionals are required to carry out to maintain the security of information. The Information Commissioner's Office (ICO) and the Data Protection Act 2018 (DPA 2018) apply to all four nations in the UK.

Key term

Common law is the part of English law derived from previous court cases. Decisions made by judges are based on examples of similar cases. It is also called 'judge-made' law or case law.

Activity

Prepare a leaflet to outline two pieces of legislation, policies or procedures relating to the management of information. A minimum of two relevant and traceable references must be included, as well as a reference list.

3.3 How the health and social care practitioner maintains security of data

The previous section outlined the duties of a health and social care practitioner to keep information secure. In this section, we look at how this is done.

Work within policies and procedures aligned with current legislative practices

Every organisation that has information must have a data protection or confidentially policy that sets out their commitment to keeping information secure. They must also have a procedure that employees are familiar with, setting out the various steps to ensure the security of data. The ICO regulates the process in the UK.

Under the Data Protection Act 2018, organisations holding data must have a **data controller** who (either alone or jointly with others) decides why and how any personal data is to be processed.

A **data processor**, in relation to personal data, refers to any person (other than an employee of the data controller) who processes the data on behalf of the data controller.

Processing, in relation to information or data, means obtaining, recording or holding the information or carrying out any operation (or set of operations) on the information, including:

- Organisation, adaptation or alteration of the information or data.
- Retrieval, consultation or use of the information or data.
- Disclosure of the information or data by transmission, dissemination or otherwise making available.
- Alignment, combination, blocking, erasure or destruction of the information or data.

(**Source: https://ico.org.uk**)

Verify identification

When using electronic systems, health and social care practitioners must verify who they are to prevent unauthorised access to data. Individual passwords identify the user which is why they must not be disclosed.

Electronic identification and trust services or '**eIDAS**' refers to services that help verify the identity of individuals and businesses online or the authenticity of electronic documents. Such services include an electronic signature, seal, time stamp, registered delivery service or website authentication certificate, designed to show that electronic data is authentic and can be trusted. The NHS is being encouraged to use more electronic systems as they can be more secure than paper-based systems.

Passwords

Passwords must be strong, kept confidential and updated regularly to prevent unauthorised access to personal data.

Consider method of transmission

Some methods of transmission are more secure than others. For example, a paper-based set of notes or a care plan carried down a corridor is not secure. Papers can come loose, or others may read information that is not covered. Fax is used in many NHS areas but this is insecure. Anyone could be at the receiving end and have access to data which should be kept secure. Data sent via unsecured electronic systems or private email is vulnerable to **hacking**. Organisations should provide safe systems for the transmission of data and practitioners have a responsibility to use them appropriately.

Environment

It is important for health and social care practitioners to consider the environment when managing information. It is poor practice to discuss patients or clients outside of the work environment and, even in the workplace, consideration must be given to what is a suitable environment. For example, a hospital corridor is not the place to ask a patient personal questions; nor is the workplace canteen the place to share information with colleagues about a case.

Need-to-know

Data protection legislation is clear that information must be shared only on a 'need-to-know' basis, given only when it is essential that someone knows something. Sometimes, it is important for health professionals to share information, for example in a case of suspected child abuse, health professionals will need to share information with the police and a social worker to protect the child from further harm.

Accessing, storing and sharing information including online and paper-based records

Every organisation must have a policy and procedure for accessing, storing and sharing information including online and paper-based records. The data controller has a responsibility to ensure this is in place, but each professional and employee is also responsible for ensuring the correct procedures are followed at each stage. Paper-based records are especially vulnerable. They can be accessed by unauthorised people, misfiled, or sent to the wrong person. Electronic records can also have these problems but usually the original information is not lost and can be retrieved. Unfortunately, with paper-based records, this may not always be the case. For example, if paper-based records regarding someone's cancer test fall down the back of the filing cabinet they may not be found for months, which could detrimentally affect the individual's life.

3.4 The tension between maintaining confidentiality and the need to disclose information

Health and care professionals are in a privileged position, caring for distressed or vulnerable people at difficult times. In such stressful states, people occasionally reveal confidential information which puts the practitioner in a difficult situation. Do they disclose the information, or keep it confidential? For example, if a young person is stabbed as part of a gang rivalry, they may tell the nurse in A&E the identity of the person who stabbed them, but do not want the police informed. If the nurse breaks confidentiality, the young person may not trust them again and will not tell them important information about their health. If the nurse does not break confidentiality, the people who stabbed the young person may stab others or attack him again. Guidance from the Royal College of Nursing is that 'in *exceptional circumstances, you may over-ride your duty of confidentiality to patients/clients if it is done to protect their best interests or the best interests of the public*' (Source: The Royal College of Nursing, 'Promoting person-centred care and patient safety: Disclosure or confidentiality', 2019. **https://rcni.com/hosted-content/rcn/first-steps/disclosure-or-confidentiality**).

There are three key issues that affect a health and social care practitioner's decision whether or not to disclose information: duty of care, consent and 'need-to-know'.

Duty of care

Duty of care refers to health and social care practitioners' responsibilities to ensure the safety and well-being of individuals and others while providing care or support.

Unit HSC M1: Equality, diversity and rights in health and social care explains that all health and social care practitioners are legally required to have a duty of care towards the individuals that they care for and support. They must:

- always act in the best interests of individuals when carrying out their responsibilities
- make sure that individuals are not placed in any danger and are kept safe from harm
- always take action to prevent harm to individuals
- only carry out the work tasks that they are able to and have the required knowledge and skills to do.

Ethical dilemmas arise between the duty of care and individuals' rights because the health and social care practitioners' duty of care may be in direct conflict with an individual's rights. Individuals may not understand the duty of care health and social care practitioners have towards them and others. Individuals and health and social care practitioners may not be able to agree on how to manage a risk safely.

Consent

Consent refers to the informed agreement to an action or decision. People must be given full information so they can make an informed decision. They must also be given information about the implications of giving or withholding consent. If consent is withheld, the practitioner must consider whether disclosure is necessary to safeguard the individual, or others, or is in the public interest. They must follow the agreed ways of working, including documenting their decision. *Unit HSC M1: Equality, diversity and rights in health and social care* discusses consent in more detail.

Need-to-know

As mentioned previously, information shared on a 'need-to-know' basis should be given only when it is essential that an appropriate person knows something, and then, only the relevant information required for the referral must be shared.

Key terms

Data controller is an individual who decides why and how any personal data is to be processed in an organisation.

Data processor is an individual who is not an employee of the data controller, who processes the data on behalf of the data controller.

eIDAS refers to 'electronic identification and trust services'. These services help to verify the identity of individuals and businesses online or the authenticity of electronic documents.

Hacking is the gaining of unauthorised access to data in a system or computer.

Description Activity

Write an article for a school newspaper describing the tension between maintaining confidentiality and the need to disclose information. A minimum of one example must be used to support the description. Use references throughout to show evidence of knowledge and understanding gained from wider reading, for example from health and social care journals. References must be relevant and traceable.

Check your understanding 3

1 What is meant by the term 'confidentiality'?
2 What is the main piece of legislation that relates to data?
3 Give three examples of how the health and social care practitioner maintains security of data.
4 Describe one example of the tension between maintaining confidentiality and the need to disclose information.

Classroom Discussion

Should the NHS and local social services use electronic systems for sharing information or should they stay with paper-based systems?

What are the advantages and disadvantages of using electronic systems and paper-based systems?

Case scenario

In the early hours of Saturday morning, Jayden is admitted to hospital as an emergency after a 999 call from a local club. He is drowsy but able to answer questions. He says he bought some drugs inside the club, but does not know what he has taken. He is 18 years old and does not want his parents to know.

1 What personal information might he be asked for?
2 What communication skills might a practitioner use to obtain this information?
3 What legislation will apply to the information he gives?
4 With your tutor, discuss aspects of confidentiality and the professional duty of care.

Read about it

Mehrabian, A., (1981), *Silent messages: Implicit communication of emotions and attitudes*, 2nd edition, Wadsworth Publishing Co Inc

Pinker, S., (2015), *The Village Effect: How Face-to-Face Contact Can Make Us Healthier, Happier, and Smarter*, Penguin Random House www.ted.com/talks/susan_pinker_the_secret_to_living_longer_may_be_your_social_life

Rideout, V., Foehr, U., and Roberts, D., (2010), *GENERATION M2: Media in the Lives of 8- to 18-Year-Olds*, The Henry J. Kaiser Family Foundation

Reduced face-to-face social interaction and increase in loneliness in adolescents: Twenge, J.M., Spitzberg, B.H., and Campbell, W.K., 2019, 'Less in-person social interaction with peers among U.S. adolescents in the 21st century and links to loneliness', *Journal of Social and Personal Relationships*, 36(6), pp.1892–1913, doi: 10.1177/0265407519836170.

Advocacy services www.nhs.uk/conditions/social-care-and-support-guide/help-from-social-services-and-charities

Care Act 2014 www.legislation.gov.uk/ukpga/2014/23/contents/enacted

Care Act 2014 factsheet www.gov.uk/government/publications/care-act-2014-part-1-factsheets/care-act-factsheets

Code of Conduct for healthcare support workers and adult social care workers www.skillsforhealth.org.uk/standards/item/217-code-of-conduct

Comedian challenging stereotypical views of disability lostvoiceguy.com

Confidentiality; NHS Code of Practice https://assets.publishing.service.gov.uk/government/uploads/system/uploads/attachment_data/file/200146/Confidentiality_-_NHS_Code_of_Practice.pdf

General Data Protection Regulation https://ico.org.uk/for-organisations/guide-to-data-protection/guide-to-the-general-data-protection-regulation-gdpr/individual-rights/

Guidance for commissioners: Interpreting and Translation Services in Primary Care www.england.nhs.uk/wp-content/uploads/2018/09/guidance-for-commissioners-interpreting-and-translation-services-in-primary-care.pdf

Health and care professions council – Regulate 16 health and care professions www.hcpc-uk.org

Health and Social Care Act 2012 www.gov.uk/government/publications/health-and-social-care-act-2012-fact-sheets

Information Commissioner's Office https://ico.org.uk/for-organisations/guide-to-data-protection/guide-to-the-general-data-protection-regulation-gdpr

Makaton information www.makaton.org

Motor neurone disease man given Yorkshire voice 5 February 2017 www.bbc.co.uk/news/uk-england-leeds-38854411

Nursing Midwifery code www.nmc.org.uk/standards/code/

Objects of reference www.oxfordhealth.nhs.uk/oxtc/good-advice/objects-of-reference

Professional boundaries www.communitycare.co.uk/2017/06/19/top-tips-managing-professional-boundaries-social-work

Professional relationships www.scie.org.uk/publications/nqswtool/professionalrelationships

Professional values www.nmc.org.uk/news/news-and-updates/nmc-and-gmc-release-joint-statement-on-professional-values

Samaritans counselling charity www.samaritans.org/active-listening

SENSE – charity for people living with complex disabilities including those who are deafblind www.sense.org.uk

Social Care code www.skillsforhealth.org.uk/images/services/code-of-conduct

Speech and language therapy www.healthcareers.nhs.uk/explore-roles/allied-health-professionals/roles-allied-health-professions/speech-and-language-therapist

The Picture Exchange Communication System
https://pecs-unitedkingdom.com/pecs/

The Power of Positive Personal Regard
Fernandez, Claudia S. P, Journal of Public
Health Management and Practice: May–June

2007 Volume 13 Issue 3 p 321–323 https://
journals.lww.com/jphmp/pages/articleviewer.
aspx?year=2007&issue=05000&article=00014
&type=Fulltext

How will I be graded?

The table below shows what learners must do to achieve each grading criterion. Learners must achieve all the criteria for a grade to be awarded. A higher grade may not be awarded before a lower grade has been achieved, although component criteria of a higher grade may have been achieved.

Grade	Assessment Criteria number	Assessment Criteria
D1	1.1	Outline types of communication. A minimum of two (2) types of communication must be outlined.
D2	1.2	Describe communication and language needs and preferences of: ● individuals ● others. Examples may be used to support the description.
D3		A minimum of one (1) relevant and traceable reference must be included.
C1	2.1	Explain the difference between a professional relationship and a personal relationship.
C2	2.3	Discuss the role of communication in building and maintaining professional relationships in health and social care.
C3	3.1	Define the term confidentiality. Examples must be used to support the definition.
B1	1.3	Explain the skills of an effective communicator. Examples may be used to support the explanation.
B2	2.2	Describe working relationships that a health and social care practitioner will have. A minimum of three (3) working relationships that a health and social care practitioner will have must be described.
B3	3.2	Outline two (2) pieces of legislation, policies or procedures relating to the management of information.
B4		A minimum of two (2) relevant and traceable references must be included. A reference list must be included.

Grade	Assessment Criteria number	Assessment Criteria
A1	3.3	Describe how the health and social care practitioner maintains security of data. A minimum of one (1) example from each of the identified areas must be used to support the description: ● storing data online securely ● storing paper-based personal records ● maintaining security through professional practice.
A*1	3.4	Describe the tension between maintaining confidentiality and the need to disclose information. A minimum of one (1) example must be used to support the description.
A*2		References must be present throughout to show evidence of knowledge and understanding gained from wider reading. References must be relevant and traceable.

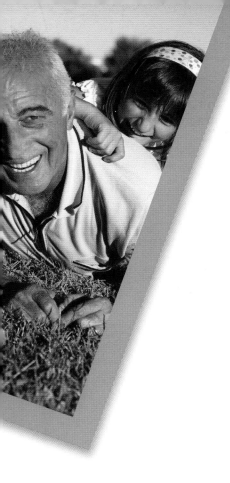

HSC M5
Working in health and social care

About this unit

Working in health and social care is a very satisfying and rewarding career. Health and social care practitioners can make positive differences to individuals' lives. In this unit, you will learn about the current legislation, policies, procedures and codes of practice that underpin working practices, as well as the essential values and principles that guide working in health and social care.

You will explore the different types of health and social care services that are available, their functions and the barriers that individuals may experience when accessing them. You will also learn more about the different job roles within the health and social care sectors, the responsibilities of health and social care practitioners and the skills, behaviours and attributes that are required. Understanding Continuing Professional Development, the sources of support for learning and development and the role of reflection will equip you with a good insight into what is required to work in this sector.

Learning Outcomes

LO1: Understand health and social care values across provision.

1.1 Legislation, policies, procedures and codes of practice in relation to health and social care:

- General Data Protection Regulation (GDPR) 2018
- Human Rights Act 1998
- Equality Act 2010
- Health and Social Care Act 2012
- Care Act 2014
- related policies and procedures
- codes of practice relevant to the sector
- current legislation as relevant to Home Nation.

1.2 Health and social care values:

- duty of care
- safeguarding

- person-centred
- partnership
- dignity
- respect
- rights
- confidentiality
- independence.

1.3 How individuals accessing health and social care services are valued:

- individual needs and preferences
- informed choice
- active support
- aids and adaptations
- health and safety
- confidentiality
- during daily routines.

→

LO2: Understand health and social care provision.

2.1 Types of health and social care services:

- statutory
- private
- voluntary.

2.2 Functions of health and social care services:

- long-term/short-term
- residential
- respite
- community
- rehabilitation
- specific service provision to meet needs
- funding
- partnership working.

2.3 Barriers to accessing health and social care services and how they may be overcome:

- communication
- cultural values and beliefs
- cost
- location
- physical access
- psychological
- lack of resources
- time.

2.4 Definition of informal care,

2.5 The role of informal carers:

- family
- friends
- neighbours
- community groups
- volunteers.

LO3: Understand the roles and responsibilities of the health and social care practitioner.

3.1 Job roles within the health and social care sectors.

3.2 The responsibilities of the health and social care practitioner:

- work within policies and procedures
- implement care values
- care planning
- risk management
- job description/person specification.

3.3 Skills, behaviours and attributes required by health and social care practitioners:

- be trustworthy
- be objective
- be patient
- be respectful
- show empathy
- show commitment
- use communication and interpersonal skills
- use initiative
- use observation skills
- show professionalism
- be able to problem solve
- be able to work as part of a team
- be a reflective practitioner.

LO4: Understand Continuing Professional Development.

4.1 Continuing Professional Development:

- staying up-to-date with sector developments
- action setting.

4.2 Sources of support for learning and development:

- formal/informal support
- appraisal/supervision
- feedback
- mentoring
- independent study
- work experience
- external agencies
- training courses
- research
- shadowing
- media.

4.3 Why Continuing Professional Development is integral to the role of the health and social care practitioner:

- up-to-date knowledge and practice
- continuous improvement
- regulatory requirements
- reflective practitioner
- application of learning.

→

LO5: Understand reflection in relation to Continuing Professional Development.

5.1 The role of reflection within Continuing Professional Development:

- reflective practitioner
- responsibility for own learning/professional growth

- ongoing review
- planning for development
- develop knowledge and skills
- self-awareness
- positive outcomes.

LO1 Understand health and social care values across provision

1.1 Legislation, policies, procedures and codes of practice in relation to health and social care

What do we mean by legislation, policies, procedures and codes of practice?

Legislation refers to the laws that are created by governments, both nationally and internationally, such as the Care Act 2014 and the Human Rights Act 1998 (you will learn more about how these relate to working in health and social care later). In the UK, these laws are then made official by parliament.

Policies and procedures are created both nationally by the government and locally by health and social care organisations; legislation forms the basis of these. An organisational policy, for example in relation to manual handling, sets out the purpose of manual handling, including how and when it is used. An organisational procedure will set out how the policy will be put into practice and the processes that health and social care practitioners must follow, including the relevant documentation they must complete.

Codes of practice are created by the health and social care sector as well as by health

and social care organisations. They set out the standards and values that are expected from health and social care practitioners. You will learn more about the values that are required for working in health and social care in AC1.2.

Why do we need legislation, policies, procedures and codes of practice?

Legislation, policies, procedures and codes of practice underpin all work in health and social care. **Figure 5.1** identifies the main reasons why they are essential when working in health and social care.

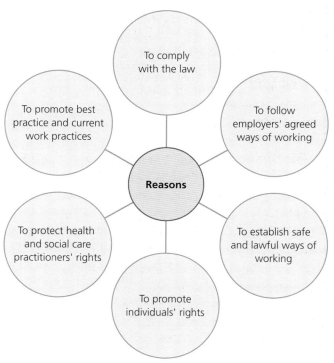

Figure 5.1 Why we need legislation, policies, procedures and codes of practice

Health and social care legislation, policies, procedures and codes of practice

There is a wide range of legislation, policies, procedures and codes of practice that are relevant to health and social care. **Table 5.1** provides some examples of the main ones.

Table 5.1 Legislation, policies, procedures and codes of practice

Legislation	Relevance to health and social care
General Data Protection Regulation (GDPR) 2018	A European Union regulation that promotes individuals' rights to have more control over how their personal information is used. The **Information Commissioner's Office (ICO)** will enforce it in the UK. Relevant to health and social care organisations because they **process** information about individuals who have care and support needs and their families, other visitors and even employees, for example the health and social care practitioners who work there. The GDPR places stringent requirements on all organisations, including health and social care organisations, who process **personal data** and special categories of data. Organisations that do not comply with the legislation risk heavy fines that will be enforced by the ICO. For example: ● When an individual or employee requests to see the personal information that is held about them (referred to as subject access requests) a £10 fee will no longer be payable and their request must be responded to within one month (previously 42 days). ● Organisations must provide individuals (adults and children) with more information about the personal data that is being processed about them. This information must be clear and easy to understand.
Human Rights Act 1998	This Act sets out the rights and freedoms that everyone in the UK is entitled to, for example the right to be treated fairly, with dignity and respect. It forms the basis of how health and social care organisations must work when providing services to individuals and others and employing health and social care practitioners.
Equality Act 2010	This Act states that people must not be treated unfairly or discriminated against because of their individual differences. It prevents discrimination and promotes equality, diversity and inclusion, which are central to providing effective and safe care and support services. It identifies nine individual differences that are protected in law from discrimination: 1 Age, for example it is unlawful to prevent an individual from making their own choices because they are considered too old. 2 Disability, for example it is unlawful to prevent an individual who uses a wheelchair to access a service because there are no disabled toilet facilities. 3 Gender reassignment, for example it is unlawful to single someone out because they are transitioning from one gender to another. 4 Marriage and civil partnership, for example it is unlawful to refuse a person a job because they are in a same-sex relationship. 5 Pregnancy and maternity, for example it is unlawful to ask an individual to leave the café where they are having lunch because the individual is breastfeeding.

Legislation	Relevance to health and social care
	6 Race, for example it is unlawful to not make information about a service available to individuals from different racial groups.
	7 Religion or belief, for example it is unlawful to not respect an individual's belief or support them to practise their religion.
	8 Sex, for example it is unlawful to refuse a health and social care practitioner training in relation to supporting individuals with personal care because they are male.
	9 Sexual orientation, for example it is unlawful to treat an individual differently when providing them with care and support because of their sexual orientation.
Health and Social Care Act 2012	This Act established a clear structure for planning, delivering and monitoring healthcare services in England. It protects individuals' rights and promotes high-quality, safe and effective services, for example: ● by establishing a voluntary register for all health care support workers and setting out the minimum standards required for practitioners working in health and social care, such as in relation to training, knowledge and skills ● by establishing Health and Wellbeing Boards that would enable different organisations, such as the NHS, adult social care services, children's services and youth services, to work together when planning and delivering services in local areas ● by establishing Public Health England as responsible for overseeing local public services.
Care Act 2014	This Act promotes the rights of individuals who are 18 and over and have care and support needs. It sets out how services must be provided, for example: ● It established Adult Safeguarding Boards to enable different organisations to work together in partnership to keep individuals safe from abuse and neglect. ● It introduced the 'well-being' principle that means that individuals' well-being must be paramount when decisions about individuals and their care and support are made. ● It further reinforced the concept of 'personalisation' in health and social care by requiring that meeting individuals' unique needs and preferences, and supporting individuals to be in control of their lives, as essential for the delivery of high-quality care and support.

Related policies and procedures

Table 5.2 Related policies and procedures

Related policies and procedures	Relevance to health and social care
A Health and Safety Policy and Procedure	Both local and national policies and procedures set out the requirements for health and social care organisations. Practitioners must follow them to comply with legislation and employers' agreed ways of working. A workplace, such as a health and social care organisation, that has five or more employees is required to have in place a written Health and Safety Policy and Procedure that: ● shows the organisation is committed to providing a safe workplace (policy) ● details the employer's, employees' and others' responsibilities ● outlines the steps that must be taken, for example reporting health and safety dangers or recording and reporting accidents.

Related policies and procedures	Relevance to health and social care
The London Multi-Agency Adult Safeguarding Policy and Procedures (2016)	This local policy established the current ways of working for all organisations who work with adults at risk from harm in London, for example the police, London Ambulance Service, local health and social care providers, housing providers and local authorities. It supports the Care Act 2014 by promoting individuals with care and support needs (who are at risk of abuse and neglect) to have greater control in their lives: to both prevent it from happening and to give meaningful options of dealing with it should it occur.
The Information Sharing Policy (2018) NHS England	This national policy was developed in line with the updated Data Protection Act and GDPR 2018. It sets out how NHS England will process all personal data about the individuals who use its services. It also sets out the requirements placed on all NHS England staff when sharing individuals' personal information within the NHS and between the NHS and other organisations.
An Infection Prevention and Control Policy and Procedure	It sets out the employer's responsibilities in relation to infection prevention and control, and can include providing information and education, such as leaflets on how infections spread and can be prevented, as well as providing equipment such as disposable aprons and gloves. It also sets out employees' responsibilities in relation to infection prevention and control, such as following their employer's policy and procedures, attending training provided and reporting all infections.
A Risk Assessment Policy and Procedure	It sets out what risks and hazards can occur in the work setting. It details how risks and hazards can be identified and then assessed, for instance, low, medium or high priority, as well as how to report and record actual and potential risks.

Codes of practice relevant to the sector

Table 5.3 Codes of practice relevant to the sector

Codes of Practice	Relevance to health and social care
The Code of Conduct for Healthcare Support Workers and Adult Social Care Workers in England	Codes of practice (or codes of conduct) provide employees with guidance on how to comply with best practice and health and social care organisations with the standards that they expect their employees to follow. The Code of Conduct for Healthcare Support Workers and Adult Social Care Workers in England is overseen by **Skills for Care** and **Skills for Health**. It establishes a set of principles or values for those who work in health and social care settings: for example, to promote and uphold the privacy, dignity, rights, health and well-being of individuals and their carers who use care and support services at all times.
The Mental Capacity Act Code of Practice	The Mental Capacity Act Code of Practice that accompanies the Mental Capacity Act 2005 sets out what must be done when representatives act or make decisions on behalf of individuals who **lack the capacity** to do so. For more information about the Act's five principles, see *Unit HSC M3: Safeguarding and protection in health and social care*.

Current legislation as relevant to Home Nation

Table 5.4 Current legislation as relevant to Home Nation

Current legislation relevant to Home Nation	Relevance to health and social care
The Children Services Co-operation Act (Northern Ireland) 2015	Each of the UK's four nations (England, Northern Ireland, Scotland and Wales) have their own legislation for working in health and social care. This Act sets out the requirements for public authorities to promote the well-being of children and young people in relation to their physical and mental health, their enjoyment of play and leisure, their learning and achievement, their living conditions, rights, and economic well-being.
The Children (Scotland) Act 1995	This Act sets out the rights and responsibilities of parents as well as the duties and powers of public authorities to safeguard and promote children's safety and welfare. Under this Act, local authorities have a duty to assess the needs of care leavers up to the age of 26.
The Social Services and Well-being (Wales) Act 2014	This Act established a National Adoption Service, giving children and young people more control over the care and support they receive. It introduced a National Outcomes Framework for setting out what children and families can expect from social services.

Key terms

Information Commissioner's Offices is the UK's independent body that upholds information rights.

Lack the capacity refers to when an individual is unable to make a decision for themselves because of a learning disability or a condition, such as dementia, a mental health need or because they are unconscious.

Personal data refers to information that is personal to an individual and can identify them, such as their name or date of birth.

Process (in relation to data) refers to the process used when holding or storing data.

Skills for Care is the sector skills council for people working in social work and social care for adults and children in the UK, as well as for the early years workforce, children and young people's services. It sets standards and develops qualifications for those working in health and social care.

Skills for Health is the sector skills council for people working in healthcare in the UK. It sets out standards and develops qualifications for those working in healthcare.

Activity

Research:
1 The changes to processing information that have been enforced by the General Data Protection Regulation (GDPR) 2018.
2 The Mental Capacity Act 2005 Code of Practice.
3 One local or one national policy or procedure relevant to health and social care.

Outline how each of the above relate to health and social care. Create a poster with your findings.

1.2 Health and social care values

Values are ideas that form the system by which a person lives their life and often a person's beliefs can develop into their values. For example, a person may value living independently, having contact with family and friends or living a **vegan** lifestyle. Health and social care working practices are underpinned by a set of values that influence how health and social care practitioners work and the approaches that they use.

Duty of care

As you will have learned, all health and social care practitioners are legally required to have a duty of care, not only towards the individuals that they provide care and support to, but also towards others that they may work with, such as individuals' families, colleagues, manager, employer and other professionals, for example the GP, social worker and pharmacist.

To uphold their duty of care, health and social care practitioners must always act in the **best interests** of individuals with care and support needs. For example, by supporting them to make informed choices by assessing the pros and cons of their decisions (you may wish to review your previous learning around positive risk taking in *Unit HSC M3: Safeguarding and protection in health and social care*). Promoting an individual's rights to, for example, privacy, dignity, respect and independence must also form part of a health and social care practitioner's duty of care. It underpins all high-quality care and support as it involves working in a person-centred way, which you will learn more about later in this unit.

Maintaining an individual's safety and taking action to prevent harm is also an important aspect of a health and social care practitioner's duty of care. For example, if a health and social care practitioner notices that the floor in the bathroom is very wet, then they must not ignore this and instead take action to prevent someone from slipping over. They must report this and ensure a danger sign is placed outside the bathroom, notifying everyone that the floor is wet and therefore slippery.

Finally, to uphold their duty of care, a health and social care practitioner must only carry out work activities that they have been trained in and have the skills and knowledge to carry out safely and skilfully. Not doing so may have serious consequences. For example, if a health and social care practitioner administers medication to an individual and they have not been trained to do so, this may result in the individual being administered their medication incorrectly. This could potentially affect an individual's **well-being** but also may result in the practitioner being dismissed from their job.

Safeguarding

Safeguarding individuals who have care and support needs, so that they can live safely and free from abuse and harm, underpins all health and social care working practices and forms part of a health and social care practitioner's duty of care. This is very important, particularly because some individuals who have care and support needs may not be able to safeguard themselves from **harm** and **abuse.** This might be because they have:

- a condition, for example dementia that means that they may not be aware of potential dangers that exist around them

- a disability, for example a learning disability that means that they may need to have potential dangers that exist around them explained to them

- been harmed or abused themselves and therefore may not be able to safeguard themselves from further harm and abuse.

You may find it useful to review your previous learning in *Unit HSC M3: Safeguarding and protection in health and social care*.

Key terms

Abuse refers to when a person is mistreated in a way that causes them pain and hurt.

Best interests refers to considering an individual's circumstances and preferences before making a decision or choice on their behalf.

Harm refers to when someone is hurt either physically or emotionally; this may be intentional (i.e. abuse) or unintentional (i.e. an accident).

Vegan refers to a person who does not eat or use any animal or by-products of animals.

Well-being refers to how a person thinks and feels about themselves, physically, mentally and emotionally.

Person-centred

Health and social care values always place the individual:

- with care or support needs at the centre of everything they do
- and their needs, wishes and preferences at the centre of everything they do
- in control of the care and support provided.

This way of working is referred to as 'person-centred' and promotes the individual's right to live their life how they want to and be in control.

Partnership

As previously discussed, a health and social care practitioner's role involves working together with individuals and others. This includes other professionals, such as social workers, physiotherapists, GPs and pharmacists. Working in partnership involves everyone working together as one team to ensure effective:

- verbal and non-verbal communication (you may find it useful to review your previous learning in *Unit HSC M4: Communication in health and social care* for more information about effective communication)
- understanding of each other's roles and responsibilities
- support of each other's ideas, views, knowledge and skills.

This leads to the development of respectful and trustworthy working relationships that, in turn, create a supportive and productive environment. The care and support provided to individuals will be more likely to meet their **holistic needs** and therefore promote their well-being.

Key term

Holistic needs involve treating an individual as a whole person and therefore meeting their range of needs, for example physical, emotional and social.

Dignity

Treating individuals with dignity is a very important health and social care value because it is essential for individuals to lead their lives as they want to. Treating individuals with dignity involves promoting individuals' self-respect and not humiliating or embarrassing them in any way. For example, if a health and social care practitioner spends some time talking with an individual to find out their views and ideas and takes these into account when planning their care and support, the individual will feel respected and valued. It is this sense of worthiness that enables the individual to then respect themselves. Promoting individuals' rights to respect, privacy and choice are also essential aspects of treating individuals with dignity.

Respect

Respecting individuals, as you will have learned, is an essential aspect of treating individuals with dignity. It involves health and social care practitioners treating individuals as unique people with their own needs and preferences. To do this effectively, the health and social care practitioner must show that they can find out and learn about individuals' differences and take these into account even when they are different to their own, i.e. this may be in relation to individuals' interests, beliefs, views, preferences.

Rights

The health and social care practitioner must be prepared to support an individual with health and care needs to understand their rights. They can do this by providing the individual with information about their rights in a format they can understand; this must include how the individual can expect to be treated by others, i.e. with dignity, privacy and respect, as well as the behaviours that are not acceptable, i.e. that cause harm, abuse or discrimination. The health and social care practitioner must also make individuals aware of their right to complain if they are, for example, unhappy about any aspect of their care and support. By making individuals aware of their rights, it will be less likely that they will be exploited, harmed or abused by others. They will be more likely to feel they can report any unwanted or unsafe working practices.

You may find it useful to review your previous learning around the factors that make individuals more vulnerable to harm or abuse

in AC3.3 of *Unit HSC M3: Safeguarding and protection in health and social care.*

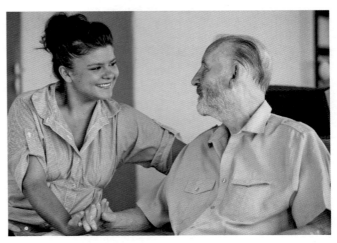

Figure 5.2 Do you know how to promote individuals' rights?

Confidentiality

Confidentiality is an essential aspect of working in health and social care and therefore a key value to uphold. It involves maintaining the privacy of individuals' information that may contain personal data, for example in relation to their care or support needs and/or sensitive information such as their health. You may find it useful to review Learning Outcome 1 of this unit regarding the current legislation in place to support individuals' rights to keep their information confidential.

Confidentiality is an important value for working in health and social care, not only for complying with current legislation, but also for showing respect towards individuals' personal information and ensuring that others, who are not authorised to do so, do not have access to it. Working in this way will mean that individuals will feel able to trust the health and social care practitioner and be more likely to confide in them. You may find it useful to review your previous learning about the boundaries of confidentiality when safeguarding and protecting individuals in AC4.3, *Unit HSC M3: Safeguarding and protection in health and social care*. It is part of the health and social care practitioner's responsibilities to maintain individuals' information safely and securely.

Independence

Promoting individuals' independence is another essential health and social care value because it involves supporting individuals to do as much for themselves as possible. It means finding out about an individual's strengths and abilities and ensuring the individual is provided with opportunities to use these. It also means reducing individuals' dependency on others by encouraging individuals to develop new skills. For example, a health and social care practitioner could promote an individual's independence when planning a shopping trip by:

- showing the individual how to budget
- organising how they are going to get to and from the shops
- providing them with information about the pros and cons of different forms of transport, for example taxi, bus, train.

Promoting independence enables individuals to reach their full potential and lead fulfilling lives.

Activity

Develop a profile for one individual with care and support needs. This can be fictitious or someone you know. For their profile, you can include brief details about their likes, dislikes, abilities, needs and preferences. Then, summarise the health and social care values that are essential for working with this individual.

1.3 How individuals accessing health and social care services are valued

Having values and being valued are two essential aspects of accessing health and social care services when you are an individual with care and support needs. Being valued can make a positive difference to an individual's life because it will enable them to continue to live how they want. You will learn more about the different types of health and social care services in Learning Outcome 2 of this unit.

Individual needs and preferences

Being treated as a unique person is essential if an individual's needs and preferences are going to be respected and if their well-being is to be promoted. For example, an individual who accesses a homecare or domiciliary service can be valued by being asked what support they feel they need to continue living in their own flat and how they would like the support provided. In this way, the support provided to the individual can be tailored to meet their individual needs and preferences. For example, the individual may require support with washing and dressing and may prefer to have a shower every morning, but may only need assistance with getting in and out of the shower and getting dressed afterwards.

Informed choice

Being supported to make informed choices is another way that a health and social care service can value an individual. For example, when an individual visits their GP for advice on how to lose weight, the GP could present the individual with a range of options they could choose from to achieve their goal, i.e. going on a diet, increasing the amount of exercise they do, attending a support group. The GP could then discuss each of the options with the individual, including what each one would involve and the pros and cons. In this way, the individual's understanding of how they could lose weight would be promoted, thus enabling them to make their own decisions and an informed choice over which option is best for them. Going through this process would enable the individual to be in control of how to achieve their goal and would provide them with a sense of self-worth, making them feel valued.

Active support

The term 'active support' refers to a person-centred approach to supporting individuals with care and support needs. It involves health and social care services ensuring that individuals lead lives that are:

- active, i.e. where individuals are active on a day-to-day basis
- meaningful, i.e. where individuals' lives are centred around their needs, preferences and goals and provide individuals with opportunities to develop their knowledge, understanding and skills
- consistent, i.e. where individuals can experience stability and comfort.

Active support enables individuals to feel valued because it involves supporting individuals, irrespective of their needs or abilities or condition, to actively participate in a range of activities and life opportunities of their choice.

Actively participating in activities on a day-to-day basis makes individuals feels valued because they will meet other people, be engaged in doing different things and have opportunities to make decisions and choices. Without active support, individuals with care and support needs may have difficulties because of their needs and/or condition to make decisions, meet others or participate in different activities. This is why this approach is essential for individuals to lead fulfilling lives.

Aids and adaptations

As all individuals who have care and support needs will have their own unique needs and preferences, the support they require from health and social care services will vary. When individuals' needs are specific, health and social care services make available aids and carry out adaptations to enable individuals to lead fulfilling lives.

Aids for individuals with care and support needs can include both technical equipment and human support.

Adaptations for individuals with care and support needs can include both physical and social adaptations that can be made to buildings and environments. **Table 5.5** includes some examples of how aids and adaptations can be used by individuals with specific needs who require care and support from health and social care services and how each of them can be of benefit and value to them.

Aids and adaptations add value to individuals' lives because they promote independence while recognising individuals' differences.

Table 5.5 How aids and adaptations can be of value to individuals

Individuals with specific needs	Examples of aids to value individuals	Examples of adaptations to value individuals
An individual with **autism spectrum condition**	The Picture Exchange Communication System (PECS) can be used by the individual to approach others and initiate communications with others through pictures. These pictures represent items or places, for example a picture of a fork and knife that can represent lunchtime or a swimming pool that can represent the individual wanting to go out to the leisure centre.	Arrange for a quiet space to be made available when meeting with the individual. A quiet environment will mean that the individual will feel more relaxed and therefore calmer. They will be more likely to engage in an activity, for example cooking, that requires them to be supported.
An individual who is deaf	A **British Sign Language (BSL) interpreter** can be accessed by the individual to communicate with others and express their views and opinions.	Ensure that the meeting room is well lit so that the individual and BSL interpreter can see people's facial expressions and gestures. Meetings could be adapted by including breaks (for the interpreter and individual) every 30 minutes.
An individual who has **dementia**	Talking Mats is an application that can be used by the individual when they have difficulties with their verbal communication. It enables them to communicate using a combination of pictures and symbols with text.	Support the individual to understand what is being communicated by speaking clearly and using short phrases. Adapt the time communications take with the individual by ensuring they do not rush the individual. Give them sufficient time to respond and interact with others.
An individual who has a learning disability	Makaton involves the use of signs, symbols and speech and can be used by the individual to communicate and interact with others.	Ensure that an **advocate** is available when the individual is making choices and decisions about their care and support.
An individual who has difficulty walking	A walking frame that is made of a sturdy, fixed aluminium frame with four legs, two wheels at the front and moulded handles on each side for grip could be used by an individual to walk on their own.	Ensure that the floor coverings in the individual's room are non-slippery and maintained well so that the individual can mobilise themselves safely and easily.
An individual who has a physical disability	A standing aid could enable the individual who requires support to stand up from where they are sitting down, for example from a chair, the toilet, their wheelchair.	Promote the individual's mobility by assisting the individual to move from one position to another. Provide training to practitioners about how to adapt their moving and handling practices.
An older individual who is recovering from a fall	A mobility scooter could be used by the individual to continue to carry out activities, for example shopping and visiting friends independently.	Provide the individual with information about the various adaptations that could be made to their home so that they can mobilise safely and independently. Adaptations could include handle bars along corridors or a stair lift.

Key terms

Advocate an independent person who represents the views, needs and interests of individuals who are unable or unwilling to do so, and supports them to express their views.

Autism spectrum condition is a lifelong condition that affects how a person perceives the world and interacts with others, i.e. they may have difficulties communicating, interacting and socialising with others.

British Sign Language (BSL) is the sign language used in the UK by individuals who have a hearing impairment. It uses a combination of hand gestures, facial expressions and body language. It is a different language to English with its own grammar and sentence construction.

Dementia is a disorder of the mental processes caused by brain disease or injury. Examples of symptoms include memory loss and/or difficulties with thinking, problem-solving or language.

Interpreters are professionals who convert spoken/oral or sign language communication from one language to another such as English to British Sign Language (BSL). Interpreters must be good listeners and be able to process and memorise words and gestures while individuals are communicating.

Health and safety

Maintaining health and safety when working in health and social care is essential for keeping everyone safe. Individuals accessing health and social care services may be more likely to have accidents, injuries and develop illnesses because they may have:

- difficulties walking, moving or positioning that may result in them slipping, tripping or falling over

- conditions that may affect how they think and feel and result in them becoming angry or distressed

- vision loss that may result in them being more likely to fall over or injure themselves

- weak immune systems as a result of health conditions that may result in them becoming ill.

An important aspect of keeping everyone safe includes being aware of how **hazards** and **risks** can occur. Assessing health and safety hazards and risks is part of high-quality care and support. It values individuals because doing so promotes an individual's:

- safety
- independence
- well-being
- rights.

Providing an environment that is welcoming and comfortable as well as safe not only safeguards individuals from being placed in danger, or at risk of being harmed or abused, but also ensures that the individual feels relaxed and content, an essential aspect for good health and well-being.

 Key terms

Hazards are dangers that have the potential to cause harm, such as an item (a broken chair), a situation (an individual who is distressed) or an activity (moving and positioning) that can be the cause of accidents, injuries, ill-health, deaths or damage.

Risks are the likelihood of harm occurring as a result of a hazard, for example an accident caused by a broken chair, damage caused by a distressed individual or a back injury caused by moving and positioning an individual.

Confidentiality

As you have already learned in AC1.2 of this unit, confidentiality is an essential health and social care value; you may find it useful to review your previous learning. Maintaining individuals' confidentiality when accessing health and social care services enables individuals to be valued, because the health and social care practitioner will be:

- supporting individuals' rights to have their personal information kept private, which will help with forming working relationships based on trust.
- preventing those who do not have permission to access individuals' personal information, which will safeguard individuals from being harmed or abused.
- providing individuals with safe care and support where the individual feels in control and has their unique needs and preferences fully met.

Not maintaining individuals' confidentiality will impact negatively on them because it could result in their personal information getting lost, misplaced or stolen. It will also impact negatively on the care and support provided because it will be difficult for the individual to trust the health and social care practitioner and therefore work in partnership with them. You may find it useful to review your previous learning in AC1.2 of this unit on the value of effective partnership working.

During daily routines

Valuing individuals does not take place in health and social care at certain times of the year or on special occasions. Valuing individuals underpins all health and social care practices. It is therefore integral to all working with individuals during daily routines from, for example, getting up in the morning to preparing a meal at lunchtime, to going out shopping in the afternoon to going to bed at night. Individuals accessing health and social care services are valued during daily routines by having their individual needs and preferences met:

- by being supported to make informed choices
- through active support
- by being provided with aids and adaptations
- by promoting their health and safety
- by maintaining their confidentiality.

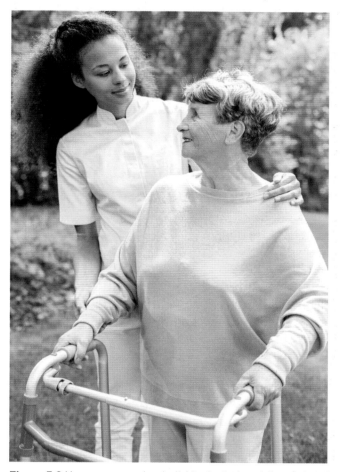

Figure 5.3 How can you value individuals during daily routines?

Description Activity

Develop a case study of an individual who has care and support needs. This can be an individual you know or a fictitious individual. Describe:

1 What their care and support needs are.
2 How they are cared for and supported by health and social care practitioners.
3 How the care and support benefits the individual.
4 How the individual is valued by the health and social care services they access.

Check your understanding 1

1 Name two pieces of legislation that are relevant to working in health and social care.
2 Name two health and social care values.
3 Describe the meaning of active support and why it's relevant to valuing individuals with care and support needs.
4 Give examples of two aids or adaptations that individuals with care and support needs can access in health and social care services.

LO2 Understand health and social care provision

2.1 Types of health and social care services

There are different types of health and social care services that provide a range of support and services to meet individuals' different needs, wishes and preferences.

Statutory

Statutory services are provided by and paid for by the UK government, for example:

- The National Health Service (NHS) provides health care services to both adults and children. It can include services such as GP surgeries, physiotherapy departments and maternity services.
- Social Services provides services and support to both adults and children. It can include services such as **domiciliary care services**, education and adoption services.

Private

Private services are not owned or managed by the UK government but are provided by organisations to make a profit. For example:

- Sheltered Housing provides self-contained accommodation with shared communal areas for older adults who would like to maintain their independence with some support. Services can include support with managing home repairs and accessing local services in the community.
- Residential Homes provide care and support to children and adults and are staffed 24 hours a day. It can include services such as support with washing, dressing and administering medication.

Voluntary

Voluntary services are not owned or managed by the UK government but are provided by non-profit making organisations. For example:

- The charity Alzheimer's Society provides information, advice, practical and emotional support for individuals and their families living with dementia.
- The **self-help group** East Midlands Open Minds provides support to isolated disabled people living in the Nottingham area.

 Key terms

Domiciliary care services refer to care and support services that are provided to individuals in their own homes.

Self-help group refers to a group of people who provide mutual support for each other on the basis of sharing a common problem, such as isolation, an illness, disability or addiction.

Activity

Create a poster that outlines the three different types of health and social care services. Give examples for each type of service.

2.2 Functions of health and social care services

Individuals' needs can vary during each life stage from childhood to adulthood. This is why different health and social care services have varying purposes and functions to meet individuals' diverse needs.

Long-term/short-term

Services that are provided both over the long term and short term can offer much needed support to both children and adults. For example, children with **special educational needs** may need long-term support to enable them to attend and make progress at school. A child who cares for their parent who has a disability may need to access a service provided over the short term, i.e. for one weekend such as a **residential short break**.

An adult who has dementia may require long-term support from a nursing home to ensure their individual needs, such as those in relation to their personal hygiene, nutrition, medical and mental health, are met. An adult who lives at home on their own and requires short-term support (up to a maximum of six weeks), to regain their independent living skills following an accident at home, can access reablement services. They enable individuals to continue to live safely at home by providing intensive, direct support, so the individual regains the confidence and skills they had prior to their accident.

Residential

Residential services, such as a care home, offer a residential setting for adults and children to live in because they are unable to live in their own home or with family. This may be because they have a disability such as autism, a condition such as dementia, or because they have mental health needs or are terminally ill. Care homes typically offer support with personal care activities such as support with eating, drinking, washing, dressing and administering medication. Some care homes provide specialist care to, for example, individuals with specific conditions such as dementia. These care homes are staffed with health and social care practitioners that have been specifically trained in dementia care. Other care homes provide both personal care and nursing care.

Respite

Respite services are provided both in individuals' homes and in the community. Respite services enable those individuals who are carers to take a break from caring, while the person they care for is looked after by someone else. For example, a respite service could involve a paid carer looking after the person being cared for while the individual goes out for the day or away for the weekend. A respite service could also involve the person being cared for being supported to attend a **day care centre** while the individual remains at home.

Key terms

Day care centre refers to a community-based setting, open during the day, where individuals can meet with others to socialise and participate in activities.

Residential short break refers to a holiday or break where individuals can socialise and take part in activities with other people their age to give them a break from their caring responsibilities.

Special educational needs refer to a child that has a disability or difficulties with learning that make it more difficult for them to learn than most children their age.

Community

Community services are provided for people who live in the local area and are usually specialist services to meet individuals' specific needs. For example, community health services such as stopping smoking, pre-natal or well-being classes. Other community-based services include teams of professionals with specialist skills. For example, in mental health care, community-based services consist of skilled professionals with expertise in mental health care, such as community psychiatric nurses and psychologists that provide information, advice, treatment and support to individuals (both children and adults) and their families who experience mental ill-health. In social care, a community-based service could provide support to individuals with learning disabilities who want to live independently, or specialist information and support to individuals who misuse alcohol and drugs.

Rehabilitation

Rehabilitation services provide specialist healthcare support to enable individuals who have lost or had their physical, mental, thinking and learning abilities lost or impaired. This might be due to an illness such as a **stroke**, an accident or treatment such as an operation and helps them to return to living an active and healthy life. There are three types of rehabilitation services:

1 **Occupational therapy** is used to rehabilitate individuals who require assistance in participating in everyday activities, for example a child with a physical disability who may require support with co-ordinating their movements so that they can feed themselves independently, or an adult experiencing **depression** following a bereavement who may need support with participating in daily activities again.

2 **Physical therapy** is used to rehabilitate individuals who experience pain or have difficulties moving around as a result of, for example, a disease such as **arthritis** or as a result of an accident. Physical therapy can include physical exercises that are designed to relive pain or improve movement, as well as rehabilitation support to enable individuals to use mobility aids to help them improve their mobility.

3 **Speech therapy** is used to rehabilitate individuals with speech-related issues to be able to use language, their voice and swallowing so that they can communicate more easily. For example, individuals who access speech therapy may have a condition such as **aphasia**, a disease such as **Huntington's disease**, or difficulties with eating or swallowing.

Specific service provision to meet needs

Health and social care services also provide specific provision to meet individuals' needs. You will have already learned about the range of services that exist to meet individuals' differing needs. In addition, other examples of specific service provision may include the provision of:

- **Advocacy services** to support individuals who may not be able to speak up for themselves due to a learning disability, mental health need or conditions such as Alzheimer's. Advocates are independent and represent only the individual's best interests, such as an Independent Mental Capacity Advocate (IMCA) when reviewing an individual's care.

- Hospice services provide care and support to adults, children and their families who have a terminal or life-shortening condition. Hospices aim to provide care and support that meets individuals' clinical, physical, emotional, social and spiritual needs.

- Memory Café services provide support, socialising opportunities and activities in a relaxed environment to individuals, their families and carers who experience memory loss.

- Recovery colleges provide education and training programmes to assist individuals who have mental ill-health to recover. They give the individual the skills and confidence they need to be in control of their lives. The programmes are developed and delivered by individuals with experience of mental ill-health and by professionals with specific expertise.

 Key terms

Advocacy services support individuals to speak up when they are unable to; they represent the individual's best interests.

Aphasia refers to a condition that affects a person's speech, understanding and use of language.

Arthritis refers to a disease that causes painful inflammation and stiffness of the joints.

Depression refers to a medical condition that causes low mood and that affects a person's thoughts and feelings. It usually lasts for a long time and affects their day-to-day living.

Huntington's disease refers to an inherited disease that stops part of the brain from working properly, causing uncontrolled movements and affecting emotions and thinking abilities.

Stroke refers to a life-threatening medical condition that occurs when the blood supply to part of the brain is cut off.

Funding

In the UK, health and social care services work together with the Department of Health and Social Care to fund the provision of care, support and treatment that individuals need. The Department of Health sets the budget for health and social care services.

At a local level, local authorities are responsible for planning, buying and monitoring care and support services; a process usually referred to as commissioning. Clinical Commissioning Groups (CCGs) are responsible for planning and buying health care services for the local communities they are responsible for. They are independent, statutory and NHS-led, working closely with NHS England and local authorities. CCGs are made up of doctors, nurses and other professionals and can buy services from any provider that can provide them within budget and can meet the required standards, i.e. NHS hospitals, voluntary organisations or private sector providers.

Partnership working

Health and social care services do not work in isolation. Individuals very often require access to care and support from more than one type of provision and service depending on their needs. As every service varies in levels of knowledge and expertise, professionals from different services often work together to provide the best possible care and support to individuals. There are different types of partnership working and the main ones are as follows:

- Multidisciplinary partnership working involves a group of professionals from different organisations who have specialist knowledge and skills working together to provide care and support to an individual. For example, Child and Adolescent Mental Health Services (CAMHS) provide specialist services to children and young people with mental health needs. It can include different professionals, for example social workers, child psychiatrists, occupational therapists and music therapists.

- Inter-agency partnership working involves different agencies working together to provide high-quality care and support to individuals. For example, as you will have learned in *Unit HSC M3: Safeguarding and protection in health and social care*, safeguarding individuals from danger, harm and abuse involves different agencies: local authorities, health organisations, housing organisations, schools, voluntary organisations, the police, health and social care providers.

- Health and social care services forums' partnership working involves individuals, their families, carers and other professionals who have experience of health and social care services working together to inform the planning and provision of services in their local areas. For example, Health and Wellbeing boards whose members include (among others) voluntary organisations and individuals who live in the local area. They will identify the health and social care services they feel their community needs and, in turn, their views will inform CCGs and local authorities when they commission services.

2.3 Barriers to accessing health and social care services and how they may be overcome

Although there are many different types of health and social care services to choose from, there are a number of factors or barriers that may prevent or make it difficult for individuals to access these. Recognising the potential barriers that exist and knowing how they may be overcome is essential for health and social care practitioners to ensure an individual's care and support needs are fully met. In this section are details about some of the main barriers and how they may be overcome.

Communication

When health and social care services communicate about their care and support provision, the information provided must be understood by those accessing their services. For example, an individual who communicates using British Sign Language may require information to be made available in a written format they can understand and may also require access to a BSL interpreter. Written and verbal communications from health and social care services must also be respectful and show professionalism. Communications that are not respectful or professional may not instil mutual trust and respect, and therefore might prevent individuals from accessing these services. You may also find it useful to review your previous learning on using effective communication in *Unit HSC M4: Communication in health and social care.*

Description Activity

Identify two health and social care services that provide specific care or support to meet an individual's needs. For each service, describe what care or support is provided and the reasons why.

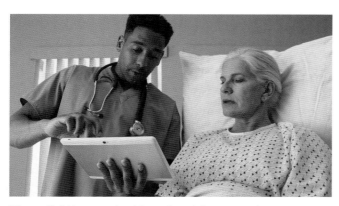

Figure 5.4 How can health and social care services communicate effectively?

Cultural values and beliefs

It is very important for health and social care services to be aware of individuals' different cultural values and beliefs and how they may influence the provision of care and support. Training, support and the sharing of best practice are good ways of raising awareness. A lack of awareness may impact negatively on individuals' well-being and prevent individuals from accessing the care and support they require. Some examples are outlined here.

- A young person from a Hispanic culture might be used to respecting the views of the older members of the family when making decisions about their care. A health and social care service will need to take this into account when planning this individual's care by also involving the individual's family when making decisions.

- An older adult may believe that it is disrespectful to question or challenge a health or social care practitioner about their care. They might prefer to be informed about what is in their best interests rather than be asked about what their preferences are.

- A woman from the Muslim faith may believe that when accessing healthcare, they must only be examined by a female healthcare practitioner; not having a female healthcare practitioner available may prevent the woman from accessing a healthcare service.

Cost

The cost of health and social care services may be too high for individuals, which could prevent them for accessing the service. Even when health and social care services are funded, there are other 'hidden' costs that have to be thought about, for example transport costs to get to the service and/or time off work by an individual's family when the individual needs support to access the service. Overcoming these costs will involve researching what services are within budget and whether there are any other opportunities to access funding to help with the costs.

Location

Where health and social care services are located may also act as a barrier to access for individuals with care and support needs. For example, sometimes specialist services, such as those in relation to children or adults with mental health needs, are located in other parts of the UK that are a considerable distance from individuals and their families. The costs of travelling to these locations, the time it takes and the arrangements that have to be made may restrict which individuals can access these. Researching what is available locally and exploring whether there is the required expertise locally could minimise this barrier.

Physical access

Providing health and social care services in inaccessible buildings, such as those where there are stairs, the lift does not work, or there are no, or limited, adapted toilet facilities, may prevent individuals with physical disabilities or mobility issues from accessing the services. The provision of ramps, widened doorways and adapted toilet facilities are examples of ways that these physical barriers can be overcome.

Psychological

Individuals' psychological needs mean that their mental and emotional health may prevent them from accessing health and social care services. For example, a young person who was abused as a child may feel failed by professionals in social services and may not want to access the support they require because they may feel angry that they were not safeguarded and protected as a child. Similarly, an older adult who lives at home on their own may not want to access health or social care services because they may fear that they will be told that they cannot continue to live on their own and must move into a care home. Health and social care practitioners have an important role to play in these situations. By developing good working relationships and providing reassurance to individuals, they ease their anxiety and support them to access the care and support they require.

Lack of resources

A lack of resources, such as qualified and experienced health and social care practitioners, time and money can mean that health and social care services can only provide some of the services that are required. As a result, individuals may have to wait for quite a long time before they can access the care and support they require. A lack of resources in health and social care provision can be overcome through partnership working when planning and delivering services to local communities. Raising awareness of the challenges and barriers that exist is very important so they must be considered at both a local and national level.

Time

When health and social care services are provided can influence who can access them. For example, if a non-smoking group is only held in the evenings, then an individual with family commitments, for example looking after a child or another family member, might not be able to access these. Similarly, providing services only during office hours (9a.m. to 5p.m.) and on weekdays but not at weekends will mean that those who are engaged in activities during the week (i.e. college, employment) may not be able to access these. Providing services in a flexible manner will mean that more individuals will be able to access the services available.

Activity

Discuss with someone you know the cultural values and beliefs that may prevent individuals from accessing one health or social care service provided in your local area. Discuss what the barriers are, the difficulties they may present and how these may be overcome.

2.4, 2.5 Definition of informal care and the role of informal carers

The care and support required by individuals is not provided solely by statutory, private and voluntary health and social care services; it is also provided by individuals who are unpaid, more commonly referred to as 'informal carers'.

Informal care can be provided by individuals' families, friends, neighbours, community groups and volunteers.

Activity

What does informal care mean to you? Write down a definition of the term 'informal care'.

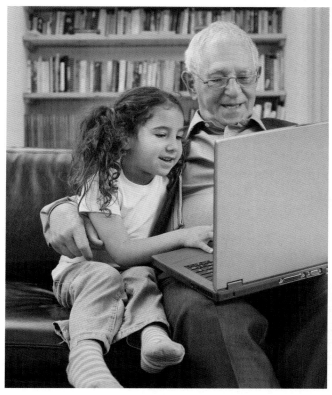

Figure 5.5 How can family benefit individuals' well-being?

Informal carers have an important role to play:

- **Family** can provide both practical and emotional care and support to individuals. For example, an individual's family may assist them with their daily activities, such as washing, dressing, eating and drinking, as well as with household tasks, such as cleaning and shopping. An individual's family can also be a source of great support and comfort because they know the individual.

- **Friends** can be the source of companionship and peer support. For example, an individual's friends may visit the individual at home or support them to socialise with others. An individual's friends can also be the people who the individual can confide in and be themselves with.

- **Neighbours** can be the source of friendship and support. For example, an individual's neighbours may visit them at home and/or take an interest in their welfare and ensure that they look out for them, particularly if the individual lives on their own or their family is away. A neighbour may also run small errands for the individual, for example buying them a newspaper or some milk if they have run out.

- **Community groups** can also be the source of friendship and peer support. For example, a community group may provide individuals with both practical and emotional support, such as assisting them to resolve a housing issue or enabling them to confide in them about loss if they have been bereaved of a family member.

- **Volunteers** can also provide individuals with valuable practical assistance, such as reading letters, but also support such as spending time with an individual who is lonely.

Informal carers are not to be underestimated as they are essential to the well-being of individuals with care and support needs. Carers UK, a national charity for carers has produced the following facts about Informal Carers:

1 in 8 adults (around 6.5 million people) are carers.

Every day another 6,000 people take on a caring responsibility – that equals over 2 million people each year.

58% of carers are women and 42% are men.

Over 1 million people care for more than one person.

(**Source:** Carers UK, 'Facts about Carers', 2015)

Description Activity

Develop a presentation that describes the role of informal carers. Include details in your presentation on who informal carers are, their roles and how they benefit individuals with care and support needs. Use examples to support your description.

 Check your understanding 2

1 Name one difference between statutory and private health and social care services.
2 Describe two different functions of health and social care services.
3 Give examples of two barriers to accessing health and social care services.
4 Define in one sentence the meaning of informal care.
5 Describe the role of family in providing informal care.

LO3 Understand the roles and responsibilities of the health and social care practitioner

3.1 Job roles within the health and social care sectors

There are a wide range of job roles within the health and social care sectors in order to meet the diverse needs of individuals and provide them with the specialist care and support they need at different life stages. Job roles in healthcare involve supporting individuals with clinical needs, while job roles working in social care involve supporting individuals with non-clinical needs.

Table 5.6 outlines some examples of job roles and their purpose across both the health and social care sectors.

Table 5.6 Job roles and their purpose across both the health and social care sectors

Health care job roles	Job role purpose
General Practice Nurse	Obtaining blood samples, dressing minor wounds, for example leg ulcers, providing child immunisations and advice. General Practice Nurses work in GP surgeries alongside doctors, pharmacists and dieticians.
Psychological Well-being Practitioner	Assessing and supporting individuals to manage their mental health, for example relating to anxiety and depression. Psychological Well-Being Practitioners work closely with other professionals, such as GPs, counsellors, housing and employment advisers.
Dietician	Providing information, support and guidance to individuals about their food and nutrition. Dieticians work in hospitals and community-based services with both individuals and groups of people.
Social care job roles	Job role purpose
Care worker	Providing support to individuals with day-to-day activities such as washing, dressing, eating, drinking and social activities. Care workers can work in a care home, a community-based service or in individuals' homes.
Activities worker	Organising social activities for individuals to participate in: these may include one-to-one and group activities. Activities workers can work in a care home, day care centre or in a community-based service.
Social worker	Providing advocacy and support to individuals and their families, including safeguarding individuals with care and support needs. Social workers can work with individuals with diverse care and support needs, working closely with other agencies, for example healthcare services, schools and the police.

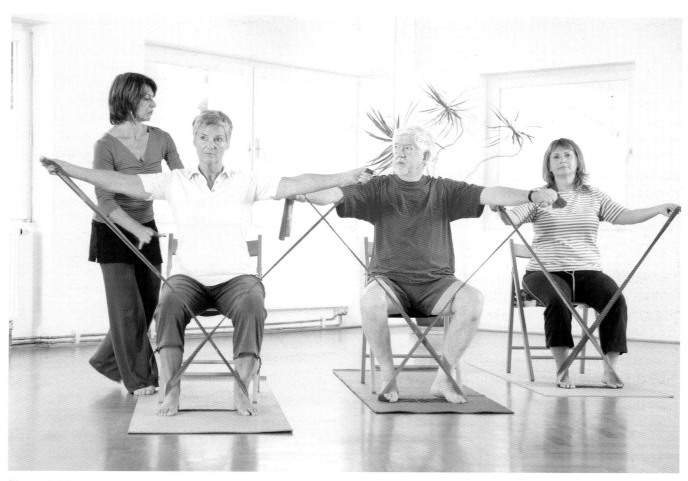

Figure 5.6 Do you have what it takes to be an activities worker?

Activity

Research the different health and social care job roles that are available. You may find it useful to visit the *NHS Health Careers* website for health care job roles and Skills for Care's *Think Care Careers* website for social care job roles.

Make an informative leaflet for those considering a career in health and/or social care that outlines two health care job roles and two social care job roles that interest you.

Key term

Job description is a document that outlines the purpose and responsibilities to be carried out as part of a job role.

3.2 The responsibilities of the health and social care practitioner

All health and social care practitioners, irrespective of which sector they work in, will have a **job description** that sets out all the responsibilities they have agreed to carry out as part of their job role. Although responsibilities will vary according to the specific job role, there are a set of responsibilities that are common to all health and social care practitioners.

Work within policies and procedures

As you will know, policies and procedures are the agreed ways of working that an employer expects a health and social care practitioner to follow on a day-to-day basis, for example in relation to safeguarding individuals by reporting concerns of unsafe practices; maintaining individuals' confidentiality by ensuring the secure handling of individuals' personal information; and promoting health and safety by identifying hazards that may place individuals and others in danger.

It is health and social care practitioners' responsibilities to work within policies and procedures because it ensures that they are:

- carrying out their responsibilities as agreed by their employer
- complying with current legislation
- carrying out their responsibilities to the best of their ability
- carrying out work activities that they have the skills, knowledge and training for.

If health and social care practitioners do not work within policies and procedures, then they will be failing in their duty of care. This is because they might be placing individuals and others in danger and not complying with legislation and their employers' agreed ways of working.

Implement care values

Implementing care values is an essential aspect of working in health and social care. It underpins all person-centred working approaches used with individuals who have care and support needs. Implementing care values ensures positive outcomes for all.

Care planning

Planning individuals' day-to-day requirements and care and support preferences (with the individual and others involved in their lives, e.g. their families) is another important responsibility that health and social care practitioners must fulfil. Care planning with individuals is an integral part of person-centred working because it:

- promotes individuals' rights to be in control of their care and support
- enables the care provided to meet individuals' unique needs and preferences
- promotes individuals' independence by enabling them to do as much for themselves as they can.

Risk management

Supporting individuals to take and manage risks enables individuals to exercise their rights to be independent, making their own choices and decisions over the risks they can take. There are many benefits to health and social care practitioners supporting individuals to take and manage risks positively. This includes individuals feeling valued, more confident in their abilities and in control of their lives. Health and social care practitioners can carry out their responsibilities in relation to risk management by:

- complying with their employers' policies and procedures for risk management
- supporting individuals to take risks by explaining to the individual what the risks are, how they can be managed and the range of measures that could be put in place to reduce the risks of danger or harm to the individual
- protecting individuals from taking risks if the risks pose a serious danger to them and/or others.

Job description/person specification

Health and social care practitioners are required to work within the agreed responsibilities that have been set out in their job description. Job descriptions describe the purpose of the job role, the responsibilities or work activities that must be carried out as part of their job role, as well as how these must be carried out. Health and social care practitioners must only carry out responsibilities that form part of their job description because these have been agreed with the employer and reflect the current expertise, knowledge and skills that the health and social care practitioner has.

A person specification is different to a job description because it details the personal qualities that are required by the health and social care practitioner to carry out their job role and associated responsibilities, for example being trustworthy, patient and respectful. Showing the personal qualities that are expected from health and social care practitioners is the basis of all high-quality care and support.

Description Activity

For one of the job roles you outlined in the activity in AC3.1, describe the associated responsibilities each one has.

3.3 Skills, behaviours and attributes required by health and social care practitioners

Working in health and social care is a specialised area of work and requires specialist skills, behaviours and attributes or personal qualities that not everyone has. **Table 5.7** describes the skills, behaviours and attributes that are required to provide effective care and support.

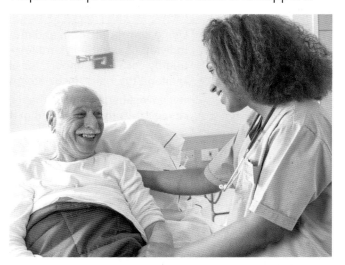

Figure 5.7 What skills and qualities does a good carer need?

Table 5.7 Skills, behaviours and attributes

Skills, behaviours and attributes	Reasons why they are required by health and social care practitioners
Be trustworthy	Enables individuals to feel relaxed and safe, for example when supporting an individual who has disclosed that they have been abused.
	Being trustworthy involves being dependable and consistent when working with individuals.
Be objective	Supports individuals so they feel they can make their own choices and decisions, for example when supporting an individual who wants to travel abroad but is unsure whether they have the confidence to do so.
	Being objective involves being fair and unbiased.
Be patient	Enables individuals with diverse needs to do as much for themselves as possible, for example when supporting an individual who has had a stroke to get dressed.
	Being patient involves being kind and supportive.

Skills, behaviours and attributes	Reasons why they are required by health and social care practitioners
Be respectful	Being respectful towards individuals who have diverse needs, cultures and backgrounds is an essential quality to have as a health and social care practitioner, for example when supporting an individual to practise their religious beliefs, such as praying at certain times of the day. Being respectful involves being understanding and tolerant of individuals' differences.
Show empathy	Showing empathy is an important behaviour to show when providing care and support to individuals, for example when supporting an individual who is finding it frustrating that they cannot make themselves understood. Showing empathy involves reassuring individuals; being able to take a step back to put themselves in individuals' situations to experience how they may be feeling.
Show commitment	Showing commitment to ensure that individuals live their lives how they want to is an important behaviour to show when providing care and support, for example planning with an individual by confirming how they want to be supported in their daily living activities. Showing commitment involves being willing and having a desire to put the individuals' needs first and at the centre of all care and support provided.
Use communication and interpersonal skills	Using communication and interpersonal skills when providing care and support to individuals and their families is the basis of working in partnership and providing high-quality care and support, for example when discussing with an individual how they can manage the risks associated with travelling independently. It involves being approachable and able to communicate information clearly and respectfully. It is the basis of all good working relationships.
Use initiative	Requires being able to think quickly and respond to unplanned situations, for example when supporting an individual who does not want to participate in an activity they have chosen because they are finding it difficult. Using initiative involves thinking on your feet and trusting your instincts.
Use observation skills	Involves observing individuals' behaviours, including what they say, don't say, do and don't do, for example when working with an individual who appears unusually withdrawn. Using observation skills involves being vigilant and factual.
Show professionalism	Embeds the care values relevant to the sector in all working practices, for example when communicating with an individual who wishes to make a complaint about an aspect of their care. Showing professionalism involves being polite and meeting the expected standards of the profession.
Be able to problem solve	Finding solutions to difficulties and seeking guidance and advice from others, for example when supporting an individual who is finding it difficult to use their new walking aid. Being able to problem solve involves being able to work in partnership with others.
Be able to work as part of a team	Involves being a good communicator and being prepared to share knowledge and expertise with others, for example when planning how to support an individual who has diverse needs. Being able to work as part of a team involves being able to work with others towards agreed goals and in line with best practice.
Be a reflective practitioner	Assess work practices honestly to learn from mistakes and make improvements, for example when reflecting on the reasons why an individual became distressed during an activity. Being a reflective practitioner involves gaining a greater insight into how working practices can be further developed to make a positive impact on individuals and others.

Classroom Discussion

Discuss the skills, behaviours and attitudes that are essential for working in health and social care. Agree on the top ten most important ones and describe why these are important.

Description Activity

For the job role responsibilities you outlined in the activity in AC3.2, describe the required skills, behaviours and attributes each job role has and detail the reasons why.

Check your understanding 3

1 Give examples of two job roles within the health and social care sectors.
2 Describe three responsibilities a health and social care practitioner has.
3 Describe two skills, two behaviours and two attributes required by health and social care practitioners.

LO4 Understand Continuing Professional Development

4.1 Continuing Professional Development

Continuing Professional Development is essential for working in health and social care and providing high quality care and support. It involves:

- identifying and documenting the skills, knowledge and experience, gained both formally and informally
- keeping a record of training and learning undertaken at work
- considering how to further develop new and existing knowledge and skills.

Continuing Professional Development involves staying up-to-date with sector developments so that work practices are current and comply with best practice, legislative and organisational requirements.

Continuing Professional Development also involves setting actions for learning and development that are clear and state exactly what must be achieved and by when, so that the goals worked towards are realistically achievable and can be recognised.

Description Activity

Produce an information handout that describes Continuing Professional Development in relation to working in the health and social care sector.

4.2 Sources of support for learning and development

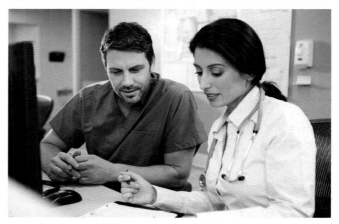

Figure 5.8 What sources of support can a mentor provide at work?

Support for learning and development of health and social care practitioners comes from a wide range of sources. **Table 5.8** outlines what these are.

Table 5.8 Sources of support for learning and development

Sources of support	Relationship to learning and development
Formal/informal support	Support is available both formally and informally within work settings, such as from the manager, employer, colleagues and others (e.g. trainers and other professionals).
	Support is also available both formally and informally outside work settings, such as from health and social care practitioners, families, friends and online forums.
Appraisal/supervision	Appraisals are conducted by employers and assess an employee's work performance, usually over one year, in relation to the work setting's aims.
	Supervision is led by managers. It involves meeting with the manager to plan and monitor professional and personal learning and development.
Feedback	Feedback from others, for example individuals, individuals' families, colleagues and managers can provide a useful insight into how work practices have impacted on them and the work setting.
	Feedback can be used to change working practices and make improvements.
Mentoring	Mentoring involves accessing guidance and advice in relation to carrying out job role responsibilities from someone more experienced.
	Mentors use their experience to offer advice in a less formal way than the manager or employer.
Independent study	Independent study can involve reading articles of interest and watching real-life documentaries.
	It also involves exploring areas of interest or expertise in more detail.
Work experience	Work experience involves spending a period of time, for example a few days or a week, in the work setting observing practitioners to gain an insight into their job roles and responsibilities.
	It can be paid or unpaid.
External agencies	External agencies can be the source of specialist information, advice and knowledge. They can also provide training.
Training courses	Training courses can further develop work practices.
	They can be one day and take place at work, or can take place over a few days. They can be delivered face-to-face or online.
Research	Research can be a useful way to explore an aspect of working in health and social care in more depth.
	Research undertaken can also form the basis of best practice.
Shadowing	Shadowing involves observing another person at work, usually someone more experienced, as they carry out their job role and responsibilities.
	It involves learning from others' work practices to model best practice.
Media	The media, including television, the radio, newspapers and the internet, can be the source of best practice stories, as well as serious failures in health and social care.
	The media presents information about different issues that influence the health and social care sector.

Activity

Design a leaflet outlining a range of sources of support for learning and development that can be used by health and social care practitioners.

4.3 Why Continuing Professional Development is integral to the role of the health and social care practitioner

Continuing Professional Development underpins the provision of safe, effective and high-quality care and support. Continuing Professional Development enables health and social care practitioners to:

- maintain up-to-date knowledge and practice. This means that their working practices are not out of date and reflect current knowledge and best practice.
- maintain their continuous improvement. This means that they can develop as professionals and make improvements to their working practices.
- comply with regulatory requirements. This means that they would be following the requirements set out in relevant legislation.
- be reflective practitioners. This means that they would be learning from their mistakes and then making changes and improvements to their working approaches.
- make applications of learning. This means that they would be able to put the learning they have gained through various sources into practice.

Case scenario

Shannon has been working as a respite worker for over 20 years and does not believe that she needs much Continuing Professional Development because she is very experienced and mentors new respite workers. Shannon also believes that as she attends all the mandatory training provided, she is fully kept up to date with current best practice.

If you were Shannon's manager, what would you say to her in relation to the importance of Continuing Professional Development?

Explain Activity

Develop a case study based on a health and social care practitioner, explaining why Continuing Professional Development is integral to their job role and responsibilities.

✓ Check your understanding 4

1 Define the meaning of Continuing Professional Development.
2 Give three examples of sources of support for learning and development.
3 Name two reasons why Continuing Professional Development is important when working in health and social care.

LO5 Understand reflection in relation to Continuing Professional Development

5.1 The role of reflection within Continuing Professional Development

Being able to reflect is an important skill to have as a health and social care practitioner as it helps with the development of knowledge, new areas of learning and working approaches. Reflection includes the following aspects:

- Reflective practitioner – enables health and social care practitioners to take a 'step back' from their day-to-day activities to examine areas of their work practice that can be improved.
- Responsibility for own learning/professional growth – enables health and social care practitioners to actively think about what learning they require to continue to develop as a professional.
- Ongoing review – enables health and social care practitioners to review their knowledge, skills and practice on an ongoing, continuous basis.
- Planning for development – enables health and social care practitioners to further develop and

improve their knowledge, skills and practice and take steps to achieve their goals.

- Develop knowledge and skills – enables health and social care practitioners to identify gaps in their knowledge and skills and make plans to further develop these.

- Self-awareness – enables health and social care practitioners to understand themselves better, gain a greater insight into the skills, behaviours and attributes they have and those that they would like to further develop or improve.

- Positive outcomes – enables health and social care practitioners to achieve positive outcomes for their own learning and development, which will directly positively influence the care and support provided to individuals.

Description Activity

Discuss the role of reflection within Continuing Professional Development using examples. Describe how it impacts upon:

1 Health and social care practitioners.
2 The care and support provided to individuals.

✔ Check your understanding 5

1 Define the term 'reflective practitioner'.
2 Give two examples of how reflection can be used to improve working practices.
3 Explain two reasons why reflection is important when working in health and social care.

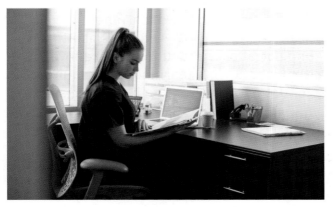

Figure 5.9 Are you a reflective practitioner?

Read about it

Care Quality Commission, 2018, 'Equally outstanding Equality and human rights – good practice resource', Care Quality Commission

Information Commissioner's Office, 2018, 'Guide to the General Data Protection Regulation', Information Commissioner's Office

Moss, B., (2015), *Communication Skills in Health and Social Care*, 3rd edition, Sage Publications Ltd

Schon, D., (1984), *The Reflective Practitioner: How Professionals Think In Action*, Basic Books

Care Quality Commission (CQC) – (information about the Mental Capacity Code of Practice) www.cqc.org.uk/sites/default/files/Mental%20Capacity%20Act%20Code%20of%20Practice.pdf

Department of Health and Social Care – (factsheets about the Care Act 2014) www.gov.uk/government/publications/care-act-2014-part-1-factsheets/care-act-factsheets

Equality and Human Rights Commission – (information about the European Convention on Human Rights) www.equalityhumanrights.com/en/what-european-convention-human-rights

Government Equalities Office – (information about equality legislation and policy) www.gov.uk/government/organisations/government-equalities-office

Information Commissioner's Office (ICO) – (information about the General Data Protection Regulation 2018) https://ico.org.uk/for-organisations/guide-to-data-protection/guide-to-the-general-data-protection-regulation-gdpr/

Skills for Care – (information about the Care Act 2014) www.skillsforcare.org.uk

The British Institute of Human Rights – (information about the Human Rights Act 1998) www.bihr.org.uk/thehumanrightsact

UNICEF – (information about the United Nations Convention on the Rights of the Child 1989) www.unicef.org.uk/what-we-do/un-convention-child-rights/

How will I be graded?

The table below shows what learners must do to achieve each grading criterion. Learners must achieve all the criteria for a grade to be awarded. A higher grade may not be awarded before a lower grade has been achieved, although component criteria of a higher grade may have been achieved.

Grade	Assessment Criteria number	Assessment of learning/What you need to show
D1	1.1	Outline one (1) piece of legislation, policy, procedure or code of practice in relation to health and social care.
D2	2.1	Outline types of health and social care services. A minimum of three (3) types of health and social care services must be outlined.
D3	3.1	Outline job roles within the health and social care sectors. A minimum of three (3) job roles must be outlined.
D4	3.2	Describe the responsibilities of the health and social care practitioner.
D5		A minimum of one (1) relevant and traceable reference must be included.
C1	1.3	Describe how individuals accessing health and social care services are valued. Examples may be used to support the description.
C2	2.3	Discuss barriers to accessing health and social care services and how they may be overcome. A minimum of three (3) barriers to accessing health and social care services must be discussed. Examples may be used to support the discussion.
C3	4.1	Describe Continuing Professional Development.
C4	4.2	Outline sources of support for learning and development. A minimum of four (4) sources of support for learning and development must be outlined.
B1	2.4 2.5	Define informal care. Describe the role of informal carers. Examples may be used to support the description.
B2	4.3	Explain why Continuing Professional Development is integral to the role of the health and social care practitioner.
B3		A minimum of two (2) relevant and traceable references must be included. A reference list must be included.
A1	1.2	Summarise health and social care values. A minimum of four (4) health and social care values must be summarised.
A2	3.3	Describe skills, behaviours and attributes required by health and social care practitioners. Examples may be used to support the description.
A*1	5.1	Describe the role of reflection within Continuing Professional Development. Examples may be used to support the description.
A*2	2.2	Describe functions of health and social care services. The description may link to the types of health and social care services outlined in D2.
A*3		References must be present throughout to show evidence of knowledge and understanding gained from wider reading. References must be relevant and traceable.

Current legislation as relevant to Home Nation.

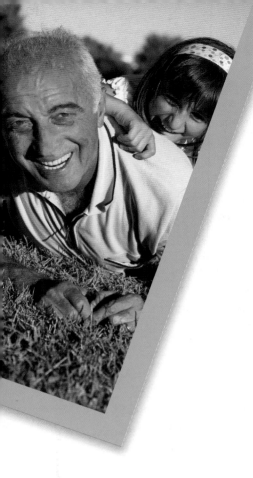

HSC 03
Creative activities in health and social care

About this unit

Creative activities encourage people to use their imagination, express themselves in original ways and learn new skills. They can offer opportunities for working independently and socialising with others, providing people with a sense of purpose and control in their life. There are creative activities to suit all ages, abilities and levels of skill. These could be artistic such as painting, sporting such as swimming or cognitive-based such as crosswords or creative writing. Such activities provide a means for people to gain a sense of achievement and belonging when participating as a part of group. They can also increase an individual's confidence and boost their self-esteem, enabling them to develop socially, emotionally, physically and cognitively and thus achieve their potential.

Creative activities are used in health and social care as a way of enabling individuals to improve their health and overall well-being. Activity that is dictated and enforced by others is not creative. Creativity involves exercising choice and using your imagination, so creative activities are about using one's own ideas, choosing what to do, how to do it and being actively involved. There are no mistakes in creative activities – just opportunities to experiment, solve problems and make your own choices.

Learning Outcomes

LO1: Understand types of creative activities within health and social care.

1.1 The purpose of creative activities:

- creativity
- life skills
- health and well-being
- therapeutic
- meet needs.

1.2 Types of creative activities:

- social
- emotional
- cognitive
- physical

- developmental
- group
- individual.

1.3 Examples of creative activities:

- as related to the types of creative activities in 1.2.

LO2: Understand how creative activities meet the needs of individuals across the life span.

2.1 How creative activities support the social, emotional, cognitive and physical needs of individuals across the life stages:

- infancy
- childhood

→

- adolescence
- early, middle, late adulthood.

Consider needs across the life stages in relation to:

- social: social skills and relationships, confidence, team-working
- emotional: self-image, self-esteem, resilience, acceptance, motivation
- cognitive: language, memory, problem-solving, imagination
- physical: coordination, motor skills, mobility, medical.

LO3: Understand the role of the health and social care practitioner in planning, implementing and reviewing creative activities within health and social care.

3.1 Legislation, policies, procedures and codes of practice in relation to planning and implementing creative activities:

- Health and Safety at Work Act 1974 and associated regulations
- Equality Act 2010
- related policies and procedures
- codes of practice relevant to sector
- current legislation as relevant to Home Nation.

3.2 Factors to consider when planning creative activities:

- aims and objectives
- resources
- risk management
- inclusive practice
- meet needs
- health and social care values
- outcomes.

3.3 The role of the health and social care practitioner when implementing creative activities:

- work within policies and procedures
- implement care values
- balance risk and challenge
- monitor
- support
- engage
- adapt activities.

3.4 Reasons for reviewing the effectiveness of creative activities:

- evaluate outcomes
- measure success
- inform future activities.

LO1 Understand types of creative activities within health and social care

1.1 The purpose of creative activities

Creative activities are not just a way of passing time or preventing boredom. They are much more important because they enhance an individual's creativity, imagination and resourcefulness. They are a way to develop **life skills** and independence, helping to restore and maintain health and well-being, both physically and mentally. Creative activities can also be therapeutic, helping people overcome traumatic experiences. Above all, creative activities meet the needs of everyone as they can offer a sense of purpose, belonging, and help to boost an individual's self-esteem. They can provide a way to develop each individual's potential to be the best that they can be at different life stages.

Creativity

Creativity is not about following instructions or orders. It is about assessing a situation, making decisions and responding to the consequences of those decisions. For example, a three-year-old child painting a picture may decide to paint the sky purple and trees black. The child has made a decision to paint, decided what to paint and what colours to use. They may decide they like the painting or they may decide they don't like it and paint all over it in black. By making decisions, choosing what to do and how to do it, and seeing the consequences, they are exercising creativity. If the child had been told they must paint a brown tree and the sky must be blue, or even told that they must paint when, in fact, they wanted to read a story, they would have no choice. This would stunt their creativity.

Life skills

Life is impacted by development and experience. The way individuals approach life is typically influenced by personal, social, interpersonal, cognitive, affective, and universal skills. They enable individuals to adapt positively to life's challenges and boost their confidence. Creative activities link to life skills, for example making bread or wood carving involves decision-making and problem-solving. It may involve communicating with others, self-awareness and coping with stress. Life skills may vary from culture to culture.

The World Health Organization Department of Mental Health (1999, p.1) identified decision-making and problem-solving; creative thinking and critical thinking; communication and interpersonal skills; self-awareness and empathy; coping with emotions and coping with stress as cross-cultural life skills. Practising these develops self-esteem, sociability, sharing, compassion, respect and tolerance.

Health and well-being

Creative activities offer a chance to relax, reduce stress, and gain confidence in one's own abilities. Work may be stressful, but being able to play the guitar or grow one's own vegetables can give a sense of well-being. The World Health Organization (1948) described health as 'a state of complete physical, mental and social well-being and not merely the absence of disease or infirmity.' This definition was amended and broadened in 1984. Health was defined as 'the extent to which an individual or group is able to realize aspirations and satisfy needs and to change or cope with the environment. Health is a resource for everyday life, not the objective of living; it is a positive concept, emphasizing social and personal resources, as well as physical capacities' (WHO, 1984). This definition focuses on a person's ability to be able to live well even if they have, for instance, a long-term or incurable illness or condition. For example, someone with diabetes may manage their condition well and this ability allows them to achieve what they want to in life.

Well-being is defined as 'the balance point between an individual's resource pool and the challenges faced' (Dodge *et al.*, 2012, p.230). If there are more psychological, social or physical challenges than an individual can cope with, they might feel overwhelmed or stressed. If there are too few challenges, they can get bored, unstimulated and lose a sense of meaning or purpose in their lives, which will negatively affect their well-being. This balance can change according to how many psychological, social, or physical resources are available to a particular individual, and how many challenges they face. Someone in good physical and mental health with a strong support network, such as family members, friends or even from organisations, may be able to cope with far more problems than someone in poor physical health who feels depressed and isolated.

Therapeutic

Therapeutic activities are those that are used as a form of treatment to restore health and are designed to reflect real-life activity. They might be physical, social or emotional in nature. For example, a person who has had a stroke may have a physical weakness on one side of their body, making it difficult for them to use a knife and fork or spoon to feed themselves. An appropriate therapeutic activity to improve their mobility might be for them to paint using a thick-handled brush or a sponge, so that they can re-learn how to control their arm movements. Once they have built up their confidence, they can then progress by choosing more delicate tools, such as a thin-handled brush or pen, eventually aiming to control a knife and fork or spoon themselves.

An example of a social and emotional therapeutic activity might involve helping an individual to develop a sense of **empathy** for others. For example, someone who has been bullying others may come to understand the impact of their behaviour by taking part in an activity where individuals list the bullying behaviours they have experienced and how it made them feel. An individual might read out an example and the victim's reaction, then say, 'A teacher saw what was happening and stopped it by saying ...' Each person in the group gets a chance to suggest what the teacher said. Next they examine what the teacher said, what they did not say, how the bully might feel, and how the victim might feel. They might suggest how the situation could be improved and how the bullying behaviour could have been prevented, to avoid it from happening again. This is a therapeutic activity because everyone is involved and has the opportunity to say how they felt and understand how others felt in a safe environment, helping to develop a sense of empathy. (Activity adapted from **www.interactiontalks.com/ bullying-role-play-anti-bullying-activities- for-teenagers/**)

Key terms

Creative activities refer to inventing and making new things. Creative means original or imaginative. Activities involve doing, not watching. Creative activities are therefore those where a person is actively involved in using their imagination to make something original.

Empathy refers to the ability to understand or feel what another person is experiencing from their point of view, i.e. putting oneself in another's position.

Therapeutic activities are those that are used as a form of treatment to restore health and are designed to reflect real-life activity.

Meet needs

Creative activities can help to meet the needs of individuals. Needs refer to the areas where we require support and will vary from person to person. They may be, for example, in relation to finding a job, learning a new skill or improving how we communicate with others. There are different types of needs that creative activities can help to fulfil, such as:

- **Social.** Individuals will have varying social needs: for example, some people may like to try out new activities, go to different places and meet new people. On the other hand, some people may be content with less social interaction. If a person feels socially isolated, creative activities can help to bring people together to participate in a pastime that they enjoy with others.

- **Emotional.** It is important that individuals feel that they can express themselves, such as their views, opinions and feelings. Everyone, whatever their age, needs to feel loved and that they belong. For example, a child taken into care or an older person forced to move into a care home may feel disorientated and potentially even rejected by their family or society. Creative activities can help them come to terms with their new situation, make friends and establish a new social group in which they belong.

- **Cognitive.** Individuals should feel that they can realise their personal potential and self-fulfilment through different life experiences. Creative activities can help a person to express their individuality. For example, someone with autism may find it difficult to read emotions from facial expressions. They could examine photos of people illustrating a range of expressions, such as smiling, frowning or surprise to show their emotions. By using paper plates and paints, the individual can then create their own masks that reflect the emotions that they have identified in the photos. Once they have built up their confidence, the range of emotions can be expanded to others such as 'worry' or 'friendly'.

- **Physical.** These are needs relating to food, shelter, maintaining body temperature and exercise and vary from person to person. For example, some individuals might have dietary needs, for example someone with diabetes might have to learn to adapt their diet in order to manage the condition properly. They may become a creative cook. Gardening is a physical creative activity that can be adapted to any age or ability, whether watering plants, growing and picking flowers or fruit. An older person might develop hypothermia, not realising when they are cold. Children or older people may sit for hours in front of a screen watching television or playing computer games, leading to a sedentary lifestyle without sufficient exercise. For older and younger people, walking or even walking football is a creative activity which can meet the needs of all.

- **Developmental.** Some individuals may need assistance to gain new skills or practise existing ones in order to go about their daily lives. Developmental needs can be met as part of a group or individually.

For example, a child learning to share and take turns in order to make friends.

The important thing to remember is that people are individuals with many different needs. Sometimes, individuals require more than one creative activity to meet their needs. An activity might meet the social needs of a person, but not their physical needs. For example, a sewing club might provide friendship opportunities that benefit the individual, but not meet their physical needs in terms of exercise or physical activity. Alternatively, one creative activity might in fact meet multiple needs. For example, a music and movement session could offer physical exercise as well as social opportunities. When planning creative

🔑 Key terms

Cognitive refers to the mind and the process of acquiring knowledge and understanding through thoughts and experiences.

Emotional relates to a person's feelings.

Holistic refers to an approach that acknowledges the whole person, rather than just one aspect of them. You should look at an individual holistically in order to meet their needs.

Life skills are skills that are necessary or desirable for full participation in everyday life, such as communication or critical thinking. They are psychosocial skills, i.e. personal, social, interpersonal, cognitive, affective, and universal skills. Life skills may vary from culture to culture.

Description Activity

Make a poster or a PowerPoint presentation of at least three slides to describe the purpose of each type of creative activity. Describe how it could meet social, emotional, cognitive, physical and developmental needs for an individual.

activities, it is important to consider the individual and their needs as a whole. Such a **holistic** approach will provide the most efficient way to meet their needs.

1.2 Types of creative activities

There is a wide range of creative activities.

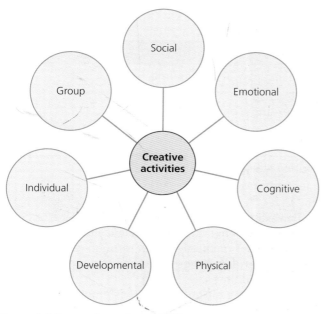

Figure 6.1 Types of creative activities

Social creative activities develop social skills and often involve people working together in groups, for example singing together in a choir.

Emotional creative activities develop a person's awareness and understanding of their own and others' emotions. These activities may be carried out in a group or could be individual activities. They may be led by a facilitator who offers alternatives for those who require guidance. For example, creative writing sessions can help individuals to explore and gain more of an understanding of their emotions, especially when reflecting on their own experiences.

Cognitive creative activities, which include memory and problem solving, can develop an individual's knowledge and understanding. These activities may be carried out in a group or individually, such as learning a new language.

Physical creative activities focus on physical needs. They may be designed to meet the specific physical needs for that individual, for example yoga practice at home helps improve balance and mobility, or they might meet the needs of a group, for example if people want to get fit they could join a walking group.

Developmental creative activities can help individuals to gain the confidence they need to learn new skills or develop existing ones that may help them with their daily lives. Activities might meet the needs of a group, for example a group of children learning to take turns; or they may meet the needs of an individual, for example an adult with Asperger syndrome may need to develop skills to enable them to interact with others. Creative role play can help them understand social expectations, for example how to have a conversation at a party.

Group creative activities have many advantages, including the opportunity to develop multiple skills at the same time, for example physical and social skills. Individuals can learn from each other through observation and discussion. The activities are also often cheaper to run as more people are involved and so contribute to covering the costs. However, there are disadvantages as they might not be able to meet an individual's specific needs. For example, someone with Asperger syndrome would not necessarily benefit from a group activity if they had not yet acquired the relevant social skills necessary to do the activity.

Individual creative activities have the advantage that they can be designed to meet specific individual needs, but individuals will not have the opportunity to develop social skills.

Activity

Create a poster outlining the different types of creative activities suitable for different ages.

groups and varying abilities. **Table 6.1** outlines some examples for each type of creative activity that you have learned about in AC1.2.

1.3 Examples of creative activities

There are a huge range of creative activities out there and many can be adapted for different age

Table 6.1 Examples of creative activities

Type of creative activity	Examples
Social (e.g. providing opportunities for interaction and making friends)	Producing and/or acting in a play or pantomime. Planning a party or event. Arts-based classes, for example painting or drawing. Crafts-based classes, for example knitting, sewing, carpentry. Gardening.
Emotional (e.g. to help individuals to explore their emotions and express themselves)	Creative writing or writing stories/poetry. Arts-based classes, for example painting or drawing. Music, for example: ● Singing in a group. For example, children might learn respect for others by singing songs from other cultures; adolescents might explore how it feels to be discriminated against through rap music; or older people may together sing songs from their younger days, exploring both happy and sad times. ● Song writing. This can help an individual to express emotions they might otherwise find difficult to put into words.
Cognitive (e.g. to develop knowledge and understanding)	Learning a new language. Travelling and/or exploring a new place or culture. Visiting a museum or art gallery. Learning a new skill, for example cooking, pottery-making, flying a kite. Activities based in nature, for example: ● Children can plant different seeds, such as sunflowers or beans, water the seedlings and watch them grow. ● Adolescents might choose and plant bulbs for spring either in bulb fibre, a spare patch of ground or even gravel in a bowl. ● Working as a group they learn to take turns, share, and negotiate with others. ● Working individually they exercise choice, make decisions, perhaps seek advice and see the results of their decisions.
Physical (can be strenuous or gentle exercises to develop physical movement and mobility)	Music, movement and dance. Tai chi, pilates and yoga. Martial arts, for example Taekwondo or capoeira. Swimming and aquarobics. For those with mobility problems, they can exercise with a chair. Children can easily express themselves through physical movement, for example pretending to be an animal and crawling or dancing.

→

Type of creative activity	Examples
Developmental (e.g. to build motor skills, aid mental developmental and help social and emotional awareness)	Creating a life story or scrap book, for example including photos of the individual and those important to them. This can help to affirm an individual's identity, especially after a major life change. Learning a song in a new language. Cutting out paper snowflakes. Cooking and baking. Designing a garden or planning what to grow in an allotment. Infants learn rapidly and labelling things round the house can help them develop vocabulary. Adolescents might choose a story in the media and tell or write the story from the viewpoint of a person of their age living there. For adults, choosing an item or memory from their childhood may help them to explore and understand their feelings. This needs to be done with caution, as not all memories may be happy and sometimes individuals do not want to remember; you must respect their wishes at all times.
Group	Singing in a choir. Writing a story or play together. Useful for social and emotional development because the activities involve interacting with others; but only address some, not all, needs.
Individual	Song writing or creating poetry. Useful for adapting to the needs of a specific individual.

Both individual and group activities are needed to help a person develop, not just as an individual but as a functioning member of society.

Key terms

Physical relates to movement. A physical creative activity could be creating a dance.

Social relates to how we interact with others. Some creative activities may be social, for example practising and learning a new language as part of a group.

Activity

Carry out your own research and outline at least five different creative activities. Ensure that you include at least one relevant and traceable reference.

Check your understanding 1

1 What is the purpose of creative activities?
2 What types of creative activities are there?

LO2 Understand how creative activities meet the needs of individuals across the life span

Creative activities meet an individual's needs throughout the different **life stages**, from infancy and childhood to old age. Babies and children are often naturally creative but it is important to remember that creativity can be developed at any age.

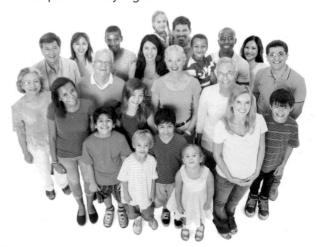

Figure 6.2 Children, young people, adults and older adults have social, physical, emotional and cognitive needs

2.1 How creative activities support the social, emotional, cognitive and physical needs of individuals across the life stages

Life stages can be divided into infancy, childhood, adolescence and adulthood. Adulthood may be divided further, into early, middle and late adulthood. Many creative activities can be adapted for these different life stages. An infant can learn nursery rhymes and create their own accompanying sounds by banging a pan lid. This helps them to learn language and rhythm. A child may make up a song and share it with others, which they sing together, developing social skills. An adult may learn to play the guitar and write their own songs or may be part of a folk group. Older people may join a ukulele group and write songs for the group to play together. Social, physical and cognitive skills develop through these activities. Emotional needs for companionship are met too.

Creative activities provide individuals with the opportunity to make their own decisions and choose what they want to do, for example deciding whether to draw, colour or paint and what they would like to illustrate. In this scenario, individuals might have to take turns collecting materials such as paper and paint, and negotiate in order to share limited resources. They might discuss with others what they want to do and listen to others expressing their views.

Infancy

Infancy refers to the state of babyhood or early childhood, usually up to the age of 2 years. An example of an age-appropriate creative activity might be making hand- or footprints for a wall display. They may choose the colour they want and whether to do a hand- or a footprint. Some may wish to do more than one print. A two-year-old may enjoy finger painting. Creative activities such as these can help to support the different needs of infancy:

- **Social.** Infants develop social skills by interacting with others, such as waiting for their turn or helping another child with an activity. In doing so, they gain confidence and learn valuable team-working skills.

- **Emotional.** Infants and children explore who they are, for example by painting a picture of themselves. They might paint a big smiley face in a circle to represent their view of their self-image. By expressing themselves creatively, they can develop their self-esteem, a sense of achievement and motivation. Negative criticism can demotivate a child, but **resilience** can be learned early on if an infant is praised for effort, not for the result. They learn acceptance of themselves and others, understanding that things may not always be perfect but they can always aim to improve.

- **Cognitive.** Infants are rapidly developing their language skills such as vocabulary, for example names of colours, and adjectives, such as words to describe their painting or environment. Memory skills are also developing quickly, for example as infants remember who has had a turn or who is next to share. They will be practising their problem-solving skills, for example as they work out how to get the right amount of paint to make a clear print, and how to avoid dripping paint all over the floor. They also will also be using their imagination, trying out other materials to make prints with.

- **Physical.** An infant's co-ordination is also rapidly developing, for example as they balance to make a footprint, or bring their hands together to spread paint on each hand. Motor skills are used, dipping the hand or foot into the paint and then guiding it to the right place to print. Mobility is also encouraged as they move between paint and paper, then go to wash hands.

Medical issues, such as an infant with delayed development, does not stop the infant from joining in such a creative activity: it can be adapted for all abilities.

Childhood

Childhood refers to the state or period of being a child, and usually ranges from 2 years to puberty. This is a long time in a child's life, during which they rapidly develop their social, emotional, cognitive and physical skills. An example of an age-appropriate creative activity might be art-based, such as a display on a topic they have covered in class, for example the environment or oceans.

- **Social.** Even though the child may work individually on their display, they can develop social skills. They will negotiate relationships and help others. Around the age of seven or eight, many children are keen to follow rules, and may even make their own rules. For example, children might establish quickly whose turn it is to give out or collect materials, or who has first turn with the glue or scissors. In doing so, they continue to build upon the confidence and valuable team-working skills they have been learning since infancy.

- **Emotional.** Children explore their world through play and by participating in creative activities, such as art, they can express their emotions and communicate how they feel. For example, they might claim they are frightened of monsters. Art gives them the opportunity to draw their monster and make it friendly instead of scary. This can help a child to understand how they are feeling, explore their emotions and develop a sense of identity. They will also learn how to manage their feelings if things do not always go to plan. For example, if the glue is not strong enough to hold their cut-out of an octopus, they can accept their frustration and try to problem-solve instead, such as using sticky tape.

It is important to note that **art therapy** is a useful tool for those children with communication difficulties, who have experienced trauma or abuse, or lived in war zones, to help them process their emotions.

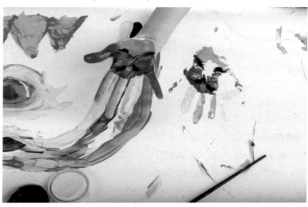

Figure 6.3 Creativity involves imagination and choice

- **Cognitive.** Children develop their cognitive skills by thinking creatively and using the appropriate language, for example what lives in the ocean or what the landscape might look like. Memory skills develop as they recall details, for example how many fins a shark has, as are problem-solving skills as they use spatial awareness to work out the layout of their display. They will also use their imagination to try out new or alternative materials to create their underwater scene.

- **Physical.** Children will be using a variety of motor skills to improve their physical co-ordination as they create their display, for example drawing, cutting different shapes with scissors and gluing materials. Mobility is encouraged as they move between different resources, for example paint and paper, then clearing up afterwards. The activity can be adapted to include all, so those with medical needs can be included according to their abilities. For example, a child with cerebral palsy might be not be able to draw a detailed picture, but they could choose from pre-cut shapes and be supported to use a glue stick to make a collage.

Adolescence

Adolescence is defined as the period following the onset of puberty, during which a young person develops from a child into an adult. During this period, adolescents undergo major hormonal changes that affect their physical and emotional development. This can be a particularly overwhelming time.

Creative activities might be helpful to alleviate stress or work through any personal issues that adolescents might be experiencing, for example making a treasure box. This involves the individual decorating a box (such as a shoe box) with items, images and things that interest them, then choosing what to keep inside it. The 'treasures' are anything that makes the individual feel good or has a positive association or memory, for example photos of their family, friends or pet; a positive school report; or just a nice thing someone said about them. These 'treasures' affirm positive aspects of the individual's identity, acting as a personal resource to draw upon whenever they feel stressed or upset.

- **Social.** While the act of making the treasure box might be an individual activity, there is scope for it to be done with others. Alternatively, sharing ideas about how to decorate or what to include with others can help to build social skills and relationships, boosting an individual's confidence. For example, an individual might realise that others, too, have similar worries or concerns to their own.
- **Emotional.** Having a store of good memories to draw upon helps the individual gain a sense of perspective. It is a reminder of positive thoughts and memories, even at a time when they might have low self-esteem or feel stressed, anxious or upset. This can be a very motivating resource, helping an individual

to build resilience and accept that bad times will also pass.

- **Cognitive.** Making a treasure box with photos of loved ones, programmes from trips to the theatre, souvenirs of museum visits or holiday snaps help to develop an individual's cognitive skills, such as memory. For children who may be in foster care, it provides a chance to retain a link to their birth families. It provides scope for imagination, thinking 'What if life had been different?' and helps problem-solving, for example 'Why did I have to go into care?'
- **Physical.** When making the treasure box, an individual will be using their fine motor skills, for example when sticking or gluing images or creating their own artwork, and developing their physical co-ordination.

In a specialist role, adolescents with emotional or behavioural issues may be helped through art therapy. This therapy is used in mental health trusts in the NHS, and is offered under the guidance of a skilled art therapist who is also a trained counsellor. An individual can use painting and drawing to express themselves and explore their emotions. Together with a trained art therapist or psychologist, they can identify issues that might hinder their ability to cope with life on a daily basis. With specialist support, they can set goals and work towards overcoming the challenges and issues they have been experiencing. Art therapy has been shown to be effective in helping those with mental health issues move forward, living a happier and more productive life.

Early, middle, late adulthood

Adulthood is the state or condition of being fully grown or mature, usually ranging from the age of 18 years to old age and/or the end of life. Within this life stage, the needs of adults will vary considerably depending on whether they are in early, middle or late adulthood.

For example, a 19-year-old individual might find that they have less contact with their friends since leaving school or college, which is contributing to their sense of loneliness. Someone in their forties might be focused on building their career or trying to keep their relationship together. Conversely, someone in their eighties might now have physical limitations on what they can do. But, regardless of the adult's life stage, there are still many opportunities for creative activities for all.

In early adulthood, creative activities could include joining a band. Social needs are met by working with others as part of the band. Emotionally there is a sense of satisfaction in creating music and cognitive needs are met as they learn new tunes, new guitar chords and write their own songs. Physically playing is very demanding, so physical needs are met. For those not into music, joining a gym can provide similar opportunities to meet social, emotional, cognitive and physical needs.

In middle adulthood, taking on an allotment or learning to garden can meet social and cognitive needs as people learn from other gardeners what grows best in different soils. Growing food and flowers is emotionally satisfying and provides an opportunity for physical exercise in digging, weeding and pruning. Some adults develop existing interests; a keen driver might join a vintage car club, attend rallies and meet socially with other enthusiasts, learn to repair their own car (cognitive needs), feel pride in rebuilding a car (emotional needs) and keep active by repairing the car.

Creative writing, photography, composing a song, rap or instrumental piece of music are all creative activities that adults can do at any life stage. Recent popularity of adult colouring books has also proved beneficial in reducing stress.

In late adulthood, reminiscence therapy can be very effective for those with memory problems. For example, adults with early-stage **dementia** often forget recent events but can still remember what happened years ago or even when they were a child. Reminiscence therapy uses the long-term memory. Working either one-to-one or in a small group, the practitioner may bring out a box of items that remind older adults of their memories. This activity works best when individuals bring their own items, but it can also work when the practitioner assembles items that appeal to sight, taste, touch, smell and sound, for example old-fashioned sweets or cosmetics such as carbolic soap.

Remembering also provides an opportunity for adults to bond and interact socially with others. It is important to note that care must be taken because some people have sad memories and do not want to remember their past. The individual should be able to choose whether they want to take part in the activity, and the practitioner must observe and monitor individuals to avoid any distress. The activity must also be risk assessed, for example check for any individual diet restrictions such as diabetes before using sweets in the activity.

An increasing number of older adults are learning to use social media to keep in touch with family and friends (social needs), learning from grandchildren how to Skype, message and use WhatsApp. This meets social and emotional needs, feeling a sense of achievement, and cognitively they learn new skills.

Key terms

Art therapy uses art to express emotions.

Dementia is a disorder of the mental processes caused by brain disease or injury. Examples of symptoms include memory loss and/or difficulties with thinking, problem-solving or language.

Life stages refer to the different phases in an individual's life. Often these are classified as infancy (0–2 years), childhood (3–5 years), late childhood (6–10 years), adolescence (11–17 years), early adulthood (18–29 years), middle adulthood (30–60 years) and late adulthood (60+ years). Different areas of study focus on different stages; for example, child care practitioners may subdivide the stages of childhood to look at each stage in more detail. Those working with older people may subdivide late adulthood stage into 60–80 years and 80+ years.

Resilience is the ability to adapt to change.

Explain Activity

Create a leaflet for a GP surgery to explain how creative activities support the social, emotional, cognitive and physical needs of individuals within one life stage. Use examples to support what you say.

Check your understanding 2

1 How do creative activities support the social, emotional, cognitive and physical needs of infants, children, adolescents and adults in early, middle and late adulthood?
2 Give two examples of each of these needs:
   ● Social
   ● Emotional
   ● Cognitive
   ● Physical.

LO3 Understand the role of the health and social care practitioner in planning, implementing and reviewing creative activities within health and social care

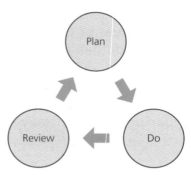

Figure 6.4 The plan, do, review cycle

The cycle of planning, implementing and then reviewing is one that helps to improve practice. Planning and implementing happens not just at the start but throughout the activity. Planning creative activities is essential if they are to succeed. A useful planning scheme asks:

● Why are you doing it? What is the aim?
● Who is it for? Who will be involved? (Staff, clients, patients, residents, visitors, etc.) Is consent required?
● What is the activity? What is involved and is it suitable for all the intended participants? What adaptations may need to be made to the activity to accommodate any diverse needs?
● When will it happen? Is it a one-off activity or is it part of a series of activities?
● Where will it happen? What equipment is needed? What are the risks?
● How will any risks be reduced or managed? How will people know if it is for them?

The **'Do'** stage is carrying out the activity as planned.

Doing the activity involves working within policies and procedures, such as obtaining informed consent to the activity from participants, following health and safety guidelines and balancing risk and challenge. It involves putting care values into practice, empowering individuals, maintaining confidentiality and treating them with respect. Throughout the activity, the organiser must monitor the situation, the participants and what else is happening in the surrounding environment. The risk assessment they did at the start may change if something changes in the environment, for instance, if a participant becomes ill.

They must provide support where appropriate, engage all participants in the activity and adapt it as necessary so that it is inclusive. For example, if a participant has difficulty hearing, the activity leader should ensure that background noise is minimised and the person with hearing impairment can see the speaker's face to lip read.

The **'Review'** stage asks:

- Did it achieve what it set out to do?
- What was the feedback from the participant(s)?
- What went well? (Both the practitioner's and participant's view)
- What did not go as planned? (Practitioner's view)
- What changes need to be made? (Both the practitioner's and participant's view)

The final review stage is particularly important because it helps with future planning, learning from any mistakes and formulating best practice.

Health and social care practitioners may be planning, carrying out and reviewing creative activities in a variety of settings. For example, a planned activity might be carried out, but the review stage identified that the chosen venue was unsuitable. Therefore, in the next planning session, changes can be made to improve the activity for next time.

Health and social care practitioners might be working with individuals and groups in the community, for example a children's home, client's home, in an office, in an NHS or private hospital, or at an adult care home. They work in hospital or community settings, such as GP surgeries and in hospitals. Creative activities may be conducted in any of these venues.

3.1 Legislation, policies, procedures and codes of practice in relation to planning and implementing creative activities

Wherever health and social care practitioners work, they must follow the policies, procedures and codes of practice that relate to planning and carrying out creative activities. These policies and procedures are based on agreed ways of working based on a legal framework, ensuring that no harm comes to those involved. Codes of practice regulate practice at all times and are based on respecting the individual and acting in their best interests.

When planning and carrying out creative activities, health and social care practitioners should ensure that all aspects of the activity are **inclusive**. They should respect the dignity of the individual, including their rights, culture, beliefs, needs and preferences, ensuring that they are able to exercise the right to choose whether or not to take part in activities. When planning an activity, the health and social care practitioner should:

- communicate effectively with the individuals involved in the activity
- maintain **confidentiality**
- ensure the individual is protected from any sort of abuse or harm.

The activity should be tailored to the needs of the individual, not the preferences of the health and social care practitioner.

Key terms

Confidentiality refers to keeping something private. It means protecting an individual's personal, sensitive or restricted information and only disclosing it with those who need to know it.

Inclusive means providing opportunities for engagement and involvement in a meaningful and satisfying way for all who wish to participate.

Health and Safety at Work Act 1974 and associated regulations

The Health and Safety at Work Act 1974 is the main piece of legislation covering occupational health and safety in the UK. When planning and implementing creative activities, health and safety is of paramount importance. Every workplace must have a Health and Safety policy and related procedures. A risk assessment must be carried out when planning any activity. This involves assessing the potential hazards that may pose harm, assessing the likelihood of harm and removing or reducing the risk. Each workplace has its own risk assessment procedures, which must be followed. Consider who will be involved and their abilities, for example if planning a group singing activity in a residential home, ask yourself the following questions:

- Will individuals be required to stand or can they sit down?
- Do any individuals have any hearing or sight problems? Do any individuals require support and/or need to be near the person leading the activity?
- Where will the activity take place?

- Will people be walking through the group or could the group be in a side room?
- How long will the activity be? Do you need to plan for comfort breaks?
- Will there be a first aider on hand in case some feels unwell?

If planning a creative activity to make something, it is important to ensure that all of the materials are suitable and safe for those taking part. Check any labels, for example some felt tip pens give off fumes. School PVA glue, glue sticks, double-sided sticky tape are safe for children and people with learning disabilities, but note that super glue is not. Scissors must also be safe and suitable for those using them. A craft knife would not be safe equipment for children or people with learning disabilities, but might be suitable for an older, more skilled adult.

Equality Act 2010

Under the Equality Act 2010, there are nine protected characteristics. It is illegal to discriminate against someone because of their:

1 Age
2 Disability
3 Gender reassignment
4 Marriage and civil partnership
5 Pregnancy and maternity
6 Race
7 Religion or belief
8 Sex
9 Sexual orientation.

For more on the protected characteristics, see *Unit HSC M3: Safeguarding and protection in health and social care*.

When planning and implementing a creative activity, consider whether it is inclusive for all taking part whatever their age, ability, gender, race, religion or belief, sexual orientation, or marital status. For example, a singing session that focuses exclusively on Christmas carols may exclude those who do not follow the Christian faith.

Related policies and procedures

Health and social care organisations will have specific policies and procedures in place, which outline how the rules should be followed by the health and social care practitioner and others. For instance, an example of a policy might be that creative activities in the dining room must take place at specific times, such as between breakfast and lunch or lunch and tea time. This is to provide adequate time for the space to be cleared for meal times. An example of a procedure might be one that specifies who can collect and set out materials; how tables are protected if there is paint or glue involved; and how the room should be left at the end of the session.

Codes of practice relevant to sector

England, Wales and Scotland have developed a code of conduct for social care. You can see the Code of Conduct for Healthcare Support Workers and Adult Social Care Workers in England in *Unit HSC M4: Communication in health and social care*.

In Northern Ireland, where health and social care is combined, there are six Standards for Conduct regarding how social care workers should behave towards service users, carers and those they work with. These are set out by the Northern Ireland Social Care Council.

The Standards of Conduct for Social Care Workers
A social care worker must:

1 Protect the rights and support the safety and well-being of service users and carers.

2 Earn and keep the trust of service users and carers.

3 Support service users to be independent and safe.

4 Respect service users' rights and keep them safe from hurting themselves or other people.

5 Behave well so that the public (people who live in the community) trust and respect social care services.

6 Make sure that they do a good job and keep learning new skills to do a good job.

(**Source: https://niscc.info/storage/resources/sociacarestandards_easyread.pdf**)

In Northern Ireland there are also six main Standards of Practice, set out by the Social Care Council, that outline how a social care worker must sufficiently carry out the responsibilities and duty of care required of their job and continue to improve their job-related skills and knowledge.

The Standards of Practice for Social Care Workers
A social care worker must:

1 Understand their job role and what they are responsible for.

2 Be good at listening and talking.

3 Provide care that is safe and puts service users at the centre of what they do.

4 Help keep people safe.

5 Follow health and safety rules at work.

6 Learn more about their job and build new skills to help them be a better social care worker.

(**Source: https://niscc.info/storage/resources/sociacarestandards_easyread.pdf**)

Current legislation as relevant to Home Nation

In England, Scotland, Wales, Northern Ireland and offshore, the current legislation relevant to planning and implementing creative activities is the Health and

Safety at Work Act 1974 and associated regulations.

The Equality Act 2010 applies to England and Wales, Scotland; section 82, 105 (3) and (4) and 199 also apply to Northern Ireland. This means that although the Equality Act applies in full to England, Scotland and Wales, there are limitations in Northern Ireland.

Activity

Produce a leaflet for health and care practitioners outlining two pieces of legislation, policies, procedures or codes of practice to consider when planning and implementing creative activities.

3.2 Factors to consider when planning creative activities

There are many factors to consider when planning creative activities if they are to be successful. These are listed in this section.

Aims and objectives

The **aim** is the overall target to be achieved. This can only be decided after assessing the needs of the individual. If, for example, a person has been diagnosed as having dementia, they and their carer might be offered the chance to attend a weekly support group or join a singing activity. The aim would be to meet people in a similar situation for mutual support. **Objectives** are the separate points that together help to achieve the overall aim. Objectives should always be SMART: specific, measurable, achievable, relevant to the overall goal, and timed. The following example illustrates how aims and objectives must be considered when planning a creative activity.

Carol runs a weekly support group for people with dementia and their carers at a local care home. The aim is to help people with dementia remember songs, join in with others and feel less socially isolated. Jack has dementia and agreed to attend the weekly support group after the GP suggested it would be beneficial for him. The aim in Jack attending is to help him and his wife, Mary, feel less socially isolated.

Jack is new to the group and Mary is not sure whether he will join in. Jack has also forgotten why he and Mary are there. Carol talks to Jack and Mary, and asks Jack if he would like to sit down and listen to the group for ten minutes. Jack agrees.

Setting small objectives, such as listening for a short while, is specific and can be measured. Jack either does it or does not. It is achievable – he is able to sit for a short while. It is also relevant, as singing helps with memory recall and has been shown to benefit people with dementia. By suggesting a timescale of ten minutes, Carol can assess whether Jack is comfortable with the activity.

Key terms

Aim is a purpose or what is intended, for example to get fit.

Objectives are specific tasks or goals, for example to get fit enough to run 5 kilometres without stopping.

Resources

It is important to consider what resources are required when planning a creative activity. A good way to check resources is to use a checklist, using the following: who, what, why, where, when and how? Using the example outlined in 'Aims and objectives', it is possible to identify the appropriate resources that are required:

- **Who is involved?** Carol has an assistant. Both are trained in dementia awareness and know how to manage the situation if an individual becomes upset. Each person taking part has their carer with them, usually a friend or relative.

- **Where is it happening?** Carol has booked a separate room in the local care home.

Toilets are nearby and no one will be walking through the room. There is plenty of space for the ten participants and chairs are arranged in a circle so they can all see Carol.

- **What is happening?** Carol has planned the activity so there is a gentle start, swaying to soft music, then a selection of songs is played using a phone attached to speakers. The audio is located well away from where people are seated. She has a variety of songs so that the participants can choose what type of music they want.

- **How is it done?** Carol faces the group and speaks clearly, ensuring that those with hearing problems can read her lips. Her tone is friendly and encouraging as she shows them what to do, humming gently to the music. Carol then demonstrates the next activity, which is clapping to music. She follows this by singing a familiar tune, encouraging all participants to join in if they feel comfortable.

- **When is it?** The singing activity is from 10–11a.m. every Wednesday. This fixed time helps those with dementia remember the day, as fixed routines help those with memory problems.

- **Why do it?** Singing releases endorphins, the 'feel good' hormone, which improves mood. Singing in a group enables individuals to meet others in a similar situation and make friends, which is the original aim of the activity for Jack (to feel less socially isolated).

Risk management

It is important to carry out a **risk assessment** when planning a creative activity at the start of every session. Many organisations have various forms of risk assessment, which are in place to identify any potential risks and hazards that could cause harm to an individual. A hazard is a potential source of harm or adverse health effect on someone, for example a trailing cable. Risk is the likelihood that a person may be harmed if exposed to a hazard. It is important to consider the following questions when dealing with risk management:

- What is the risk or likelihood of the hazard causing harm?
- Is it high, medium or low risk?
- What might be the consequences of the risk or hazard?

For example, the physical environment might change from session to session, for example someone has moved the furniture or equipment, which might now be a tripping hazard or blocking a fire escape. Sometimes, a person's physical or mental condition may be the hazard. They may be anxious or confused. The risk is the likelihood of harm to themselves and/or others if their condition (the hazard) is not managed appropriately. This may mean that the environment might have to change to accommodate them or the planned activity has to be postponed.

It is important to remove, or at least reduce, the risk by dealing with the hazard. For example, a trailing cable is a high risk if it is on the floor and people are moving around the room. It can be moved out of harm's way so that the planned activity can continue.

 Key term

Risk assessment is the identification of hazards, assessing the likelihood of harm from those hazards and reducing the risk of harm from them.

Inclusive practice

Inclusive practice involves health and social care practitioners working in ways that respond to individuals' unique needs and preferences. They should support individuals so that they have a meaningful role in society and develop a sense of well-being. Inclusive practice enables health and social care practitioners to provide high-quality care and support that is unique to the individual, safe and effective.

Reflect on the section on equality earlier in this unit, and in *Unit HSC CM1: Equality, diversity and rights in health and social care*. Does the planned activity meet the requirements of the Equality Act 2010? Does it exclude anyone with protected characteristics, such as their age, disability, sex, etc.? Always check that any planned activity is equally open and available for everyone who wishes to join in. With a little thought, most activities can be adapted to be inclusive.

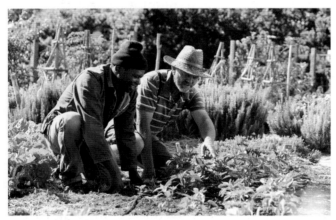

Figure 6.5 Creative activities can be adapted for all ages and abilities

Meet needs

Creative activities should take into account an individual's social, emotional, cognitive and physical **needs**. When planning a creative activity, the health and social care practitioner will need to consider whether it meets specific or multiple needs of the individual or group. For example, singing is a creative activity promoted by the Alzheimer's Society. This is because singing has a range of benefits for those with the condition, such as:

- **Social**, for example meeting new people; teamwork by singing together.

- **Emotional**, for example bringing pleasure; boosting self-esteem and confidence (which might have been lost to dementia).
- **Cognitive**, for example language, memory and problem-solving.
- **Physical**, for example breathing.

All individuals are unique with their own set of preferences and needs, so they might not all enjoy the same activity: it might be a matter of finding a different activity to meet their specific needs.

Health and social care values

These are explained in detail in *Unit HSC M5: Working in health and social care*. The values are a guide for health and social care practitioners and include the following:

- duty of care
- safeguarding
- person-centred care
- partnership
- dignity
- respect
- rights
- confidentiality
- promoting independence.

These values must be embedded in every aspect of planning an activity. Respect for the individual means listening to them and their preferences, ensuring that activities are inclusive for all and that confidentiality is maintained. Above all, the activity must be planned with the individual, not for the individual, so person-centred care is always maintained with the individual's beliefs, preferences, needs and wishes in mind.

 Key term

Needs may be social, emotional, physical or cognitive.

Outcomes

An outcome is a result or effect of an action. When planning a creative activity, the outcomes must be considered to measure whether or not the activity has been successful and, if not, what must be changed at the review stage. Outcomes must be related to the original aim of the planned activity. Using the example of Jack attending the weekly support group for dementia, the aim was to help Jack feel less socially isolated by meeting new people. If the activity changed to a more solitary one, such as an individual singing lesson, this will not provide the same opportunities for Jack and the planned outcomes will not be achieved. If, for example, Jack did not like the group singing activity, he might like a different group activity such as an art class at the day centre. In this case, although the activity changed, the outcomes for Jack can still be achieved.

Explain Activity

Prepare a poster to explain at least three factors to consider when planning creative activities. Use examples to support what you say.

3.3 The role of the health and social care practitioner when implementing creative activities

The health and social care practitioner has many different roles and responsibilities, which they must be aware of and adhere to at all times. In relation to implementing creative activities, they must always ensure that they carry out the responsibilities listed in this section.

Work within policies and procedures

Health and social care practitioners must be aware of their work organisation's specific policies and procedures when implementing the creative activity, as well as the policies and procedures of their own employer if this differs from the place where they are working. For example, the signing in procedures might be different depending on the location; the way to contact a first aider might also vary.

Implement care values

Health and social care practitioners must put care values into practice wherever they are. Care values were explained in *Unit HSC M5: Working in health and social care* and in the previous section of this unit. If they work in different places, they might see poor practice in action but should not copy it. Rather, they should demonstrate good practice and report poor practice. A practitioner planning a singing activity would demonstrate a duty of care by knowing the abilities and condition of people in the group. Safeguarding would include checking that nothing in the activity is likely to upset people or trigger any adverse effects. Person-centred care comes from knowing each individual and their preferences, respecting their wishes and treating them with dignity and respect. They have a right to participate or withdraw from the group. They may explain in confidence why they do not wish to sing a particular song – this must be kept private. Independence is encouraged by the practitioners involving the participants in choosing the songs, playing the music and running the session.

Balance risk and challenge

It is important that health and social care practitioners balance risk and **challenge** when implementing a creative activity. They should follow best practice, but this does not necessarily mean removing all risk: it means assessing risk appropriately and taking the relevant precautions to protect the individual from any potential harm while fulfilling their needs. For example, Sam, who is 20 years old and has learning difficulties, wants to learn to swim. His support worker recognises this is a challenge for Sam who has always been afraid of water. As a professional, the health and social care practitioner should help Sam to find a course of swimming lessons with an instructor who can adapt their methods to meet his needs, rather than try and put Sam off the idea by saying it's too risky for him.

Monitor

Health and social care practitioners must continually **monitor** the creative activity, not just review the outcomes at the end. They should reflect during the activity, and ask themselves questions in order to improve it, such as:

- Is the individual enjoying the activity?
- Is the individual settling in well or are there any particular points where they appear to be distressed and/or anxious?
- Does the activity need to be structured differently, i.e. into bitesize chunks or perhaps include more comfort breaks?

Support

Effective health and social care practitioners should provide individuals with ongoing support but, at the same time, be careful not to completely take over and remove the individual's right to make their own decisions. For example, the aim of a cooking activity might be to encourage an individual to choose a recipe and carry out the instructions for themselves. However, if the health and social care practitioner steps in and makes decisions for that individual, for example which recipe or ingredients, then the aim will not be achieved.

Engage

Health and social care practitioners should always engage with the individual, not

the activity. Sometimes, eye contact and a reassuring smile is enough. At other times, a simple enquiry such as 'How's it going?' is enough. If a person is becoming upset or frustrated with the activity, a practitioner may intervene and provide encouragement, support and/or suggest a short break.

Adapt activities

Not all creative activities work out as planned. Sometimes, it is necessary to change them in order to meet the overall aim and meet individual needs. For example, singing might not work out for Jack at the weekly support group, but he might prefer to listen to music with others and then discuss it in a music appreciation group. Or, he might find the same opportunity for friendship in a gardening club. The needs of the individual are of prime importance.

3.4 Reasons for reviewing the effectiveness of creative activities

Creative activities are only effective if they are planned, implemented, monitored and reviewed. Unless an activity ends with a review, it remains unfinished. When reviewing a creative activity, it is important to consider the following:

- Look back at the original aim and objectives.
- Was the aim achieved? Were the objectives met?
- Was the aim clear? Were the objectives SMART?
- What could be done to improve the aims and objectives for next time?

Evaluate outcomes

After an activity has taken place, it is important to evaluate the outcomes to measure its effectiveness. This can be done by reviewing the aims and measuring the outcomes to determine the extent they have been achieved. How do the outcomes reflect whether or not the aims of the activity been met? Perhaps they have been met partially and, if so, in what way?

A good way to do this is to get feedback from those taking part. This can sometimes be gauged through body language, such as smiling faces. Others may wish to give anonymous feedback. Depending on the abilities of participants, they could be given a piece of paper with a smiley face and sad face and asked to mark which they felt after the event, or they could be offered the chance to write what went well and what did not and post it in a suggestions box. Feedback from others is the most useful type of feedback and gives material for reflective practice. What you think worked well might not have been so good for others, and they may even suggest improvements.

Measure success

It is easy to measure whether an activity has been effective if SMART objectives have been set. For example, using the SMART objectives to focus on Jack's aim of feeling less socially isolated:

- **Specific:** did Jack and Mary make friends?
- **Measurable:** if so, how many friends did Jack and Mary make?
- **Achievable:** has this aim been achieved? If not, what needs to change to make sure it can be?
- **Relevant:** could this aim be met in the chosen activity, i.e. was it relevant?
- **Timely:** was the aim achieved in the time allocated?

Inform future activities

Measuring success is important to know whether or not it is worth implementing the same activity or whether changes have to be made to meet individuals' needs. For example, if an art class is proving popular with lots of people going every week, then it can be offered to other individuals who might benefit from it. Alternatively, if fewer and fewer people attend every week, it is worth examining the reasons why and either experimenting with changes (e.g. holding the class at a different time or in a more accessible location) or stopping the class entirely.

Key terms

Challenge means setting a goal which can be reached with a little effort.

Inform means to advise or guide.

Monitor means to keep an overview.

Description Activity

You have been asked to write a short guide for new health and social care practitioners who are about to go on placement and carry out creative activities. Describe the role of the health and social care practitioner when implementing creative activities. Use examples to support (not to replace) your description.

Use at least two relevant and traceable references and include a reference list.

Explain Activity

Add a section to your guide in which you explain, with examples, at least three different reasons for why it is necessary to review the effectiveness of creative activities.

Use at least three different sources to show evidence of knowledge and understanding gained from wider reading. Sources must be relevant and referenced using a traceable method, such as Harvard referencing.

Case scenario

AB has lived in a Residential Home since she fell and broke her hip last year. She used to be a translator for court procedures. She is an alert, 70-year-old woman, but has no close family that live nearby, and she misses her grandchildren. The programme of activities at the residential home is as follows:

Monday afternoon: Bingo
Tuesday afternoon: Watch television
Wednesday afternoon: Hairdresser
Thursday afternoon: Bingo
Friday afternoon: Quiz
Saturday and Sunday: Family visits

Questions

1. Is this a varied programme of activities that would meet a wide range of the residents' needs?
2. Are social, emotional, cognitive and physical needs catered for within this programme?
3. What suggestions could you make to improve the variety in this programme? Name some activities that will help to meet individual's social, emotional, cognitive and physical needs.
4. Suggest two activities specifically for AB and give reasons for your choice.

 Classroom Discussion

What is the role of the health and social care practitioner in planning, implementing and reviewing creative activities?

 Check your understanding 3

1. Select an activity for a given age range. Create a spider diagram to show how the activity is creative and what the benefits of the activity are in relation to developmental areas for individuals within the age range.

   When you have done this, explain it to your tutor and the rest of your group and invite feedback.
2. Explain how you would adapt your chosen activity across an individual's lifespan.
3. What factors must a health and social care practitioner consider when planning these activities?
4. What factors must be considered when implementing these activities?
5. Why should the health and social care practitioner review after each activity?

Read about it

Anti-discriminatory practice and protected characteristics www.equalityhumanrights.com/en/equality-act/protected-characteristics

Art therapy positivepsychologyprogram.com/art-therapy/

Art therapy in West London mental health unit www.westlondon.nhs.uk/patients-and-carers/treatments/art-therapy/

Code of Conduct social care www.skillsforcare.org.uk/Document-library/Standards/National-minimum-training-standard-and-code/CodeofConduct.pdf

Community care – (online journal for social care) www.communitycare.co.uk

Dodge, R., Daly, A., Huyton, J. and Sanders, L., 2012, 'The challenge of defining wellbeing', *International Journal of Wellbeing*, vol. 2(3), pp.222–235, doi:10.5502/ijw.v2i3.4 [accessed online 21 December 2018]

Health and safety www.hse.gov.uk/simple-health-safety/index.htm

Health care careers – (speech and language therapy assistant) www.healthcareers.nhs.uk/Explore-roles/wider-healthcare-team/roles-wider-healthcare-team/clinical-support-staff/speech-and-language-therapy-assistant

Anti-bullying activity for teenagers to address bullying wrongdoing www.interactiontalks. com/bullying-role-play-anti-bullying-activities-for-teenagers/ [accessed online 21 December 2018]

Men's sheds to combat isolation for older men menssheds.org.uk/

NHS website – (exercise for older people) www.nhs.uk/live-well/exercise/exercise-as-you-get-older/

Nursing Times – (online and print journal for nursing and health care) www.nursingtimes.net

Nursery World journal for childcare – (available online and in print) www.nurseryworld.co.uk

World Health Organization, 1999, 'Partners in Life Skills Education: Conclusions from a United Nations Inter-Agency Meeting', World Health Organization www.who.int/mental_health/media/en/30.pdf [Accessed 21 December 2018]

Singing for the brain www.alzheimers.org.uk/get-support/your-support-services/singing-for-the-brain

Social skills for children with autism www.autism.org.uk/about/communication/social-children.aspx

The role of social work assistants nationalcareers.service.gov.uk/job-profiles/social-work-assistant

World Health Organization, Constitution of the World Health Organization as adopted by the International Health Conference, New York, 19–22 June 1946; signed on 22 July 1946 by the representatives of 61 States (Official Records of the World Health Organization, no. 2, p. 100) and entered into force on 7 April 1948. In Grad, Frank P., 2002, 'The Preamble of the Constitution of the World Health Organization', *Bulletin of the World Health Organization*, 80 (12): 982

World Health Organization. Regional Office for Europe, 1984, 'Health promotion: a discussion document on the concept and principles: summary report of the Working Group on Concept and Principles of Health Promotion', Copenhagen, 9–13 July 1984 (ICP/HSR 602(m01)5 p). Copenhagen: WHO Regional Office for Europe.

How will I be graded?

The table below shows what learners must do to achieve each grading criterion. Learners must achieve all the criteria for a grade to be awarded. A higher grade may not be awarded before a lower grade has been achieved, although component criteria of a higher grade may have been achieved.

Grade	Assessment Criteria number	Assessment Criteria
D1	1.2	Outline types of creative activities.
	1.3	Give examples of creative activities.
		A minimum of four (4) examples of creative activities used in health and social care settings must be included.
D2	1.1	Describe the purpose of creative activities.
D3		A minimum of one (1) relevant and traceable reference must be included.
C1	3.1	Outline two (2) pieces of legislation, policies, procedures or codes of practice in relation to planning and implementing creative activities.

Grade	Assessment Criteria number	Assessment Criteria
C2	3.2	Explain factors to consider when planning creative activities. A minimum of three (3) factors to consider when planning creative activities must be explained.
B1	3.3	Describe the role of the health and social care practitioner when implementing creative activities. Examples may be used to support the description.
B2		A minimum of two (2) relevant and traceable references must be included. A reference list must be included.
A1	2.1	Explain how creative activities support the social, emotional, cognitive and physical needs of individuals within one (1) life stage.
A*1	3.4	Explain the reasons for reviewing the effectiveness of creative activities. A minimum of three (3) reasons for reviewing the effectiveness of creative activities must be explained.
A*2		References must be present throughout to show evidence of knowledge and understanding gained from wider reading. References must be relevant and traceable.

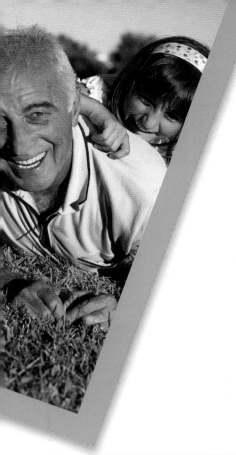

HSC 09
Mental health and well-being

About this unit

This unit provides an introduction to the topic of mental health and well-being. It starts by looking at what we mean by mental health and ill-health, then examines the legislation and policies relating to mental health and well-being. The unit explores different types of mental ill-health, how they affect people and considers how others might react to people with mental ill-health. It examines how people can look after their own mental health and well-being and what help is available to them and others involved. Finally, the unit considers how health and social care practitioners and national strategies can both promote and support mental health and well-being.

Learning Outcomes

LO1: Understand types of mental ill-health.

1.1 Definition of:

- mental health
- mental ill-health.

1.2 Types of mental ill-health:

- mood disorders
- personality disorders
- cognitive disorders
- anxiety disorders
- psychotic disorders
- substance-related disorders
- eating disorders.

LO2: Understand legislation and policies in relation to mental health and well-being.

2.1 Legislation and policies in relation to mental health and well-being:

- Health and Social Care Act 2012
- Equality Act 2010
- Mental Health Act 2007, Mental Health Act 1983
- Mental Capacity Act 2005 (MCA)
- Human Rights Act 1998

- Mental Health: Priorities for Change 2014
- The Mental Health Strategy for England 2011
- current legislation and policy as relevant to Home Nation.

LO3: Understand the impact of mental ill-health on individuals and others.

3.1 The impact mental ill-health can have on individuals and others:

- confidence
- self-esteem
- relationships
- dependence
- finances
- employment
- environment
- isolation
- discrimination.

3.2 Public attitudes towards mental ill-health:

- understanding
- acceptance
- integration
- tolerance.

LO4: Understand how to support and promote mental health and well-being.

4.1 How an individual can promote their own mental health and well-being:

- monitoring and self-awareness
- diet and exercise
- accessing support, information and guidance
- lifestyle choices
- hobbies and interests
- relationships.

4.2 Support available to individuals and others:

- community resources
- substance misuse services
- support group, networks
- rehabilitation
- IAPT services (Improving Access to Psychological Therapies)
- crisis services.

4.3 The role of the health and social care practitioner in promoting mental health and well-being:

- duty of care
- safeguarding
- care planning
- person-centred practice
- referral
- encouraging self-referral
- information, advice, guidance
- positive relationships
- activities
- risk management.

4.4 National strategies to promote mental health and well-being:

- Closing the gap: priorities for essential change in mental health (Department of Health 2014)
- No Health Without Mental Health (Department of Health 2011)
- strategies relevant to Home Nation.

LO1 Understand types of mental ill-health

Mental ill-health is an umbrella term for a variety of conditions that negatively affect the mental health of individuals. Some conditions might last for a short while; others last longer. It is important to be clear what we mean by the terms 'mental health' and 'mental ill-health'.

1.1 Definition of mental health and mental ill-health

Mental health is not just the absence of mental disorder. It is defined by the World Health Organization (WHO) as 'a state of well-being in which every individual realizes his or her own potential, can cope with the normal stresses of life, can work productively and fruitfully, and is able to make a contribution to her or his community.' (WHO, 2014). Mental health is positive.

Mental ill-health is an emotional or psychological disorder that hinders the individual from making the most of their abilities, making it difficult for them to cope with the stresses of life. It prevents them working effectively and prevents them from contributing to society.

1.2 Types of mental ill-health

Sometimes, an individual with mental ill-health may also be experiencing physical ill-health too. In the next section, we explore the different types of mental ill-health, but be aware that there are many more not mentioned here. Mental disorders are classified in Chapter 5 of the *International Statistical Classification of Diseases and Related Health Problems (ICD)*, published by the World Health Organization.

Mood disorders

Everyone experiences mood changes, sometimes feeling happy or sad. Such mood changes are normal and are part of what it is to be human. The term 'mood disorders' in mental ill-health refers to more than just ordinary mood changes. These mood disorders are also referred to as 'affective disorders'. According to ICD 10th edition (ICD-10), mood disorders are often related to stressful events. There is a change in mood or 'affect' which varies from depression to extreme joy, causing a change in the person's level of activity. Mood disorders tend to recur. Examples of mood disorders include bipolar affective disorder, manic and depressive episodes, and cyclothymia (a mild form of bipolar disorder).

Bipolar affective disorder involves mood swings that range from extreme highs (mania) to extreme lows (depression) and that last for weeks or even months. The depressive phase involves the person feeling despair, a lack of motivation, difficulty in sleeping, having illogical thoughts and in extreme cases experiencing hallucinations. In the manic phase, they might be full of energy, talk very quickly, and have lots of new ideas and some illogical thoughts. They may act impulsively, for example spending a lot of money and getting into debt. Such mood swings may make it difficult for them to hold down a job, but in some areas of work such as the creative arts, the manic aspect of bipolar disorder may stimulate creativity. During the periods between mania and depression, a person might appear to be stable. Some people have rapid cycling with no stable period between mood swings. Others experience a mixed state of mania and depression at the same time, i.e. being overactive yet depressed (**www.nhs.uk/conditions/bipolar-disorder/symptoms**).

Personality disorders

According to ICD-10, personality disorders tend to persist, with behaviours related to the person's lifestyle, how they relate to themselves and others. These behaviours may appear early in life or develop later and are often very different from how the average person in that culture thinks and relates to others. The behaviour patterns are stable and may make it difficult for them to get on with others.

There are different types of personality disorder. With borderline personality disorder, a person may have disturbed thoughts, behave impulsively and have difficulty controlling their emotions. Their relationships may be intense, unstable and they are frightened of being abandoned, yet their behaviour drives others away.

Someone with anti-social personality disorder may have problems managing their emotions, get frustrated easily and may be quick to get angry. They blame others when things don't go how they want, and may be verbally and physically aggressive or even violent (**www.nhs.uk/conditions/personality-disorder**).

Cognitive disorders

Cognition refers to development of the mind. Cognitive disorders are often first noticed when children do not reach expected developmental milestones. ICD-10 classifies cognitive disorders as 'disorders of psychological development'. These include:

- speech and language disorders
- disorders of motor skills related to delayed neurological development
- a failure to develop particular skills, such as reading or basic arithmetic.

A child may show some or all of these developmental problems.

Pervasive developmental disorders involve problems in interacting with others and in patterns of communication, such as maintaining a conversation. The child may also have a limited range of interests. Autism is a spectrum of disorders typically diagnosed before the age of three years, when there is impaired development in social interaction, communication and when there is repetitive behaviour. There may be sleeping and eating disturbances. Asperger syndrome is one type of autism.

Anxiety disorders

Another word for anxiety is 'worry'. Anxiety occurs in several conditions, for example panic disorder, phobias such as claustrophobia, post-traumatic stress disorder (PTSD) and social anxiety disorder (social phobia). With generalised anxiety disorder (GAD), which can be long-term, people feel anxious all the time about different things. They never seem to relax, may have problems concentrating or sleeping, and may feel dizzy or have heart palpitations.

Psychotic disorders

Psychosis occurs when people perceive things differently from those around them. This might involve hallucinations or delusions. Someone having a hallucination hears, sees, feels, smells or tastes things that aren't there. They may hear voices or see things that others cannot. Delusions are strong beliefs not shared by others, for example believing everyone is trying to harm them. The person's behaviour changes as a result of their hallucinations or delusions. A psychotic episode can be severe and distressing for the individual and those who care for them.

Substance-related disorders

Psychoactive substances are substances that, when taken, affect the cognition of the brain. Examples include tobacco, alcohol, caffeine, stimulants and sedatives, hallucinogens, cocaine and opioids. Ecstasy tablets, or MDMA in its powder form, is an illegal psychoactive substance. Sometimes, psychoactive substances are prescribed for the individual by a doctor, for example morphine or tramadol. Both opioids may be prescribed for pain relief but all psychoactive substances are addictive and can cause dependency. The individual may crave a specific psychoactive substance such as tobacco, alcohol, or diazepam. Other users may be addicted to opioids, such as heroin, morphine, or fentanyl or to cannabinoids. When people who are addicted cannot get the substance, they experience withdrawal symptoms such as agitation and irritability. In extreme cases, they have uncontrollable shaking, convulsions and may become delirious. Psychoactive substances affect memory and can cause an early type of dementia.

Hallucinations, seeing things which are not there, and delusions, such as believing they can fly, are two effects of psychoactive substances. There is a synthetic cannabinoid known as 'Spice' that alters the individual's mood and causes hallucinations or paranoia. Ecstasy can result in emotional 'highs' or intense fear in a 'bad trip'. Alcohol can heighten feelings of jealousy or paranoia. Paranoia may persist long after the individual has stopped taking the substance.

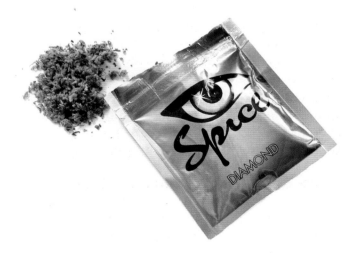

Figure 7.1 Spice alters mood and causes hallucinations

Any of these substances can have detrimental physical effects and result in sudden death. For example, **binge drinking** raises blood alcohol levels and can cause alcohol poisoning, and even death. Ecstasy affects the body's temperature control mechanism causing overheating and collapse. Street drugs which are unregulated may be contaminated with chalk or flour, or alternatively, may be pure and in much higher concentrations than are safe. Pure street drugs are a contributory factor in accidental drug overdose. The method of taking drugs can cause disorders too. Injecting drugs may cause blood vessel collapse, resulting in gangrene and the need for limb amputation. Dirty needles may also spread infections, leading to diseases such as hepatitis or liver failure.

Some people take more than one psychoactive substance, for example taking ecstasy then alcohol. The effects are unpredictable and can have a lasting impact on physical and mental health, resulting in long-term brain damage or even death.

Eating disorders

Eating disorders occur when abnormal or disturbed attitudes towards food take over an individual's life. They can make an individual feel unable to fulfil their potential or cope with the stresses of everyday life. They become obsessed with weight, body shape and appearance, eating too much or too little to become their perceived ideal size or weight. This may not be the healthiest weight and may be influenced by many factors, for example peers, fashion or social media. There are many types of eating disorders:

- **Anorexia nervosa** involves an obsessive desire to keep weight as low as possible by not eating, by exercising too much (or both). Anorexia is less common than other eating disorders.

- **Bulimia nervosa** is when an individual binges on food then makes themselves sick, uses laxatives, restricts what they eat, and/or exercises too much to prevent weight gain.

- **Binge eating disorder (BED)** refers to an individual regularly eating amounts of food to feel uncomfortably full, often feeling a sense of losing control during the binge, and then feeling guilt or shame during or after the binge.

- **Other specified feeding or eating disorders (OSFED)** are not the same as anorexia, bulimia or binge eating disorder, but include an unhealthy relationship with food and are the most common eating disorders (**www.nhs.uk/conditions/Eating-disorders**).

Key terms

Binge drinking refers to drinking lots of alcohol in a short space of time or drinking to get drunk.

Mental health refers to 'a state of well-being in which every individual realizes his or her own potential, can cope with the normal stresses of life, can work productively and fruitfully, and is able to make a contribution to her or his community.' (WHO, 2014).

Mental ill-health refers to an emotional or psychological disorder that hinders the individual from making the most of their abilities, and makes it difficult for them to cope with the stresses of life. It prevents them working effectively and from contributing to society.

Activity

Create an information booklet that defines mental health and mental ill-health, using references to help you. Provide information outlining at least three different types of mental ill-health, using at least one relevant and traceable reference. Make sure that you include an accurate reference list (bibliography) at the end of the booklet.

Check your understanding 1

1 What is the difference between mental health and mental ill-health?
2 Describe three different mental disorders.
3 Why is binge drinking dangerous?

LO2 Understand legislation and policies in relation to mental health and well-being

The UK government is responsible for providing the National Health Service (NHS). As part of this responsibility for health, the government tries to prevent people getting ill, provides services when they are ill and also services to help them recover their health. One way the government does this is to make laws (legislation) and policies (plans) about health.

2.1 Legislation and policies in relation to mental health and well-being

Legislation and policies can change as new research finds better ways to treat people. It is very important to use the most recent, up-to-date versions of legislation and policies.

Health and Social Care Act 2012

The Health and Social Care Act 2012 reorganised the NHS, giving local authorities power to commission (buy) and provide public health services. It changes some aspects of previous laws, bringing in ways that health and social care can work together in order to meet needs in their local area. Some areas have a higher proportion of elderly people, while others have more young people: their needs will differ. The 2012 Act gives local areas the power to provide services needed in their area. It introduces changes in how health and social care is commissioned, providing and placing a legal duty on the NHS to treat mental and physical health as equally important. The government has pledged to achieve this by 2020.

A major criticism of the Act is that it has two opposing purposes. On the one hand, it encourages a split between those buying care and those delivering care, and on the other hand, there is a requirement to bring services together and integrate them. This leads to an increase in **bureaucracy**. A further criticism is that mental health is still not on an equal footing with physical health in terms of provision of services.

The Act created:

- **Clinical Commissioning Groups (CCGs)** – public bodies made up of doctors, nurse specialists, lay people and others.
- **Health and Wellbeing Boards (HWBs)** which consist of CCGs and local authorities. HWBs produce a Joint Strategic Needs Assessment (JSNA) and a Joint Health and Well-being Strategy (JHWS). They provide services and commission services from private providers. Local authorities and CCGs share some of their budgets as part of the Better Care Fund. One example is that in London, a specialist nurse and a paramedic in a car with blue lights attend situations where someone has a mental health crisis. This reduces the number of emergency admissions.
- NHS Commissioning Board (NHSCB), now **NHS England** – a national body holding CCGs to account and commissioning specialist services.
- **NHS Improvement** oversees trusts and monitors spending in the NHS.
- **Healthwatch England (HWE)**, part of the Care Quality Commission (CQC), represents views of patients, service users and the public.
- **NHS Digital** provides data for monitoring how services are doing.

Equality Act 2010

The Equality Act 2010 makes it illegal to treat people unfairly. It provides individuals with protection against discrimination, particularly those with specific characteristics. This is discussed in *Unit HSC M1: Equality, diversity and rights in health and social care*. In terms of mental health, the protected characteristic relating to disability is most relevant where a person with physical or mental impairment, which has a 'substantial and long-term adverse effect' on that person's ability to carry out normal day-to-day activities, is protected under this Act.

Mental Health Act 2007, Mental Health Act 1983

The Mental Health Act (MHA) 2007 updates the MHA 1983 and it applies to England and Wales specifically. It sets out processes and safeguards for patients so they are not incorrectly detained or treated, but it also outlines how those with serious mental disorders can be treated without consent where necessary so they do not harm themselves or others.

The 2007 amendments include:

- A single definition of 'mental disorder'.

- To be '**sectioned**' or detained, a person must be suffering from a mental disorder that needs assessment or treatment in a hospital for their own health or safety and for the protection of others.

- Replaces the role of 'approved social worker' with 'approved mental health professional'. The professional does not have to have a social work qualification. They still need specific training but can be a psychologist, occupational therapist or psychiatric nurse.

- A patient applying to have another person, not their nearest relative, represent them if they think their nearest relative is not suitable.

- Introducing **Community Treatment Orders** to allow some patients with mental health disorders to be discharged into the community. They are supervised by a community psychiatric nurse to ensure they continue their medication or therapy. This supervision helps to avoid the 'revolving door' pattern of re-admission, where previously, patients wouldn't be supervised and would potentially stop their treatment. They would then become ill again and would have to be re-admitted to hospital.

- Electroconvulsive therapy (ECT) cannot be given without consent unless it to save an individual's life or to prevent their condition getting worse. ECT also cannot be used if the individual has made an advance decision or a person holding Lasting Power of Attorney (LPA) on their behalf has refused the treatment in the best interests of the patient.

- Ensuring that hospital accommodation for patients aged under 18 admitted with a mental disorder is suitable for their age. Previously, they were put on adult wards.

- Ensuring that independent mental health advocates (IMHAs) are allocated to 'qualifying patients' with a mental disorder. Mental health professionals must tell individuals that they have a right to an IMHA. Qualifying patients are:

  - detained in hospital under the MHA

  - subject to a Guardianship Order under the MHA

  - subject to a Community Treatment Order in the community

  - discussing with their doctor the possibility of neurosurgery or any surgical operation on the brain tissue

  - or under 18 years old and discussing with a doctor the possibility of ECT.

The current Mental Health Act was reviewed in December 2018. Recommendations are to improve choice and autonomy so that people are supported to express their needs and understand their rights. Patients are treated as individuals and their care involves no unnecessary restriction on their freedom.

Mental Capacity Act 2005 (MCA)

This Act helps provides guidelines as to whether or not an individual has the ability or **capacity** to make decisions for themselves. The MCA applies to people working in health, social care and other sectors who support and treat those aged 16 and over, living in England and Wales, and who are unable to make all or some decisions for themselves. It ensures that those who are able can make their own decisions. When a person is unable to do this, their best interests must be followed, i.e. the option chosen must be the one that allows them the most freedom. For more information about the MCA, see *Unit HSC M3: Safeguarding and protection in health and social care*.

There is a two-part assessment when deciding whether a person has the capacity to make their own decisions. The first part requires evidence of mental disturbance or impairment, while the second part is the test.

Part 1: There must be evidence that the person has an impairment or disturbance in the functioning of the mind or brain. The impairment means they cannot meet the next part of the test (part 2).

Part 2: This is the functional test that determines whether the person:

- understands the information relevant to the decision
- retains the information long enough to make a decision

- uses and weighs up the information to make a decision
- communicates their decision by any means.

If they cannot meet *any one* of these requirements because of the mental impairment then they lack capacity *for the specific decision at this time.* The test relates to a specific time. They may be able to meet the requirements at a different time, for example when they are less agitated. Communication by any means could be by blinking if, for example, that is their only way of communicating. It does not have to be verbal communication.

An important part of the Mental Capacity Act 2005 deals with **Deprivation of Liberty** safeguards. Deprivation of liberty means detaining people against their will, for example not allowing residents of a care home to go out.

The Mental Capacity Act 2005 brought in the role of the Independent Mental Capacity Advocate (IMCA). IMCAs represent people where there is no family or friend able to represent them. They must be independent so that they are not influenced by the needs of the service, for example a nurse cannot be the IMCA for a patient because there is a conflict of interest. The NHS might need the bed for an emergency, and a nurse might be influenced by this need, rather than what is best for the patient. IMCAs are a legal safeguard for people who lack the capacity to make specific important decisions such as where they live and what treatment options to choose.

The Mental Capacity Act 2005 also clarified advanced planning and decision-making so that people can leave instructions about what they want to happen to them if they become unable to make decisions. Under this Act, a person can give **Lasting Power of Attorney (LPA)** to someone to make financial decisions for them in case they lose capacity. They can also give LPA to someone to make decisions on their behalf about their health and welfare.

The Act provides for advance decisions made by an individual for when they are unable to say what specific treatments they do not want, for example a person may not want to be resuscitated if they have a heart attack. These are legally binding on the medical profession. Advance statements allow people to say what care they want (but are not legally binding), for example devout Catholics may wish to have a priest visit them in hospital.

Human Rights Act 1998

The **Human Rights Act** comes from the European Convention on Human Rights and protects everyone in the UK. It came into force in the UK in October 2000. Public authorities must obey the Human Rights Act. If your human rights have been breached, or broken by any public body, you can go to court in the UK to have your rights respected.

Of the 16 human rights, key ones relating to mental health issues include the right to life, freedom from torture and inhuman or degrading treatment, freedom from slavery and forced labour, right to liberty and security, freedom of thought, belief and religion. People with mental health issues are vulnerable. They are often stigmatised, may be locked away and abused. Some people think that those with cognitive disorders should not be allowed to marry and have children, which is why the right to marry and start a family is an important human right for those with mental ill-health.

Mental Health: Priorities for Change 2014

This policy document applies specifically to England and explains how changes in local service planning and delivery will make a difference to the lives of people with mental health problems. It supports the government's mental health strategy 'No Health Without Mental Health'. It sets out 25 priorities for change in four key areas. These are:

1 Increasing access to mental health services.

2 Integrating physical and mental health care.

3 Starting early to promote mental well-being and prevent mental health problems.

4 Improving the quality of life of people with mental health problems.

While this document identifies many of the problems experienced by people with poor mental health, and expresses plans to improve the situation, issues still remain. For example, demand for services is increasing and some buildings are unsuitable. The Care Quality Commission (CQC) published 'The state of care in mental health services 2014 to 2017' and identified several areas of concern, including:

- Concerns about 'locked rehabilitation wards', which are wards in psychiatric hospitals which are locked to prevent individuals going out. They are meant to be places where individuals are rehabilitated and helped to get back in the community, but due to poor care individuals are kept locked up. One person was locked up for 21 years at Birmingham and Solihull Mental Health NHS Foundation Trust (**www.theguardian.com/society/2019/apr/23/nhs-mental-health-patients-locked-in-secure-ward-rehabilitation-years**).

- Variation between wards in how frequently staff use restrictive practices and physical restraint to de-escalate challenging behaviour.

- The negative impact of staffing shortages.

- Poor quality clinical information systems.

- Commissioning of crisis care services.

The Mental Health Strategy for England 2011

The government launched a mental health strategy 'No Health Without Mental Health' in England in 2011 as a response to the increase in young people with mental health problems and increase in dementia and depression in the ageing population.

No Health Without Mental Health is a strategy for people of all ages. It sets out six objectives to improve the mental health, well-being and outcomes for those with mental health problems. It states that mental health is everyone's business and good mental health and resilience are fundamental to physical health, along with achieving potential.

The six shared objectives are:

1 More people will have good mental health.

2 More people with mental health problems will recover.

3 More people with mental health problems will have good physical health.

4 More people will have a positive experience of care and support.

5 Fewer people will suffer avoidable harm.

6 Fewer people will experience stigma and discrimination.

Current legislation and policy as relevant to Home Nation

NHS Five Year Forward View, October 2014

This policy document sets out the need for further change in England in the NHS with a focus on prevention of ill-health, more emphasis on public health and more care delivered locally where possible. The aim is to break down barriers between health and social care and between hospital and care in the community, ultimately saving money and reducing the £30 billion overspend in the NHS.

Scotland

The Mental Health (Care and Treatment) (Scotland) Act 2003 is the Scottish equivalent of the Mental Health Act 1983. The Mental Health (Scotland) Act 2015 clarifies the Mental Health (Care and Treatment) (Scotland) Act 2003, which specifies the:

- right to independent advocacy services
- circumstances in which a person may be detained against their wishes
- compulsory treatment orders.

Northern Ireland

The Mental Capacity Act (Northern Ireland) 2016 came out of the Bamford Review, a legislative framework that reviewed the law, policy and provision affecting people with mental health needs in Northern Ireland.

 Key terms

Bureaucracy refers to the administrative procedures that help run an organisation. Some people call bureaucracy 'red tape'.

Capacity refers to the ability to understand information, retain it, make and communicate decisions.

Community Treatment Orders allow some patients with mental health disorders to be discharged into the community and supervised by a community psychiatric nurse, as part of the Mental Health Act. These patients can be recalled to hospital if they stop taking their medication.

Deprivation of liberty refers to detaining people against their will.

Lasting Power of Attorney (LPA) is a way of giving someone else power to decide what is in the best interests of the person. There are two types: financial, and health and welfare. LPAs are appointed to make decisions about an individual's welfare, including healthcare, property and affairs.

Sectioned refers to the detention of an individual suffering from a mental disorder which needs assessment or treatment in hospital for their own health or safety and for the protection of others.

It defines terms such as 'lacking capacity' and 'best interests decision-making', bringing mental health law and mental capacity law together in one law. It defines the High Court's role in making decisions on a person's behalf, and their ability to appoint deputies to act on someone's behalf. The Act outlines safeguards currently in place to protect the care, treatment and personal welfare of those who lack capacity and provides for Independent Mental Capacity Advocates where support is needed with best interests decision-making.

Activity

Create a poster that outlines one piece of legislation or policy in relation to mental health and well-being. The information should identify the document specifically relating to mental health and well-being, whether it is legislation or policy, and should highlight the key points and a reference for further information.

✓ Check your understanding 2

1 Describe the difference between legislation and policy.
2 Name the Acts that specifically relate to mental health.
3 Give an example of a national strategy.
4 Give an example of a policy for mental health.

LO3 Understand the impact of mental ill-health on individuals and others

Mental ill-health doesn't just affect the **individual** who is experiencing it, but also their carers, colleagues, family members and anyone close to that individual. Mental ill-health may be short term or long term, mild or severe, but it affects people socially, emotionally, physically, and financially. Sometimes, relatives might feel ashamed, especially in some cultures where mental health issues carry a **stigma**. They may worry that they might develop a mental health problem too and feel uncertain about how to cope. Sometimes, families pretend there isn't a problem and adapt their behaviour to try to avoid dealing with the situation.

3.1 The impact mental ill-health can have on individuals and others

Different types of mental ill-health may have different impacts. Mood disorders and personality disorders might make a person's behaviour unpredictable. Cognitive disorders might make them slower in understanding situations. People with anxiety disorders may be too worried to make decisions and colleagues may find this frustrating. Psychotic and substance-related disorders may mean they miss time from work or education. Eating disorders may restrict an individual's social life as they might be too anxious to eat in front of **others**. The impacts of mental ill-health on individuals and others are listed in this section.

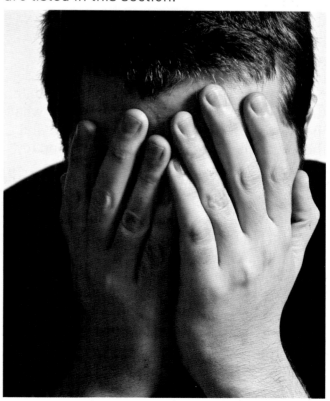

Figure 7.2 Mental ill-health can cause a loss of confidence, low self-esteem and isolation

Confidence

Mental ill-health can undermine an individual's confidence. Extreme mood swings or sudden panic attacks can lower a person's perceived ability to cope with life. Not being in control of one's moods or behaviour, or having hallucinations, can be very frightening. Others might lose confidence in the person, for example a seemingly capable business person may have a sudden panic attack when talking to clients, who might then lose confidence in their abilities and withdraw their business.

Self-esteem

Losing confidence and not being able to control one's moods can lead to a loss of self-esteem. Self-doubt creeps in. Someone with dependency issues, for example drug or alcohol dependency, might feel they have let others down and feel worthless. Low self-esteem may make them less able to interact with others.

Relationships

Loss of confidence and low self-esteem also affect how we behave towards others. Instead of greeting a friend, we may walk past them and hope they have not noticed. In turn, they may feel rejected and wonder what they have done wrong. Friendships cool and then in addition to loss of confidence and low self-esteem, the person finds themselves socially isolated. Someone with a cognitive disorder may find it difficult to make friends. Those with autism might not interpret social cues such as eye contact and body language correctly, and fail to pick up that the other person does not want to talk.

Dependence

Dependency happens when an individual cannot function without the help of someone or something. It involves a loss or potential loss of independence. Alcohol, drugs and even nicotine can cause cravings that dominate everything else for the affected individual. They might make excuses and attempt to hide their addiction. Sometimes, dependency leads to criminal behaviour, such as shoplifting, in order to pay for their addiction. An individual with dependency issues could also be homeless and see no other option but to beg or steal. Family members may lose contact for a variety of reasons and this in turn may lead to further health-related concerns.

Finances

Mental ill-health can make it difficult for an individual to hold down a job. If the individual has a partner and children, and they are the main earner, the family may lose their home if rent or mortgage repayments are not paid. Mental ill-health also means it might be difficult at times to meet the requirements for claiming benefits or understanding the requirements for universal credit.

Employment

Similar to the financial effects of mental ill-health, employment might be difficult for individuals who are suffering. Some employers may be understanding, for example if a person has early onset dementia, an employer can adapt the job or find them a different role in the organisation. Addictions and mood or personality disorders are more difficult to understand, and so an employer might not be as flexible when an individual's behaviour is unpredictable in the workplace. However, there is protection from discrimination under the Equality Act 2010 which lists disability as a protected characteristic. Disability is 'physical or mental impairment which has a substantial and long-term adverse effect on that person's ability to carry out normal day-to-day activities' (**www.equalityhumanrights.com**).

Another example of difficulties regarding mental ill-health and employment involve the interview process, which can be very challenging. For example, those on the autistic spectrum might be highly skilled but find interviews difficult to manage, especially when communicating with others. One technology employer, SAP, allows individuals to make a Lego robot instead of having a formal interview. In this way, they are assessing the individual's skills while attending to their mental health needs. Another firm, Auticon, allows employees to use headphones to block out noise and use messaging apps instead of verbal communication. If they are feeling stressed, they can have 'anxiety days off' (BBC, 2019).

Environment

The environment can affect those with mental ill-health, such as anxiety disorders, for example a person with anxiety may be more likely to have a panic attack in a crowded store. Some people with autism find socialising in an office difficult since communication can be a struggle. For someone with dependency issues, such as alcoholism, socialising in a public place where alcohol is readily available might make it difficult to avoid temptation. For someone with an eating disorder, a family meal could be very stressful as they worry about comments or judgements from others. A busy supermarket may not be the best place for a parent to take an autistic child and may make the parent reluctant to take the child shopping. A partner of someone with panic attacks may avoid taking them on crowded public transport.

Isolation

Isolation refers to being alone, which can make an individual with mental ill-health feel worse. This isolation might be self-imposed, for example an individual with depression may not want to see their family, friends or meet others. Sometimes, those with mental ill-health issues find themselves isolated by others. Friends and family might find it hard to cope with their mood swings or dependency issues. Employers and colleagues may be intolerant of their differences and isolate the individual by ignoring them and/or their needs.

Discrimination

Discriminating, i.e. treating a person differently because of their disability, is illegal but it still happens. People are not defined by their mental ill-health: they are their own person with a unique set of beliefs, preferences, wishes and needs. However, rather than seeing the individual for themselves, others see the disability. As a result of this, many with mental ill-health face discrimination and find it difficult to achieve goals that others might not find as challenging, for example getting a job, or if they have one when they become ill, finding it hard to keep a job. They might also be excluded from friendship groups. For example:

Jeff has dementia. His friends at the golf club avoid him because he asks repetitive questions and forgets what was said, which they find irritating. Sometimes, Jeff does not recognise them.

Amina has bipolar disorder and at times is hyperactive, but at other times, is deeply depressed. Her family avoid taking her to social events because her behaviour is unpredictable and they don't know how best to manage the situation.

In addition to the problems caused by their illness, they face the added problems caused by discrimination. This makes it even more difficult for them to regain their health, realise their own potential, cope with the normal stresses of life, work productively and fruitfully, and make a contribution to their community.

MIND and Rethink Mental Health joined forces on the 'Time To Change' campaign which aims to raise public awareness and end mental health discrimination (**www.time-to-change.org.uk**).

Description Activity

Write a factsheet or prepare a group presentation describing the impact mental ill-health can have on individuals and others. Provide detailed information to describe how mental ill-health can affect individuals and others, using referenced examples to support what you say and give a reference list at the end.

3.2 Public attitudes towards mental ill-health

Just because someone has mental ill-health does not mean they are unintelligent: however, many assume that lack of intelligence goes with mental health problems. Public attitudes towards mental ill-health are often negative, based on fear, a lack of understanding and misinformation. Powerful prejudice is challenged through education and promotional campaigns. This supports everyone's mental health and raises awareness of mental ill-health in others, which helps to break down barriers.

For example, an individual experiencing a psychotic episode might behave unusually. Others cross the street to avoid them and avoid eye contact in case the person becomes violent. Unpredictable behaviour associated with mood or personality disorders may make others feel they are unreliable. Some members of the public have little sympathy for those with substance-related disorders, anxiety disorders or eating disorders, as there's a perception that these are self-imposed problems, i.e. that the individual could choose to behave differently if they really wanted to. Some people might assume that all cognitive disorders are inherited. In some cultures, people believe that mental ill-health is caused by witchcraft and so avoid the cursed individual.

Occasionally, there are positive attitudes towards those with mental ill-health, especially towards creative artists. Beethoven, the German pianist, suffered from extreme highs and lows in his mood which contributed to his musical compositions. Vincent van Gogh, the Dutch artist, painted his most famous pictures while staying in a mental hospital: they are regarded as some of the best in their field. More recently, celebrities such as Lady Gaga and Ruby Wax have talked about their own mental health issues, inspiring others to pursue better mental health.

Understanding

Charities such as MIND and Rethink Mental Illness do a lot to increase the public's understanding of mental ill-health by providing information and support for everyone, whether it is for friends, family or individuals with mental ill-health. For example, MIND host an online support group and Rethink Mental Illness organise local support groups for those with mental ill-health and their carers. Both charities promote a greater understanding of mental health and mental ill-health. The NHS also provides information online and sets out its plans for increasing awareness of mental illness by 2020. This includes providing better services so that mental and physical health are seen as equally important in the health sector.

Acceptance

One in four adults and one in ten children experience mental illness. Everyone knows someone who has had or will be affected by mental illness. Unfortunately, mental illness remains a stigma in many societies. If someone has a physical illness such as cancer, they get a lot of sympathy. If they have a mental illness, they may be avoided. Charities such as MIND and Rethink work to overcome this and to gain acceptance for those with mental illness. World Mental Health Day promotes awareness of mental health annually, enlisting support from famous people to increase acceptance of those with mental ill-health.

Integration

Mental illness can result in homelessness, which in turn can make mental illness even worse. In England and Wales, Streetlink, a charity partly funded by the government and by St Mungo's charity, enable members of the public to report concerns they have about anyone sleeping rough. Outreach workers then contact the individual and connect them to local services, including housing and medical care to support them. Sheltered housing is one way that people with mental ill-health can integrate back into society. The organisation 'Homeless' provides information about accommodation and health care, linking to sheltered accommodation. Once an individual has a home, they can register for a GP and have access to regular health care.

If the individual is well enough, having a job can provide structure to their life, along with the chance to meet new people and earn money. Those who are too unwell to work may be able to claim benefits, but the best way to integrate into society is to have a purpose. Gaining or regaining employment after a period of mental illness varies according to the individual, the nature of their employment and the impact of the illness. Sometimes, a person will change their employment, especially if their previous job was stressful. They might do voluntary work for a while so they establish a routine for their life, and then progress to part-time work before considering a full-time job. The Rethink website has links to local support, for example they offer an eight-week self-help course with support to access education, volunteering roles, employment opportunities and local peer support groups.

For those in full-time employment, mental illness can disrupt their working life. Employers have a legal duty to make reasonable adjustments to help employees continue to do their jobs. This may include flexible working hours so that the individual can attend therapy sessions, or offering a quiet area to work when they are stressed.

Tolerance

Tolerance and acceptance come when people have more of an understanding about mental ill-health. The Mental Health Foundation runs a campaign each year to raise awareness of mental health issues such as stress. For 2019, the campaign focuses on the idea of accepting yourself for who you are. Campaigns like this raise the public's awareness about mental ill-health issues and can help to increase their understanding in relation to mental health being as important as physical health. This removes the feeling of fear and people then become more tolerant of themselves and others.

Activity

Write an article for a school or college newspaper discussing the public attitudes towards mental ill-health. Include positive and negative public attitudes towards mental ill-health and use examples to show how positive public attitudes impact on people with mental ill-health. You should use two different references, referencing in the text and at the end.

Key terms

Individual(s) refers to person(s) accessing health and social care services.

Others refers to parents/carers, family, friends, colleagues, external partners and health and social care practitioners.

Stigma is a mark of disgrace associated with a particular quality or characteristic such as having mental ill-health or a disability.

Check your understanding 3

1 Give three ways that mental ill-health can impact on an individual.
2 Give three ways that public attitudes can help people with mental ill-health.

LO4 Understand how to support and promote mental health and well-being

Mental health and well-being is just as important as physical health. We know a lot about physical health, for example that eating too much sugar and fat is bad for you as it can lead to excess weight gain. Many try to control the amount of sugar and fat they consume because they do not want to become obese or develop diabetes. As a society, we are just beginning to understand the impact of what we do and how it affects our mental health.

4.1 How an individual can promote their own mental health and well-being

There are many things we can do to keep mentally healthy and prevent getting ill by considering the following factors.

Monitoring and self-awareness

Learning to understand yourself, or developing **self-awareness**, is a good way to maintain mental health. If you know you get stressed in certain situations, such as in interviews, you can learn different ways to lower stress such as using deep breathing and relaxation techniques. Monitoring yourself can give clues about what triggers certain behaviours. How we think affects how we feel and our feelings affect how we behave. For example:

Jed dislikes a work colleague. He doesn't know why, but he avoids the person, leaves them out of important communications and is generally not very kind towards them. Jed isn't happy with his own behaviour but cannot explain it. His boss calls him into the office and asks Jed why he is behaving like this as it is disrupting the team. Jed takes some time to think why he dislikes this person and realises it is because he reminds him of a school bully who made his life a misery. He thinks this person is like the school bully. This affects how he feels towards them (feelings) and how he behaves towards them (behaviour). Once Jed realised that his behaviour is based on his thoughts, he can see that this work colleague may look like the school bully but there are lots of differences. He begins to see the good points in his colleague. As his thoughts change so do his feelings, and in turn, his behaviour. He feels ashamed of his previous behaviour and tries to be friendly.

Developing an awareness of how you think, feel and behave and then monitoring it is an important way to maintain your mental health. It puts you in control of your feelings and your behaviour.

Mindfulness is another way to develop self-awareness. It is a skill that can be learned and the more you do it, the better you become at doing it. Mindfulness has proved helpful in relieving depression, anxiety and stress. It helps people be more self-aware, feel calmer and more able to choose how to respond to thoughts and feelings. It is useful in coping with negative unhelpful thoughts and in helping people be kinder to themselves. Mindfulness focuses on the body and breathing. By slowing and relaxing breathing, a person becomes calmer and more aware of any tensions, therefore feeling more in control of how to relax and let them go. Focusing on the moment allows all the other stresses to fade for a moment so it is easier to get things in perspective.

Key terms

Mindfulness is the ability to focus on the present moment, being aware of what is happening in your mind, body and surroundings, without judging or worrying about what might happen in the future or what has happened in the past.

Self-awareness is being able to see yourself as others see you and being aware of your own behaviours, motivations and feelings.

Diet and exercise

A healthy balanced diet low in fat and refined carbohydrates, such as sugar, along with sufficient vitamins and minerals, is the basis for physical and mental health. Some helpful guidance for a healthy diet includes:

- Half the plate should always be filled with vegetables.
- At least five portions of fruit and vegetables should be eaten each day.
- Water, rather than fizzy drinks, and regular meals provide the fuel our bodies need.
- Carbohydrates, for example wholemeal bread or pasta, provide our bodies with energy.
- Proteins, for example beans, eggs, milk, cheese, fish, chicken and meat help to build muscles.

Too much food, especially sugar, can lead to obesity, high blood pressure and diabetes. Too little food means the body is malnourished and cannot fight infections.

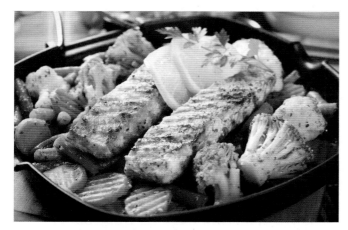

Figure 7.3 A healthy diet promotes good mental health

Exercise also helps to keep our bodies and minds healthy. A brisk walk in the park, or working on a plan such as the NHS 'Couch to 5K' fitness programme releases natural chemicals in the body, such as endorphins and serotonins which improve mood and help to avoid mental illnesses such as depression.

Accessing support, information and guidance

Support, information and guidance is available from a variety of sources. Arguably, the most common source of support is the internet but it is important to use only reliable websites. The NHS has advice and guidance including an A–Z of mental health, with advice for carers and for those with mental health issues. MIND and Rethink Mental Illness are two voluntary organisations with websites that have links to local support, information and guidance on mental health issues. MIND has links online for those needing urgent help. There are 135 local MIND centres offering advice on supported housing, crisis helplines, drop-in centres, employment and training schemes, counselling and befriending. Rethink Mental Illness has similar services. Both campaign for better public awareness of mental health.

Lifestyle choices

Lifestyle choices are decisions that an individual makes about how to live and behave, according to their attitudes, tastes and values. Whether an individual decides to take drugs, drink alcohol, socialise with those that do, or to focus on trying to look like the latest fashion model, are all choices that can impact on mental health. Psychoactive substances cause chemical changes in the brain, and may cause long-term side effects, for example there is a confirmed link between cannabis use and psychotic illness (**www.nhs.uk/news/mental-health/cannabis-linked-to-psychosis**).

Recent studies show that social media and the internet have more of a negative effect on girls than boys and that girls are more unhappy with their physical appearance and life on a whole. One report found that 22 per cent (over a fifth) of 14-year-old girls self-harm in the UK, when self-harm includes a wide range of behaviours including drug and alcohol abuse, as well as physical self-harming (**www.nhs.uk/news/mental-health/nearly-quarter-14-year-old-girls-uk-self-harming-charity-reports**). Recent recommendations have included limiting time spent on social media to improve mental health.

Mood disorders are linked to disrupted sleep patterns, so it is important to get enough sleep. There is evidence that good sleep at night and activity during the day is linked to better mental health. Turning off screens an hour before bedtime and having a quiet, dark, cool bedroom helps better sleep. Having enough physical activity during the day also helps sleep (**www.nhs.uk/news/mental-health/body-clock-disruptions-linked-mood-disorders**). Shift workers who work night-time or irregular hours, for example airline crew and health workers, may have more mood disorders because of their disrupted sleep patterns.

Hobbies and interests

Having a hobby and/or a variety of interests contributes to good mental health. Activities may include:

- Exercise, for example walking, swimming and cycling. They not only boost mental health but improve physical health too.

- Creative activities, for example drawing, writing, song writing. They help to focus thoughts away from harmful behaviours and towards boosting positive self-esteem.

- Learning a new skill, for example playing an instrument or learning to cook, add an extra dimension to life and provide opportunities to meet other people and socialise in a positive way.

Hobbies and interests are available for all levels of ability. For example, gardening, even on a small scale (for example, a window box in a flat, or digging an allotment) bring people in touch with nature and the natural cycle of life, enabling them to put issues in perspective.

Mindfulness and meditation have value in improving mental health. A study by Otago University, New Zealand found that students using mindfulness apps improved depressive symptoms, resilience, mindfulness, and college adjustment, and those who continued to use the apps were more likely to maintain improvements in mental health (**https://link.springer.com/article/10.1007/s12671-018-1050-9**).

Relationships

Relationships influence mental health. Stable, happy relationships contribute to good mental health, while unstable relationships contribute to poor mental health. A person in an abusive relationship is more likely to have low self-esteem and poor mental health than a person in a supportive relationship. Relationships where one person constantly undermines the other are harmful to both. It is important to recognise when relationships are destructive and how to change bad patterns. To do this may require support from a relationship counsellor.

Positive social ties, whether it be family, friends or as part of a community, provide emotional support which can reduce unhealthy behaviours and boost a person's sense of self-esteem. For example, Jess moved to a new town for work. At first, she did not know anyone and was lonely. She began to doubt whether she could do the new job. Her confidence sank and she began to get depressed. She kept in touch with her mum and an old school friend, both of whom reminded her of what she had achieved so far and boosted her confidence. Her mum suggested she join a local exercise group, which she did. She gradually met more people and made new friends. Emotional support provided by social ties enhances psychological well-being, and reduces the risk of unhealthy behaviours and poor physical health.

Sometimes, a person who has been in a stable, happy relationship becomes mentally unwell and their partner struggles to understand why they have changed. Service men and women suffering post-traumatic stress disorder (PTSD) might become withdrawn or angry, finding it difficult to sleep and may have recurrent nightmares. This can affect their relationship with their family. If they do not get outside help, this stress can lead to relationship and family break up. There is a high proportion of ex-servicemen compared to other careers ending up homeless due to mental health issues.

Description Activity

Create a poster in which you describe, using examples from reliable sources, two different ways that individuals can promote their own mental health and well-being. Two different references should be used and referenced in the text and at the end.

4.2 Support available to individuals and others

While there is a lot that people can do for themselves, in terms of lifestyle choices, sometimes additional help is needed. This is provided through local and national services. Some are provided by the state, others by voluntary or charitable organisations. Some services might even be private, i.e. paid for by the individual themselves.

Community resources

Child and Adolescent Mental Health Services (CAMHS) are the NHS services that assess and treat young people with emotional, behavioural or mental health difficulties. Support covers depression, eating disorders,

self-harm, abuse, violence or anger, bipolar, schizophrenia and anxiety. Local NHS CAMHS services around the UK have teams of nurses, therapists, psychologists, support workers and social workers, and other professionals.

The general practitioner (GP) is the first person in the line of community resources. GPs often see people with depression or stress. They then refer the individual on for specialist help. In England, the NHS provides community-based adult mental health services locally for those with mental health issues (**www.england.nhs.uk/mental-health/adults/cmhs**).

For individuals experiencing their first episode of psychosis, they might see their GP first or could be admitted as an emergency to hospital. They are then referred on for further treatment. The **early intervention in psychosis standards (EIP)** require more than half of those admitted to begin treatment within two weeks of referral because early intervention improves the chance of recovery.

Key term

Early intervention in psychosis standards (EIP) are a set of standards published by the Royal College of Psychiatrists that guide practitioners in the early treatment of people with psychosis. The standards bring together the latest research and evidence from best practice to say how people with psychosis should be cared for.

Substance misuse services

Substance misuse usually refers to drug abuse. It is the use of a drug where the person uses the substance in amounts or in ways harmful to themselves or others. Some drugs are legal, others are not. Illegal drugs are not regulated and may vary in strength and be contaminated by other materials. Alcohol, cannabis, street drugs such as spice, ecstasy,

MDMA and crystal meth are just some of the drugs which may cause addiction.

The GP is usually the first place to go for help. GPs may offer treatment at the practice or refer the person to a local drug service. Some people do not want to talk to their GP. They can refer themselves to the local drug treatment service and find out where their local services are from the Talk to Frank drugs helpline.

The NHS offers help in the form of psychological treatments and medication. Psychological treatments may include counselling, cognitive behavioural therapy (CBT) and family therapy. Medication may be used, substituting a less harmful drug for the one the individual is using. Methadone is often used to help people reduce their dependency on opioids, but methadone itself causes addiction. Detoxification, i.e. weaning the person off opioid drugs like heroin, may be offered. The person may also be referred to self-help support groups like Alcoholics Anonymous and Narcotics Anonymous where they can meet people with similar experiences.

The NHS Substance Misuse Provider Alliance includes eleven NHS trusts from across England. They are NHS drug and alcohol treatment providers working collaboratively with service users, carers and other organisations and pool ideas to improve services (**www.nhs-substance-misuse-provider-alliance.org.uk**).

In addition to NHS services, charities and private drug and alcohol treatment organisations also offer help. Private treatment may be expensive. Adfam is a national UK charity supporting those affected by someone else's substance use. They support frontline workers in drug and alcohol sectors working with family members and carers, as well as families themselves, providing a list of useful organisations to support families (**https://adfam.org.uk**).

Support group, networks

Support groups and networks can be face-to-face or online and are separate from NHS services. They offer support from others, not necessarily health professionals, who have had similar experiences and understand their issues. The NHS also has a list of support groups which can be found online.

Some examples of support groups and networks include:

- MIND, one of the most well-known mental health charities providing support.
- Campaign against Living Miserably (CALM) for men aged 15 to 35.
- No Panic, a voluntary charity offering a helpline and a course to help those with panic attacks and obsessive compulsive disorder (OCD).
- PAPYRUS is the national charity dedicated to the prevention of young suicide. As well as a website, they provide confidential support and advice to young people through a helpline, HOPELINEUK.
- Alcoholics Anonymous (AA) is a support group for people who wish to stop drinking. They organise local face-to-face support groups, as well as online groups and operate a telephone helpline. They offer a twelve-step programme to recovery.
- Narcotics Anonymous (NA) similarly offer support meetings face-to-face or online but also offer a service for those in prison. Like AA, they also offer a twelve-step programme.

Rehabilitation

Rehabilitation aims to keep people as independent as possible so they can live their lives and, wherever possible, return to work. In the report 'Commissioning Guidance for Rehabilitation (March 2016)' the NHS advises to use a **holistic** and person-centred approach, recognising the interaction of mental and physical health. It proposes a six-stage process of rehabilitation from high dependence to independence.

The process begins with acute complex specialised rehabilitation, for example in complex psychosis units. As the person improves, they may be moved to a ward in a general mental hospital. Later, they may return to live in the community with support from a community psychiatric nurse and trained staff, who helps them to develop a healthier lifestyle. Structured peer support, for example through a voluntary support group, provides further support. Finally, the person becomes independent, using community assets to pursue hobbies and a healthier lifestyle such as parks, outdoor gyms, swimming pools and leisure facilities. They achieve physical and mental health together.

This is the ideal. Unfortunately, in practice this does not always work. Those with complex psychosis, whose needs are more than can be met by general mental health services, may often be cared for a long way from home and support networks and far away from the support services they need when discharged. The Care Quality Commission have asked the Department of Health and Social Care and NHS England to use local health and care systems to reduce the number of patients placed in out-of-area mental health rehabilitation wards.

Key terms

Holistic refers to an approach that acknowledges the whole person, and therefore meets their range of physical, emotional and social needs.

Rehabilitation is the process of restoring someone to health or normal life through training and therapy after addiction, or illness.

IAPT services (Improving Access to Psychological Therapies)

Clinical Commissioning groups offer psychological therapies through **IAPT services (Improving Access to Psychological Therapies)** pathway. If people have a long-term condition (LTC) such as diabetes or heart problems, this treatment may also combine physical health care for long-term conditions with psychological therapies. This is then called the IAPT-LTC pathway.

This holistic approach to care means that someone needing psychological therapy, such as counselling for depression, should at the same time be able to get any physical care needed, such as advice about their diabetes care. This **joined-up approach** to care is better for individuals but requires practitioners to work together across specialities. For example, at the Oxford Health NHS Foundation Trust, psychological well-being practitioners and cardiac rehabilitation nurses work together to support people with depression and cardiac problems (**http://positivepracticemhdirectory.org**).

Crisis services

During a mental health **crisis**, a person may feel:

- unable to cope
- emotionally distressed
- anxious
- may self-harm
- experience hallucinations and/or hear voices.

People with mental ill-health are more likely to hurt themselves than others. In this situation, the person needs expert help. They may have a crisis line number from a health professional and a care plan that states who to contact for urgent care. If the situation is life threatening, they or others nearby can call 999 or the person can go to A&E. For urgent concerns about children and young people, vulnerable adults or people with learning difficulties, social services are the best contact. There is always an emergency social worker on duty and the number is on the local council website.

In a crisis, when someone is experiencing a psychotic episode, self-harming or threatening or attempting suicide, the Crisis Resolution and Home Treatment services (CRHT) may be needed. CRHT are a 24-hour service. Often, the police or hospital A&E staff contact the team on behalf of the person having an acute crisis. CRHTs try to avoid hospital admission for the individual, and try to review them at home or in a crisis house, providing support so they can stay at home. CRHTs are also involved in planning a person's discharge or temporary leave if they have been hospitalised. The team support people as they leave hospital and work with the community mental health team to try to prevent the person having a relapse.

Crisis houses have a small number of beds and are sometimes used short-term instead of admitting a person to hospital. People are usually referred from mental health services. They are also used if a person's home is unsuitable. They provide a safe environment where a vulnerable person or one in danger of committing suicide can be treated (**www.nhs.uk/using-the-nhs/nhs-services/ mental-health-services/dealing-with-a- mental-health-crisis-or-emergency**).

Effective support for people experiencing mental crisis requires organisations to work together. In 2014, Crisis Care Concordat was set up by the government and the mental health charity MIND. It created local working agreements between the police, social care, mental health and ambulance services. The Concordat focuses on four areas:

1 Access to support before crisis point, i.e. making sure people with mental health problems can get help 24 hours a day and

that when they ask for help, they are taken seriously.

2 Urgent and emergency access to crisis care, i.e. making sure that a mental health crisis is treated with the same urgency as a physical health emergency.

3 Quality of treatment and care when in crisis, i.e. making sure that people are treated with dignity and respect, in a therapeutic environment.

4 Recovery and staying well, i.e. preventing future crises by making sure people are referred to the appropriate service.

(**Source: www.crisiscareconcordat.org.uk**)

 Key terms

Clinical Commissioning Groups (CCGs) are local public bodies made up of doctors, nurse specialists, lay people and others such as service users. They commission (buy) care services from private and NHS providers to meet the needs of their local community.

Crisis refers to a sudden severe onset of symptoms that can be harmful to the individual and others.

IAPT services (Improving Access to Psychological Therapies) provides psychological therapies to people with anxiety disorders and depression. In many cases people can refer themselves to this service.

Joined-up approach is when services work together, for example a social worker from social services and a GP from primary care may support a person with addiction issues.

Description Activity

Using a variety of sources, describe in detail one type of support available to individuals with mental ill-health and others who support them. Describe the support offered, who can access it and how they can access it. Provide contact details for each source. At least two different references should be used and referenced in the text and at the end.

4.3 The role of the health and social care practitioner in promoting mental health and well-being

Health care practitioners such as doctors and nurses, including mental health nurses, physiotherapists, psychologists and health care assistants, work in NHS hospitals and the community. Social care practitioners such as social workers and social work assistants work in the community. Because health care is organised nationally and social care is organised by local councils, the two sets of practitioners do not always work together, and may be unaware of developments within their geographical area. In addition to these professionals, police, youth workers and teachers may also be involved with people with mental health issues. However, health and social care practitioners may be the only ones with specialist training in mental health.

Duty of care

In *Unit HSC M1: Equality, diversity and rights in health and social care,* the duty of care is explained in detail. **Duty of care** refers to health and social care practitioners' responsibility or duty to ensure the safety and well-being of individuals and others while providing care or support.

The Mental Capacity Code of Practice is the code that supports the Mental Capacity Act 2005. It sets out how those who work with individuals who lack capacity should apply the principles of the Act, such as the support that can be provided to an individual who is unable to make a decision, what information should be provided to individuals and how. There is also a code of conduct provided by the Nursing and Midwifery Council which was updated in 2018. For more information, see *Unit HSC M4: Communication in health and social care.*

As part of prioritising people, social workers, nurses, midwives and nursing associates must make sure that people's physical, social and psychological needs are assessed and responded to appropriately. They must act as an advocate for the vulnerable, challenging poor practice and discriminatory attitudes and behaviours relating to their care. They must act in the best interests of people at all times while balancing this with the requirement to respect a person's right to accept or refuse treatment. They must ensure they get properly informed consent and document it before carrying out any action, keep to all relevant laws about mental capacity that apply in the country in which they are practising, and ensure that the rights and best interests of those who lack capacity are still at the centre of the decision-making process. For further information about duty of care, see *Unit HSC M1.*

 Key term

Duty of care refers to the health and social care practitioner's legal obligation to ensure the safety and well-being of individuals and others, such as their colleagues and visitors, while providing care and support.

Safeguarding

Social workers, nurses, midwives and nursing associates must ensure that they work within the limits of their competence, exercising professional 'duty of candour' and raising concerns immediately whenever they come across situations that put patients or the public at risk. They must take action to deal with any concerns where appropriate. They must accurately identify, observe and assess signs of normal or worsening physical and mental health in the person receiving care, referring them on when necessary. They must act without delay if they believe that there is a risk to patient or public safety, for example if a patient threatens to harm themselves or others.

Health and social care practitioners must take all reasonable steps to protect vulnerable people or those at risk from harm, neglect or abuse. They must share information if they believe someone may be at risk of harm, in line with the laws relating to the disclosure of information, and they must know and follow the relevant laws and policies about protecting and caring for vulnerable people.

Care planning

Care planning is not done to someone, but it is discussed, planned and agreed with them. Care planning should consider all of an individual's needs, not just what services are available. The plan should be made with them and reviewed regularly, especially after any change. According to the English Mental Health Act Code of Practice and guidance from the National Institute for Health and Care Excellence (NICE), a care plan should be made with the individual on admission to a mental health unit, including planning for discharge. It needs to be reviewed after admission and before for discharge. Care plans should also consider the person's strengths and aims for their future with the support of services.

In England and Wales, the care plan should identify how the social worker, community mental health team and GP will work together to support the person after discharge. It should assess risks, plan for any problems following discharge and provide the contact details of who to talk to if they need help. Individuals should be given at least 48 hours' notice of the discharge date and care arrangements discussed with those involved in their care. Anyone considered at risk of suicide should be followed up within 48 hours of discharge.

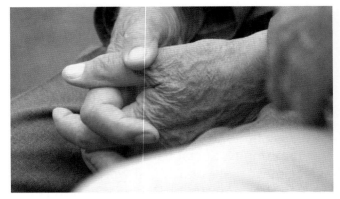

Figure 7.4 Counselling is often part of treatment

In England, the Care Programme Approach (CPA) is for people with severe or complex mental health problems and those who need support from a number of agencies. People who are currently (or were) recently sectioned under the Mental Health Act 2005 should be supported under the CPA. They should have:

- support from a CPA care co-ordinator
- a full assessment of needs, including all the supporting services
- a written care plan, which includes plans for risks and what should happen in case of a crisis
- ongoing review of care, including a full review of all the support from all services at least once a year
- consideration of ongoing need for CPA support
- consideration of the need for advocate support
- support for identified carers. They should be told of any rights they have to have their needs assessed while giving care.

Care planning depends on the individual's condition and needs. It may include:

- medical treatment needed for mental and physical health, including medication

- identifying risks to the individual's well-being and safety and to the safety of others
- identifying the process to follow in case of crisis
- needs related to alcohol or drug problems
- personal circumstances including family and carers
- financial circumstances
- housing needs
- employment, education and training needs.

Person-centred practice

All codes of practice in health and social care identify that the individual must be at the centre of care. This means that their needs must be identified and plans made to meet their needs, otherwise the plan is bound to fail. The opposite of person-centred practice is service-led practice, where what services are offered determine what care is given and individual needs are often not a priority.

Everyone in need of care should have a care plan that considers all their needs as discussed earlier. Each organisation has their own format but every care plan should consider physical, as well as mental, needs. For example, a person desperate to escape an unhappy relationship and admitted to a crisis house must have their need for safety and security identified and plans made for their safe discharge into the community: they should not be discharged back to the home with the abusive partner.

Referral

Health and social care practitioners are responsible for referring people needing mental health support to the appropriate services at the right time. A midwife or health visitor may be concerned about a new mother with depression and refer the woman to the GP. A GP as a health care practitioner is often the first person someone sees if they have mental health issues. A GP may refer someone with depression for counselling, or if they are in crisis, they might refer them to mental health services as an emergency admission.

Encouraging self-referral

Where possible, individuals should be empowered to recognise when they need help and refer themselves. Some mental health services that allow self-referrals are services for drug problems and alcohol problems, as well as psychological therapies (IAPT) services. Details are available locally in GP surgeries, pharmacists and online. The Samaritans have a free confidential service and telephone support 24 hours a day, 365 days a year, on 116 123. If the situation is not life-threatening, the individual can call NHS 111 or book an emergency GP appointment.

Information, advice, guidance

Health and social care practitioners offer information, advice and guidance and can also signpost to other sources of help, such as local support groups, depending where an individual is in the process of recovery and rehabilitation. Hospital out-patient departments often have details of local support groups. National charities such as MIND, Rethink and the Mental Health Foundation are just three organisations which practitioners may suggest that offer information, advice and guidance online.

Positive relationships

Health and social care practitioners have a role in promoting positive relationships as part of helping people with their mental health. However, practitioners must maintain professional boundaries. The General Social Care Council's Code of Conduct 5.4 states that social care workers should not form inappropriate relationships with clients, while 5.8 states they should not behave in a way, in work or outside work, which would call into question their suitability to work in social care. Within those boundaries, practitioners can support people to have positive relationships. The code of conduct for health care support workers and adult social care workers in England, the Nursing and Midwifery code for nurses, midwives and nursing associates, and the standards of the Health and Care Professionals Council all reflect these values.

Research by Gilburt, Rose and Slade (2008) showed that practitioners who communicate effectively, are culturally sensitive and do not use **coercion**, and convey a sense of trust which results in patients experiencing the hospital as a place of safety in terms of risk from other patients and staff.

 Key term

Coercion is the action of persuading someone to do something by using force or threats.

Activities

Part of a therapeutic programme of recovery includes a variety of activities. Good mental health is about learning to manage emotions, both positive and negative, and being able to form and maintain healthy relationships with others. It is also about coping with and managing change. Health and social care practitioners can help individuals with their mental health by working with an individual to plan activities.

Physical and mental activity promotes physical and mental health. For example, singing as part of a group, or alone, reinforces memory. A person with dementia may attend a day centre with their carer and join in singing activities combined with gentle exercises. Some care homes invite nursery schools to bring their classes into

care homes so that old and young can share activities. Social contact between generations promotes good mental health: older people are happy to see young people, and young children learn empathy by meeting older people.

For people with depression or anger issues, keeping a mood tracker and recording emotions every two hours helps with recognising their mood and what triggers certain emotions. Mindfulness exercises, such as focusing on one sense for one minute, for example 'How many things can you hear?', can promote calmness at any age.

Someone with social anxiety might need help with social situations, so a health and social care practitioner might support them by providing a gentle introduction to social interaction, for example walking with them in the park so they get used to other people. A support worker may help someone with a cognitive impairment in sheltered accommodation to plan a short holiday, and support workers will accompany the group as carers. The role of the practitioner is to support the individual during these activities and help them towards independence. Activities must be part of a planned programme agreed with the individual and must address their needs.

Risk management

Health and social care practitioners are responsible for assessing and managing risks to those in their care and to members of the public. All activities must be risk assessed. This involves assessing:

- Who might be involved in the activity.
- Where the activity will take place.
- When and how the activity will work.
- Potential hazards, i.e. assessing the likelihood of harm and reducing that harm.

For example, it might be dangerous for a person with dementia to go to the park alone because they might get lost, but going to the park with a support worker would reduce the risk of harm.

Managing risk when a person has mental health issues follows the same principles of risk management. It must consider the individual's needs and preferences, and must balance the risk of harm to the individual and others against the opportunity for the individual to develop an improved mental health. The person's condition may vary from day to day, so risks must be assessed on an ongoing basis. An activity that is suitable for an individual when they are stable might not be suitable if they are in crisis, so the activity might need adapting. Someone in a manic state may benefit from relaxing music, whereas the same person in a depressive state might benefit from music that lightens their mood. Each organisation has its own procedure for risk assessment and this must be followed at all times.

In *Unit HSC M1: Equality, diversity and rights in health and social care*, risk management and the health and social care practitioner's role is outlined in more detail. In *Unit HSC O3: Creative activities in health and social care*, there are more details regarding risk management when planning activities.

Explain Activity

Put together a careers file that explains the role of health and social care practitioners in promoting mental health and well-being. Ensure that you use examples and include more than one type of health and social care practitioner.

Use a range of sources to support what you say and reference your sources.

4.4 National strategies to promote mental health and well-being

In addition to what health and social care practitioners do as part of their practice, there are national plans or strategies which the government has put in place to improve mental health and well-being.

Closing the gap: priorities for essential change in mental health (Department of Health 2014) is the same document as Mental Health: Priorities for Change 2014. It explains how changes in local service planning and delivery will make a difference to the lives of people with mental health problems. For more details see Learning Objective 2 in this unit.

No Health Without Mental Health (Department of Health 2011) is a strategy to improve mental health and well-being. For more details see Learning Objective 2 in this unit.

Strategies relevant to Home Nation
Scotland

The Scottish Mental Health Strategy 2017–2027 published in 2017 by the Scottish government focuses on:

- Prevention and early intervention.
- Access to treatment and joined-up, accessible services.
- The physical well-being of people with mental health problems.
- Rights, information use, and planning.
- Data and measurement.

It is part of a range of measures the Scottish government is taking to create a Fairer Scotland. In the Scottish government's 2020 Vision for Health and Social Care, delivery, integrated care and prevention, anticipation and supported self-management are emphasised. The Scottish government's

Health and Social Care Delivery Plan places equal importance on mental and physical health and the need to address underlying conditions, such as housing and unemployment, which affect health.

Northern Ireland

Northern Ireland published Mental Health in Northern Ireland: Overview, Strategies, Policies, Care Pathways, CAMHS and Barriers to Accessing Services (2017). It highlights relevant strategies and policies specific to mental health, mental illness and suicide for Northern Ireland. It describes the care pathway for treating mental health problems, with specific reference to child and adolescent mental health services (CAMHS). Key documents include the Bamford Review of Mental Health and Learning Disability, a series of 11 reports published by 2007, reviewing law, policy and provisions affecting people with mental ill-health or a learning disability. The Northern Ireland Executive has also made 'Improving Mental Health' an indicator in the Draft Programme for Government 2016–2021.

Check your understanding 4

1 How can a person promote their own mental health and well-being?
2 What support is available to individuals and others?
3 What is the role of the health and social care practitioner in promoting an individual's mental health and well-being?

Case scenario

Sam is 15 years old and worried that she is not attractive and that she is not clever enough to pass her exams. She is worried about letting her parents down as they have high hopes for her. She has so much to revise and nothing seems to stay in her head. When she feels really down, she binges on crisps and chocolate and has put on weight, which makes her feel even more depressed. She spends a lot of time in her room at home, away from her little brother and sister, and avoiding her mum who always seems to be nagging her. To make matters worse, her mum and dad have split up, and her dad has moved away so she doesn't see him much. One night, after a particularly bad argument with her mum, she locks herself in her room and considers ending it all.

1 What immediate help could Sam get?
2 Which professionals might help Sam?
3 What help might they offer?
4 What could Sam do to help herself and improve her own mental health?

Classroom Discussion

What support is available for mental health for your age group? You may need to do some research before the discussion. Consider both local and national support and the different ways of getting support, such as online or telephone support. How likely might someone of your age use the support? What might put them off? What might encourage them to use the support?

Activity

Create a poster that outlines one national strategy to promote mental health and well-being. The information should identify the strategy and summarise the key points, and a reference for further information should be provided.

Read about it

Gilburt, H., Rose, D. and Slade, M., 2008, 'The importance of relationships in mental health care: A qualitative study of service users' experiences of psychiatric hospital admission in the UK', *BMC Health Services Research*, Vol. 8, Number 1, p. 1, available at https://bmchealthservres.biomedcentral.com/articles/10.1186/1472-6963-8-92

Haddon, M., 2008, *The Curious Incident of the Dog in the Night-time*, Vintage (for an insight into Asperger's and autism)

Examples of good practice

Campaign against mental health discrimination www.time-to-change.org.uk

Improved Access to Psychological Therapies and Long term physical health conditions; IAPT-LTC services http://positivepracticemhdirectory.org/nccmh/talking-space-plus-iapt-oxford-healthcare-nhs-foundation-trust-nccmh

The firm whose staff are all autistic www.bbc.co.uk/news/technology-46538125

Charities for mental health

ADFAM for families with addiction https://adfam.org.uk

Alcoholics Anonymous www.alcoholics-anonymous.org.uk

Children's Society – (children's well-being) www.childrenssociety.org.uk/good-childhood-report

FRANK – (drug advice) www.talktofrank.com

Homelessness and mental health www.homeless.org.uk

Mental health foundation www.mentalhealth.org.uk

MIND www.mind.org.uk

Papyrus preventing suicide in young people https://papyrus-uk.org

Rethink Mental Health www.rethink.org

Streetlink – (to refer homeless people to services) www.streetlink.org.uk

The Campaign Against Living Miserably (CALM) – (a movement against male suicide) www.thecalmzone.net

Young minds mental health issues https://youngminds.org.uk

NHS

Cannabis and psychosis www.nhs.uk/news/mental-health/cannabis-linked-to-psychosis

Child and Adolescent Mental Health Services www.nhs.uk/using-the-nhs/nhs-services/mental-health-services/child-and-adolescent-mental-health-services-camhs

Help for drug addiction www.nhs.uk/live-well/healthy-body/drug-addiction

Improved Access to Psychological Therapies www.england.nhs.uk/publication/the-improving-access-to-psychological-therapies-iapt-pathway-for-people-with-long-term-physical-health-conditions-and-medically-unexplained-symptoms

Mental health and children www.nhs.uk/news/mental-health/nearly-quarter-14-year-old-girls-uk-self-harming-charity-reports/

Mental Health conditions www.nhs.uk/conditions

Mental health crisis www.nhs.uk/using-the-nhs/nhs-services/mental-health-services/dealing-with-a-mental-health-crisis-or-emergency

Mental Health Services www.england.nhs.uk/mental-health

Mood disorders and body clock disruption www.nhs.uk/news/mental-health/body-clock-disruptions-linked-mood-disorders

NHS help for substance misusers www.nhs-substance-misuse-provider-alliance.org.uk

Royal College of Psychiatrists – (information about mental disorders) www.rcpsych.ac.uk/mental-health/problems-disorders/personality-disorder

Policy, planning, strategy

Better Care Fund www.england.nhs.uk/ourwork/part-rel/transformation-fund/bcf-plan

Closing the gap: priorities for essential change in mental health https://assets.publishing.service.gov.uk

CQC Mental health services 2014–2017 www.cqc.org.uk/publications/major-report/state-care-mental-health-services-2014-2017

How the NHS works www.kingsfund.org.uk/audio-video/how-does-nhs-in-england-work

Mental Health; priorities for change www.gov.uk/government/publications

NHS Five Year Forward View www.england.nhs.uk

NHS Guidance on rehabilitation www.england.nhs.uk/wp-content/uploads/2016/04/rehabilitation-comms-guid-16-17.pdf

No Health without Mental Health, 2011 www.gov.uk/government/publications

Northern Ireland Mental Health strategies and policies www.niassembly.gov.uk/assembly-business/committees/2016-2017/committee-for-health/research-papers-2017/mental-health-in-northern-ireland-overview-strategies-policies-care-pathways-camhs-and-barriers-to-accessing-services

Scotland's Mental Health Strategy 2017–2027 www.gov.scot/publications/mental-health-strategy-2017-2027

Talk to Frank – (self-referral drugs helpline) www.talktofrank.com or by calling the Frank drugs helpline 0300 123 6600

The Mental Health Crisis Care Concordat – (organisations working together to improve support for people in mental health crises) www.crisiscareconcordat.org.uk

The mental health strategy for England www.gov.uk/government/publications

Laws

Equality Act 2010 and Human Rights Act www.equalityhumanrights.com

Health and Social Care Act 2012 www.legislation.gov.uk/ukpga/2012/7/contents/enacted

Mental Capacity Act 2005 www.scie.org.uk/mca/introduction/mental-capacity-act-2005-at-a-glance

Mental Health Act www.scie.org.uk/publications/guides/guide15/legislation

Problems with Health and Social Care Act 2012 www.kingsfund.org.uk

World Health Organization www.who.int

How will I be graded?

The table below shows what learners must do to achieve each grading criterion. Learners must achieve all the criteria for a grade to be awarded. A higher grade may not be awarded before a lower grade has been achieved, although component criteria of a higher grade may have been achieved.

Grade	Assessment Criteria number	Assessment Criteria
D1	1.1	Define: • mental health • mental ill-health.
D2	1.2	Outline types of mental ill-health. A minimum of three (3) types of mental ill-health must be outlined.
D3		A minimum of one (1) relevant and traceable reference must be included.
C1	2.1	Outline one (1) piece of legislation or policy in relation to mental health and well-being.
C2	4.4	Outline one (1) national strategy to promote mental health and well-being.

Grade	Assessment Criteria number	Assessment Criteria
B1	3.2	Discuss public attitudes towards mental ill-health.
B2	4.1	Describe how an individual can promote their own mental health and well-being.
		A minimum of two (2) ways an individual can promote their own mental health and well-being must be described.
B3		A minimum of two (2) relevant and traceable references must be included. A reference list must be included.
A1	3.1	Describe the impact mental ill-health can have on individuals and others.
A2	4.2	Describe support available to individuals and others.
		A minimum of four (4) types of support available to individuals and others must be described.
A*1	4.3	Explain the role of the health and social care practitioner in promoting mental health and well-being.
A*2		References must be present throughout to show evidence of knowledge and understanding gained from wider reading. References must be relevant and traceable.

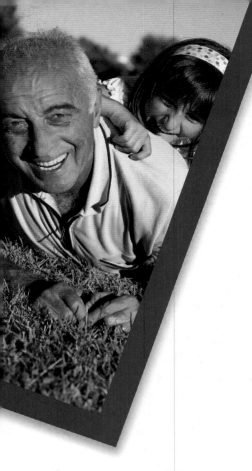

HSC 010
Nutrition for health and social care

About this unit

The aim of this unit is to provide learners with the knowledge and understanding of nutrition for health and social care.

This unit is about the nutrients and food groups that make up a healthy diet, and what the current guidelines and recommendations are to help plan a healthy diet across all the life stages, from infants to adults. Dietary intake has an impact on our health and well-being, so the factors which influence what we choose to eat are crucial in remaining healthy. Health and social care practitioners have an important role in promoting a healthy diet, influencing people to make the right choices so they remain healthy.

Learning Outcomes

LO1: Understand nutritional needs across the lifespan.

1.1 The main food groups:

- starches/whole grains
- meats, poultry, fish, nuts and seeds
- fruits and vegetables
- dairy
- fats.

1.2 The components of a healthy diet:

- nutrients (carbohydrates, protein, fat) and food sources
- vitamins and minerals and food sources.

1.3 Current nutritional guidelines for a healthy diet:

- World Health Organization
- National Health Service
- Department of Health
- National Institute for Health and Care Excellence
- Reference intakes.

1.4 Nutritional needs across the life stages:
Nutritional needs:

- balanced diet for growth and health
- nutrient and hydration requirements.

Life stages:

- infants
- children
- adolescence
- early, middle and late adulthood (consider: males, females, pregnancy).

LO2: Understand the impact of diet on health and well-being.

2.1 Factors which influence dietary intake:

- special dietary requirements (intolerances; allergies; medical; religious/cultural, preparation)
- socio-economic
- cost
- location
- life stage
- level of activity

→

- preferences
- availability
- ill-health.

2.2 The impact of dietary intake on health and well-being.

- balanced diet: (growth and development, energy, increased immunity) versus unbalanced diet (illness, disease, malnutrition, obesity)
- long-term and short-term impacts.

LO3: Understand how the health and social care practitioner promotes a healthy diet.

3.1 How initiatives promote healthy eating:

- local, national, global initiatives
- current initiatives as relevant to Home Nation.

3.2 How the health and social care practitioner promotes a healthy diet:

- education
- informed choices
- empowerment
- modelling
- access and availability
- nutritional planning.

LO1 Understand nutritional needs across the lifespan

This section will focus on the main food groups and the components of a healthy diet, including the current nutritional guidelines that should be followed. As we grow and transition through the life stages, from infancy to adulthood, our nutritional needs will change, i.e. a balanced diet for growth and health, as well as nutrient and hydration requirements.

1.1 The main food groups

The food we eat can be divided up in to five main food groups: starches/whole grains, meats, fruits and vegetables, dairy and fats. More information about each food group is listed in this section.

Starches/whole grains

This group consists of:

- Bread
- Rice
- Potatoes, yams and plantain
- Cereals, for example oats, maize, wheat, pearl barley, cornmeal
- Pasta and noodles
- Whole grains, for example couscous, quinoa, millet, spelt.

These starchy foods should make up approximately one-third of the food we eat. They are a good source of energy. The wholemeal or wholegrain product, for example brown rice or wholemeal bread, should be chosen when possible because it is higher in **fibre**. Fibre is found in the cell walls of vegetables, fruit, pulses and cereal grains. The fibre cannot be broken down by the digestive system so passes through the intestine, absorbing water and increasing in bulk. This process helps strengthen the muscles of the intestines and push out undigested food.

Meats, poultry, fish, nuts and seeds

This group consists of:

- Meat, for example beef, lamb
- Poultry, for example chicken, turkey
- Game, for example duck, goose, pheasant
- All types of fish, for example salmon, cod, mackerel
- Nuts, for example peanuts, walnuts, hazelnuts
- Beans, for example kidney, black, baked
- Pulses, for example chick peas, lentils
- Seeds, for example sunflower, sesame.

These foods are good sources of protein and some, such as beans, seeds and pulses, are lower in fat.

Fruit and vegetables

Fruit and vegetables should make up just over a third of the food we eat each day. Vegetables provide B-group vitamins, vitamin C and fibre. Green vegetables also provide iron and calcium.

Fruits contain a variety of micronutrients, especially vitamin C. They are also a good source of fibre.

For healthy eating, it is recommended as part of your five a day, two servings come from fruits and the other three from vegetables. These should each be 80 g servings for adults.

Dairy

This group refers to food products containing or made from milk, and examples include:

- Milk
- Cheese
- Yoghurt, crème fraiche
- Dairy alternatives, such as soya or almond milk.

Dairy foods are good sources of protein, vitamins and minerals and should be eaten every day to keep bones and teeth strong.

Fats

The body uses fat as a source fuel, and fat is the major storage form of energy in the body. This group consists of:

- Oils, for example sunflower, olive
- Soft spreads
- Butter, lard, margarine.

Fats are needed in the diet for warmth and energy but in very small quantities, as an excess of fat storage is unhealthy and can lead to different health complications, such as obesity or diabetes.

Saturated fats are solid at room temperature and are generally found in animal products such as red meat, butter, lard and in pastries, cakes and biscuits. They have been linked to heart disease as they can lead to a build-up of fatty deposits in and around the heart.

Unsaturated fats are liquid at room temperature and are found in oils, nuts, seeds, and oily fish. Research suggests that unsaturated fats are healthier than saturated fats as they may lower blood cholesterol and reduce the risk of heart disease.

Activity

Prepare a poster showing the five main food groups and some of their sources.

1.2 The components of a healthy diet

Nutrients

Nutrients are the vital components which make up food. The food you eat should provide your body with the nutrients it needs to stay alive and be healthy. Each nutrient has a specific function and is found in different food sources. **Macronutrients** are needed by the body in large amounts, for example protein, fat and carbohydrates. **Micronutrients** are needed by the body in small amounts, for example vitamins and minerals.

Sources and functions of macronutrients

Table 8.1 Sources and functions of macronutrients

Nutrient	Sources	Function	
Protein	Meat, poultry, game All types of fish Nuts Beans – kidney beans, baked beans Pulses – chick peas, lentils Seeds – sunflower, sesame	Growth, repair and maintenance of tissues. A secondary source of energy.	
Fat	Oils, for example sunflower, olive Soft spreads Butter, lard, margarine	Provides energy. Keeps the body warm. Protects organs. Provides essential fatty acids and the fat-soluble vitamins A, D, E and K.	
Carbohydrate starches	Starchy sources of carbohydrates, such as: ● Potatoes ● Cereal and cereal products such as bread, pasta and rice ● Root vegetables. Sugary sources of carbohydrates – all types of sugar, including: ● Treacle, golden syrup ● Honey, jam, marmalade.	Energy for movement and growth. Chemical reactions and processes.	

Sources and functions of vitamins

Sources and functions of minerals

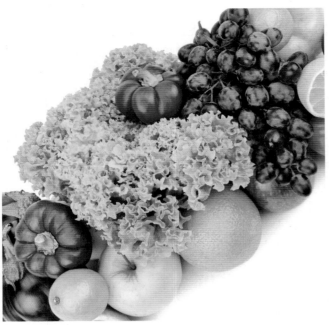

Figure 8.1 Sources of vitamins

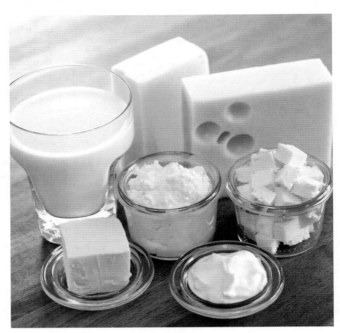

Figure 8.2 Sources of minerals

Table 8.2 Sources and functions of vitamins

Vitamin	Sources	Function
A	Animal sources, for example eggs, oily fish, milk, butter, liver, cheese. Plant sources, for example spinach, carrots, sweet potatoes, butternut squash, cantaloupe melon, papaya.	Helps vision in dim light; protects the body as it is an **antioxidant**.
D	Sunshine, milk, eggs, **fortified** breakfast cereals, fat spreads.	Prevents bone diseases; develops and maintains bones and teeth. Helps the body to absorb calcium.
E	Green peas, beans, broccoli, spinach, vegetable oils.	Protects the body; it is an antioxidant.
K	Green leafy vegetables, vegetable oils, cereal grains.	Helps blood to clot and maintains bone health.
B1 Thiamin B2 Riboflavin B3 Niacin	Fortified breakfast cereals, milk, flour and bread, eggs.	Releases energy from food; helps the nervous system.
B6 Pyridoxine	Vitamin B6 is found in lean meat, eggs, chicken, fish, beans, nuts, whole grains and cereals, bananas and avocados.	Vitamin B6 is involved in the metabolism and the maintenance of the immune system, including the formation of antibodies.
Folic acid	Fortified breakfast cereals, broccoli, sprouts, chick peas, spinach, and peas.	Reduces the risk of nervous system faults in unborn babies. Folic acid is needed to make new DNA and to allow the body to make immune cells in response to infection.

→

Vitamin	Sources	Function
B12	Meat, eggs, milk and cheese, salmon and cod, fortified breakfast cereals.	Maintains the nerves, makes blood and releases energy. Vitamin B12 works with Vitamin B6 to make new DNA and protein, which is used to make new immune cells.
C	Citrus fruits, blackcurrants, broccoli, red and green peppers, strawberries.	Makes and maintains healthy connective tissue; helps wounds to heal; helps the absorption of iron in the body.

Table 8.3 Sources and functions of minerals

Mineral	Sources	Function
Calcium	Nuts, bread and fortified cereals, cheese, milk, green leafy vegetables, soya and tofu.	Builds strong bones and teeth.
Iron	Meat, eggs, fortified cereals, bread, green leafy vegetables, nuts, dried fruit.	Makes haemoglobin in red blood cells to carry oxygen around the body.
Sodium (salt)	Cheese, salted nuts, smoked fish, bacon, ready meals, tinned food.	Maintains water balance in the body.
Fluorine	In some areas, it is added to drinking water, sardines, seafood, and tea.	Prevents tooth decay.
Iodine	Red meat, sea fish and shellfish, cereals and grains.	Makes the hormone thyroxine, which maintains a healthy metabolic rate.
Phosphorus	Red meat, dairy foods, fish, poultry, brown rice, oats.	Maintains bones and teeth with calcium; releases energy from food.

Key terms

Antioxidants protect cells from harmful substances.

Fibre is a substance found in the cell walls of vegetables, fruit, pulses and cereal grains. It is an essential component of a healthy diet.

Fortified refers to a food that has vitamins or minerals added to it to improve its nutritional value, for example breakfast cereals and bread.

Macronutrients are required by the body in large amounts, for example protein, fat and carbohydrates.

Micronutrients are required by the body in small amounts, for example vitamins and minerals.

Nutrients are the vital components which make up food. Each nutrient has a specific role in the body, for example the growth of bones.

Description Activity

Briefly describe the function of protein, fat, carbohydrate, vitamins and minerals in the diet, using relevant examples.

1.3 Current nutritional guidelines for a healthy diet

It is important to make an informed choice for a heathy and balanced diet. Published guidelines are a useful source of information to enable us to make these choices.

World Health Organization

The World Health Organization (WHO) has an important role in providing scientific advice, advising how to address **malnutrition** and support the health and well-being of every individual throughout their life. Malnutrition is a deficiency, excess, or imbalance of nutrients that causes adverse effects on health and well-being. Some key facts WHO have recognised are:

1 Adequate nutrition is a crucial part of health and development.

2 Malnutrition remains a risk to human health, whether it be undernutrition or overnutrition.

3 A healthy diet helps to protect against malnutrition and diseases, such as diabetes, heart disease, **stroke** and cancer.

4 An unhealthy diet and lack of physical activity are leading global risks to health.

The advice and information on nutritional guidelines is used by government, as well as the public and private sectors. Governments have a central role in creating a healthy food environment that enables people to adopt and maintain healthy dietary practices. Some of the effective actions taken include:

- Increasing incentives for producers and retailers to grow, use and sell fresh fruit and vegetables.

- Reducing incentives for the food industry to continue or increase production of processed foods containing high levels of **saturated fats**, trans-fats, free sugars and salt/sodium.

- Ensuring the availability of healthy, nutritious, safe and affordable foods in pre-schools, schools, other public institutions and the workplace.

Some of the ways they also encourage consumer demand for healthy foods and meals are:

- Promoting consumer awareness of a healthy diet.

- Developing school policies and programmes that encourage children to adopt and maintain a healthy diet.

- Educating children, adolescents and adults about nutrition and healthy dietary practices.

- Encouraging culinary skills, including in children through schools.

- Supporting labelling that ensures accurate, information on nutrient contents in foods.

- Providing nutrition and dietary counselling at primary healthcare facilities.

- Promoting appropriate infant and young child feeding practices.

WHO Member States have agreed to reduce the global population's intake of salt by 30 per cent by 2025. They have also agreed to halt the rise in diabetes and obesity in adults and adolescents as well as in overweight children by 2025.

With many countries now seeing a rapid rise in obesity among infants and children, in May 2014, WHO set up the Commission on Ending Childhood Obesity. In 2016, the Commission proposed a set of recommendations to successfully tackle childhood and adolescent obesity in different contexts around the world.

In May 2018, WHO identified the reduction of salt/sodium intake and elimination of industrially-produced trans-fats from the food supply as part of their priority actions to achieve the aims of ensuring healthy lives and promote well-being for all, at all ages (**www.who.int/news-room/fact-sheets/ detail/healthy-diet**).

National Health Service

The National Health Service (NHS) has advice, tips and tools on helping people make better choices about health and well-being. They provide information about:

- Food groups in the diet.
- Fruit and vegetables, i.e. '5 a day'.
- Starchy foods in your diet.
- Milk and dairy foods, i.e. how to choose the lower-fat varieties.
- Beans, pulses, fish, eggs, meat and other proteins.
- Oils and spreads.
- Eating less saturated fat and sugar.

They also have a section online focusing on how individuals can lose weight. In this section, it is possible to check whether you are a healthy weight by calculating your **Body Mass Index (BMI)**. BMI is a measure that uses your height and weight to work out if your weight is healthy. It divides a person's weight in kilograms (kg) by their height in metres squared (m²).

There are recipes and weight loss plans available online, for example a 12-week diet and exercise plan to help lose weight and how to develop healthier eating habits.

Department of Heath

The Department of Health aims to help people live more independent and healthier lives for longer. Public Health England is an agency sponsored by the Department of Health and Social Care and it aims to protect and improve the nation's health and well-being, and reduce health inequalities.

Public Health England has produced eight tips for eating well. These include:

1 Base your meals on starchy foods.
2 Eat lots of fruit and vegetables.
3 Eat more fish, including a portion of oily fish each week.
4 Cut down on saturated fat and sugar.
5 Try to eat less salt, less than 6 g a day for adults.
6 Get active and try to be a healthy weight.
7 Drink plenty of water.
8 Don't skip breakfast.

Public Health England have also produced the Eatwell Guide which has been developed to show how eating different foods can make a healthy and balanced diet. It divides food into groups and shows the percentage of each food group needed for a healthy varied diet. This balance of foods does not need to be eaten every meal, but over the course of a day or two. For example:

- **Fruit and vegetables** – 40 per cent (5 portions per day are recommended)
- **Starchy carbohydrates** – 38 per cent
- **Protein** – 12 per cent
- **Dairy and alternatives** – 8 per cent
- **Oils and spreads** – 1 per cent

The Eatwell Guide also provides other information, such as:

- Foods high in fat and/or sugar are not in the main segments as they should be eaten less often and in small amounts.
- You should drink 6–8 glasses of liquid a day. These drinks could include water, lower fat milk, sugar-free drinks, tea and coffee. Fruit juices and smoothies are high in sugar, so only a maximum of 150 ml a day is recommended.
- A traffic light food label is included. The green label shows healthy choices.
- The average energy needs of men and women are included so that adults are reminded that all foods and drinks contain energy.

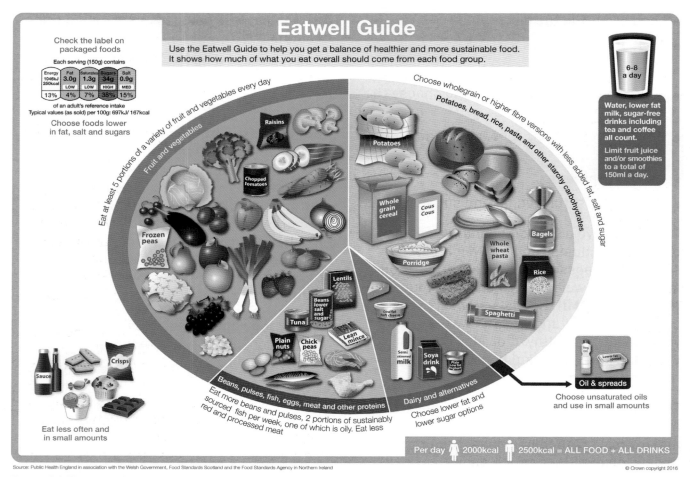

Figure 8.3 The Eatwell Guide

National Institute for Health and Care Excellence

The National Institute for Health and Care Excellence (NICE)'s role is to improve outcomes for people using the NHS and other public health and social care services. It provides a range of information services, evidence-based guidance, advice, and quality standards for health, public health and social care practitioners. Their guidance can be used by the NHS, local authorities, employers, voluntary groups and anyone who delivers care, and promotes well-being.

An example of a quality standard is QS98 – Maternal and Child Nutrition. This standard focuses on disadvantaged families and those with low incomes. It sets out improvements in nutrition for pregnant women and those trying to get pregnant, babies, children under 5 years, and the mothers and carers of young children. It describes how high-quality care can be improved in priority areas. The following topics are covered:

- Eating healthily while pregnant.
- Structured weight loss programmes.
- Breastfeeding.
- Advice on weaning.
- The 'Healthy Start' scheme, in partnership with the NHS.

For further information visit **www.nice.org.uk**

Reference intakes

Reference intakes are the maximum amount of calories and nutrients you should eat in a day. They are now displayed on food labels in a format such as the one shown in **Figure 8.4**.

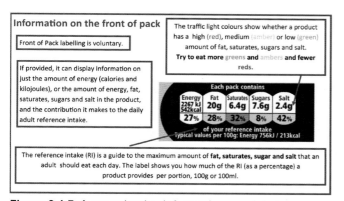

Figure 8.4 Reference intake: information on a label

Source: British Nutrition Foundation **www.nutrition.co.uk**

Daily reference intakes for adults are:

- Energy: 8,400 kJ/2,000 kcal
- Total fat: less than 70 g
- Saturates: less than 20 g
- Carbohydrate: at least 260 g
- Total sugars: 90 g
- Protein: 50 g
- Salt: less than 6 g

Reference intakes give consumers an idea of how much energy and other nutrients they should be eating each day. Unless the label says otherwise, reference intakes are based on an average-sized woman doing an average amount of physical activity. Specific reference intakes for both males and females at different life stages vary. This aims to prevent people with lower energy requirements eating more than they need. It is also a way of ensuring that the information on labels is consistent.

Key terms

Body Mass Index (BMI) is a calculation that is used to determine whether a person's weight is healthy in proportion to their height.

Malnutrition is a deficiency, excess, or imbalance of nutrients that causes adverse effects on health and well-being.

Saturated fats are fats from animal sources, for example butter and lard. They can be harmful to health as they have been linked to cardiovascular diseases.

Stroke refers to a serious, life-threatening medical condition that occurs when the blood supply to the brain is cut off.

Activity

You have been asked to develop an eating plan for an elderly patient in hospital. Summarise at least two current nutritional guidelines for a healthy diet that will help when developing the plan.

Reference daily intakes for some nutrients

Table 8.4 Reference daily intakes for some nutrients (**Source:** DEFRA Manual of Nutrition, 12th Edition, 2012)

	Boys 11 to 14 years	Girls 11 to 14 years	Men 19 to 50 years	Women 19 to 50 years
Protein (g)	42.1	41.2	55.5	45
Calcium (g)	1000	800	700	700
Iron (mg)	11.3	14.8	8.7	14.8
Vitamin C (mg)	35	35	40	40

1.4 Nutritional needs across the life stages

The nutritional needs of each individual will vary depending on their life stage. For example, a diet that is suitable for a child will not be suitable for an older person as they will have different nutritional needs. The nutritional needs will be outlined for each life stage in this section.

Nutritional needs

There are a number of different factors which affect an individual's nutritional needs.

The snacks, meals and drinks that you eat every day make up your diet. Your diet should include a variety of foods to ensure you get all the nutrients you need to stay healthy. No single food can supply all the nutrients you need. This is why you need a balanced diet containing lots of different foods, so that your diet provides all of the nutrients and energy your body needs.

You need a balanced diet for:

- Growth and repair of cells.
- Energy for physical activity.
- Protection from illnesses and diseases.
- Body processes, such as metabolism, breathing, digestion, transmitting nerve impulses, and maintaining body temperature.
- Stopping you feeling hungry.
- Well-being as eating is an enjoyable experience.

Nutrient requirements and the components of a healthy diet are discussed in section AC1.2.

Hydration requirements

Your body is made up of approximately 70 per cent water. Every cell and tissue in the body contains water so it is essential to life. **Hydration** is the supply of water required to maintain the correct amount of fluid in the body. **Dehydration** occurs when your body loses more water than you take in. To stay healthy, it is important to replace the water you lose when you breathe, sweat and urinate.

The functions of water include:

- cooling the body
- removing waste from the body
- swallowing food, i.e. it is an important component of saliva which helps with the digestive process.

How much fluid you need depends on many factors such as your age, diet, the amount of physical activity you do and the temperature of the environment. Most people need approximately 1.5 to 2 litres of water a day, which is about 8 average size glasses.

Besides water, you can get the fluid you need from soft drinks, milk and fruit juices. We get 70–80 per cent from drinks and drinking water. The remainder comes from food; fruit and vegetables contain a lot of water.

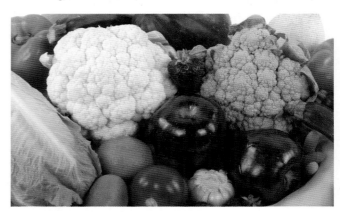

Figure 8.5 Foods that contain water

When your body does not have enough water, you become dehydrated. One of the first signs of dehydration is feeling thirsty. The impact on the body of dehydration is:

- Dark urine and/or not passing much urine when you go to the toilet
- Headaches
- Lack of energy
- Feeling lightheaded.

However, drinking too much water can also be harmful. The condition is called **water intoxication**. Water intoxication is extremely rare. The symptoms are:

- Headache
- Nausea and vomiting.

Severe cases can produce more serious symptoms, such as:

- Increased blood pressure
- Confusion
- Double vision
- Drowsiness
- Difficulty breathing.

Key terms

Dehydration occurs when the body loses more water than it takes in.

Hydration is the supply of water required to maintain the correct amount of fluid in the body.

Water intoxication is the condition when you drink too much water. Drinking too much water can be harmful.

Life stages

This section looks more closely at the nutritional needs of different life stages, ranging from infants and children to adolescence and early, middle and late adulthood, as well as the differences between males, females and those who are pregnant.

Infancy

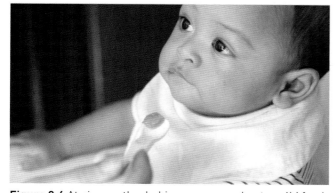

Figure 8.6 At six months, babies are weaned onto solid food

Infancy refers to the period of babyhood or early childhood (0–2 years). During the first 4 to 6 months of life, babies go through a period of rapid growth and development. Breast milk (or infant formula) contains all the nutrients required during this period. Breastfeeding is recommended by the Department of Health, especially for the first six months of life, and should ideally continue for the first year. The process of introducing solid foods into a baby's diet is called **weaning**. Most babies are weaned at six months old.

During the early months of life, babies draw upon iron stores they have accumulated before birth but these stores are rapidly depleted. It is important that the diet given during weaning contains enough iron to meet the baby's needs for growth and development. Requirements for protein and B vitamins also increase between 6 and 12 months. Young children go through rapid growth spurts, as well as normally having a very active lifestyle.

As children's stomachs are small, they cannot eat large meals at one time and so need to eat regular smaller meals, as well as snacks and drinks throughout the day to provide sufficient energy and nutrients. The Eatwell Guide should not be followed strictly for young children, as they benefit from foods such as whole milk that will provide more energy and the important fat-soluble vitamin D, which is needed for the absorption of calcium to strengthen bones and teeth.

Childhood

Childhood refers to the period of being a child (3–8 years). School children are growing fast and should be physically active every day, which increases the need for more energy (calories) in the diet. Their diet should be varied, following the principles of the Eatwell Guide, in order to ensure that they are consuming the foods they need to provide the nutrients and energy during this time of rapid growth and development. Because school children are not as active as in the past and due to an increase in the consumption of fatty/sugary foods, in 2016/17, one in five children in Year 6 and one in ten children in Reception were classified as obese (source: NHS Digital 'Statistics on Obesity, Physical Activity and Diet – England, 2018 [PAS]').

As a child's energy requirements increase, there is a greater need for protein, all vitamins (except vitamins C and D) and all minerals (except iron). Vitamin D will be synthesised in the skin following exposure to sunlight. The vitamin C and iron requirements do not need to change when a child is growing.

If children do eat foods and drinks containing sugar, it is best to have them only at meal times. Eating sugary foods frequently between meals can cause dental decay. Snack foods such as cakes, biscuits, crisps, chocolate and sweets are often high in sugar and saturated fat, and low in certain vitamins and minerals, so their consumption should be limited.

To achieve a high-energy intake, children should be eating small, frequent meals consisting of energy-rich foods. This may be necessary for younger children (4–6-year-olds), who do not have large enough stomachs to cope with big meals. Children's weight gain should be gradual and in line with height increases, so that they grow to be an acceptable weight for their height.

Milk and dairy products remain essential for tooth and bone development and, together with vitamin D, help to make bones stronger.

Adolescence

Adolescence refers to the period following the onset of **puberty**, during which a young person develops from a child into an adult. Puberty is the process during which there is a spurt of physical growth leading to an increase in height and weight, changes in body composition and sexual development.

Adolescents should follow the guidelines of the Eatwell Guide to ensure a good balance of foods and nutrients. While adolescents have rapid growth spurts, an increase in energy may not be needed by all. It will ultimately depend upon their current body weight. According to a study by UCL Institute of Education (IOE), one in five young people born in the UK at the turn of the century was obese by the age of 14, and a further 15 per cent were overweight.

Adolescent boys develop a higher proportion of new muscle tissue compared to girls so their protein requirements are higher. They are also usually taller and bigger than girls, which increases their calcium requirements for development of bones.

Adolescent girls require more iron than boys to compensate for the blood lost during menstrual periods.

It is important that adolescents continue to eat as healthily as possible during these years as they are critical for growth, especially some nutrients, for example calcium and vitamin D. This is because bones are still growing and although the skeleton is not fully formed until the late 20s, most of the minerals are laid down in the adolescent years to reach peak bone mass.

Early and middle adulthood

Adulthood refers to being fully grown or mature, and can be divided into early (19 to 45 years), middle (45–65 years) and late (65 years+) stages.

The adult's diet is very important even though they have stopped growing. Adults still need a well-balanced diet to ensure they have the correct nutrients in the right quantities. The Eatwell Guide should be followed by adults to ensure the right balance. At the adult stage of life, nutrients are needed for energy requirements, to maintain and repair body tissue and for normal bodily functions.

Table 8.5 The nutrient and energy needs of adolescents

Nutrient and energy needs	Reasons why they are important to adolescents
Protein	There is a greater need for protein due to rapid growth. Boys need more protein than girls as they have a higher proportion of muscle tissue.
Calcium and Vitamin D	For healthy bone and teeth development. Boys need more calcium than girls as they are usually a bigger build.
Iron and Vitamin C	To prevent iron deficiency anaemia by keeping the red blood cells healthy. The vitamin C helps the body to absorb iron. Adolescent girls need the most iron as they are menstruating.
B group vitamins	To release energy from carbohydrates.
Energy	Energy needs increase as the child gets older. Children are growing fast and should be physically active every day, which increases the need for more energy (calories) in the diet.

Nutrients that are especially important for adults are the mineral calcium and vitamin D. Vitamin D helps the body's absorption of calcium which ensures bones stay strong.

The mineral iron is also important to maintain as it can be low in adult diets, especially adult females who lose iron during menstruation. Vitamin C helps the body's absorption of iron, which is why the adult diet should contain a high proportion of fruit and vegetables.

In the UK, adults are more likely to be at risk of overnutrition than undernutrition. The dietary energy required by an adult should equal exactly the energy required for body maintenance and physical activity.

There are some key differences between adult males and females aged between 19 and 49 years old.

The nutrients that are especially important for women's health include iron due to menstruation and calcium to keep bones strong and prevent osteoporosis.

Men tend to have a larger body overall in terms of both height and weight, and will also have a greater muscle mass. This means that they will also have increased caloric needs compared to women and therefore need to eat more on a daily basis compared to women.

Pregnancy

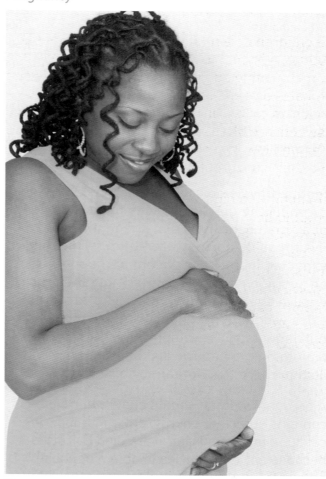

Figure 8.7 A pregnant woman

A woman's nutritional needs change during pregnancy because her diet must provide for the growth and development of the

Table 8.6 The nutrient and energy needs of adults aged 19 to 49

Nutrient	Males	Females
Protein	55.5 g	45 g
Vitamin A	700 mcg	600 mcg
Vitamin B1	1.0 mg	0.8 mg
Vitamin B2	1.3 mg	1.1 mg
Vitamin B3	17 mg	13 mg
Vitamin B6	1.4 mg	1.2 mg
Vitamin B12	1.5 mcg	1.5 mcg
Folic acid	200 mcg	200 mcg
Vitamin C	40 mg	40 mg
Vitamin D	Not stated as it is assumed it will be met by sunlight	Not stated as it is assumed it will be met by sunlight
Calcium	700 mg	700 mg
Phosphorus	550 mg	550 mg
Sodium	1,600 mg	1,600 mg
Potassium	3,500 mg	3,500 mg
Iron	8.7 mg	14.8 mg
Iodine	140 mcg	140 mcg
Zinc	9.5 mg	7.0 mg
Magnesium	400 mg	270 mg

foetus. Physiological changes occur, for example the uterus changes from the size of a small pear in its non-pregnant state to five times its normal size at full term. The expected increase in weight of the mother in an average pregnancy is 9–12 kg. She must ensure she has enough energy to carry the extra weight of pregnancy and sufficient nutrients to aid development of the foetus. Maintaining a healthy diet in pregnancy will also prepare the woman for birth.

A pregnant woman should ensure her diet contains sufficient energy, protein, iron, calcium, folate and vitamins C and D. This is because any deficiencies in obtaining these nutrients may lead to a reduction in the woman's own stores of nutrients. There are increased requirements for some, but not all, nutrients during pregnancy. Women intending to become pregnant or who are pregnant are advised to take supplements of folic acid (also called folate) for the first 12 weeks of pregnancy. This is to reduce the risk of neural tube defects in the developing foetus. Neural tube defects occur when the development of the spine or brain is incomplete, for example spina bifida and anencephaly. Additional energy and thiamine are required only during the last three months of pregnancy. Mineral requirements do not increase, although iron supplements may sometimes be given if the woman's iron stores are low.

Late adulthood
There is very little difference between the nutritional requirements of most adults and those in late adulthood (i.e. 65+ years) or the elderly. However, as we get older we tend to become less active, so the main difference is that energy expenditure decreases. The elderly are the fastest

growing sector in society, so ensuring they receive an adequate diet is of increasing relevance. The personal circumstances and state of health of older people also needs to be considered, because this can affect what they are able to eat.

As there is a reduction in physical activity, energy requirements decrease gradually. The requirement for vitamins remains the same but an elderly person's diet is more likely to be deficient in vitamins C, D and folate. Elderly people may not consume enough green leafy vegetables, which would account for the lack of folate in their diet. Those who are housebound may be lacking in vitamin D due to limited exposure to sunlight, so foods rich in vitamin D and calcium should be included in the diet. Vitamin C deficiency may result if a person has difficulty in peeling fruit and vegetables. An elderly person's diet will benefit from the recommended amounts of iron, zinc and calcium. Zinc is needed for a healthy immune system and to help with wound healing of pressure sores and leg ulcers; a lack of zinc may be a factor in causes of dementia.

Adequate intakes of calcium should be included in the diet of those in late adulthood for good bone health. Those individuals who are healthy should restrict saturated fat intakes but fat restrictions are less likely to be beneficial in those over 75. Fat restriction is not appropriate for people who are frail, have experienced recent weight loss or those with a very small appetite. Some very elderly people may suffer with constipation and bowel problems due to reduced gut mobility and inactivity, but the consumption of cereals can help with this. Dehydration can also interfere with digestion (which can lead to constipation) so drinking a variety of fluids will maintain water intake and reduce the risk of dehydration.

Check your understanding 1

1 State one reason why young children should not be given large meals.
2 Explain why teenagers have an increased need for protein in their diets.
3 Identify three starchy foods which have health benefits to us.
4 Describe three functions of water in the body.
5 Explain how the Eatwell Guide helps people make informed choices about their diet.

Key terms

Puberty refers to the physical and emotional transition when a child becomes a young adult. This process is characterised by a spurt of physical growth leading to an increase in height and weight, changes in body composition and sexual development.

Weaning is the process of introducing solid foods into a baby's diet.

Outline Activity

Prepare a leaflet for potential new parents which summarises the nutritional needs of a pregnant woman.

LO2 Understand the impact of diet on health and well-being

The diet you eat affects how healthy you are. Generally, if you follow the principles of the Eatwell Guide and do not over- or under-eat, you will achieve a healthy, balanced diet. If you do not have a healthy diet you can become ill.

2.1 Factors which influence dietary intake

Many factors influence people's diets, not just the nutritional needs of the body. These factors are outlined in **Figure 8.8**.

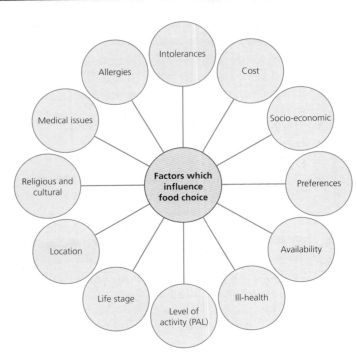

Figure 8.8 Factors which influence food choice

Intolerances

Some people have a sensitivity to certain foods, which can give them symptoms such as nausea, abdominal pain, joint aches and pains, tiredness and weakness. This is called a **food intolerance**.

Allergies

A food allergy is when an individual has an allergic reaction to a specific food. Foods that may cause an allergic reaction are shellfish, nuts, eggs and strawberries.

Medical

Some people cannot eat certain foods without becoming ill: they might have an intolerance or an allergy, but other people have specific medical conditions. This means that they cannot eat certain foods, or that they are already ill. Examples of medical factors that influence dietary intake are listed here.

Table 8.7 Two examples of food intolerance

Lactose intolerance	An individual who is lactose intolerant cannot digest the sugar in milk called lactose. As a result, it gets broken down in the stomach by bacteria, which causes abdominal pain, nausea, diarrhoea and flatulence.
	They need to avoid all dairy products such as milk, cheese, yoghurt, butter, cream and any processed food which contains dairy products.
Gluten intolerance	Gluten is a protein present in a number of cereals, including wheat, rye, oats and barley, as well as flour, baked products, bread, cakes and pasta. An individual who is gluten intolerant cannot digest gluten found in these food products.
	Coeliac disease is a bowel disease; people with coeliac disease have this sensitivity or intolerance to gluten. An individual suffering from coeliac disease is called a coeliac. Symptoms of the disease include: ● Weight loss (because a coeliac cannot absorb food properly) ● Diarrhoea ● Lack of energy, which may also leave people tired and weak ● Loss of appetite and vomiting ● Children may not gain weight or grow properly ● General malnutrition, as a coeliac cannot absorb enough nutrients. Individuals with coeliac disease need to follow a strict gluten-free diet.

Table 8.8 Food allergies

Food allergies	People with food allergies need to be really careful that they do not eat these foods by mistake. If they do, they may experience symptoms such as: ● An itchy sensation inside the mouth, throat or ears. ● Swelling of the face, around the eyes, lips, tongue and roof of the mouth. ● In some severe cases, it can bring about an anaphylactic shock, which could be fatal unless an epi-pen containing adrenalin is used.

Obesity

Obesity or being **obese** means being very overweight. One in four UK adults and one in five UK children are obese, which is higher than any other country in Western Europe.

If you are obese, then losing weight is better for your health. To do this, it is advised that you have a healthy diet following the Eatwell Guide, reducing the energy (calories) in your diet, reducing your fat and sugar intake, and watching your portion sizes. This guidance is also applicable if you are suffering from **coronary heart disease** or high blood pressure. You should also reduce your salt intake.

Osteoporosis

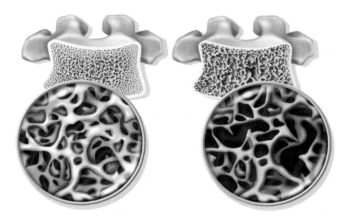

Figure 8.9 Osteoporosis

Osteoporosis is a condition that weakens bones, making them fragile and more likely to break. It can be caused by a lack of vitamin D and calcium from early childhood through to the late 20s in early adulthood. Eating a healthy diet that includes sufficient levels of calcium and vitamin D, as well as exercising, can help to prevent osteoporosis.

Diabetes

Diabetes is a condition where the sugar in a person's blood gets too high. There are two types of diabetes:

- Type 1 diabetes occurs when your immune system attacks and destroys the insulin-producing cells of the pancreas.

Scientists think it is caused by genes and environmental factors.

- Type 2 diabetes is the most common type of diabetes in the UK. It causes the level of sugar (glucose) in the blood to become too high. It is caused by problems with a chemical in the body (hormone) called insulin. It is often linked to being overweight or inactive, or having a family history of type 2 diabetes.

Diabetics should follow the Eatwell Guide and ensure they eat regular meals throughout the day. Their diet should consist of eating mainly starchy carbohydrates, such as wholegrains, which release sugar more slowly into the bloodstream.

Recovering from illness or an operation

When recovering from illness, your body needs to repair itself. Any type of illness can cause low energy and a loss of appetite, leading to a lack of nutrients and subsequent weight loss. Choosing foods that provide your body with the right nutrients is essential for returning to full health. Foods high in protein and vitamin C are essential, as they provide energy from starchy carbohydrates.

Religious, cultural and preparation

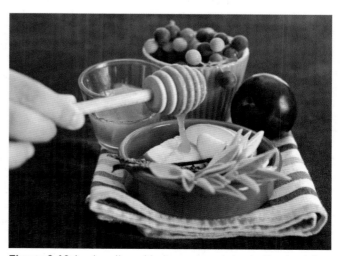

Figure 8.10 Apples dipped in honey to celebrate the Jewish New Year, Rosh Hashanah

Many cultural and religious groups have specific rules and guidelines regarding acceptable foods, food combinations, preparation of food, eating patterns and eating behaviours. Food is very important for many different faiths, and some of these are outlined in **Table 8.9**.

Table 8.9 Food guidelines and rules for various faiths

Religion	Guidelines and rules regarding food preparation, food combinations, eating patterns and behaviour
Judaism	Do not eat shellfish or pork. Do not eat dairy and meat in the same meal – they only eat meat that has been slaughtered in a specific way in order to be called **kosher**. At Passover, a celebratory meal is eaten including matzah, a type of unleavened flatbread. At Rosh Hashanah (the Jewish New Year), a celebratory meal is eaten with apples dipped in honey. Yom Kippur is a day of fasting and prayers when families eat before the sun sets and then fast for 24 hours. Hanukkah is the festival of lights, where a lot of food is eaten to celebrate, including different types of fried foods.
Hinduism	Do not eat beef or any beef products. The cow is considered to be a sacred animal. Use milk, because no animal is killed during the process. Many are vegetarians, which comes from the principle of 'Ahimsa' (i.e. not harming). Do not drink alcohol.
Islam	Do not eat pork. Do not eat seafood without fins or scales, for example crab, prawns. Do not eat meat that is not **halal**, meaning that it has been slaughtered in a very specific way. Do not drink alcohol. During Ramadan, Muslims do not eat during daylight hours over a month-long period. To celebrate the end of Ramadan, they have a three-day festival called Eid where special food is eaten.
Sikhism	Do not eat beef or any beef products. The cow is considered to be a sacred animal. Many are vegetarians. Many will not eat Halal or Kosher meat, as they believe the animals are not killed humanely. Devout Sikhs do not drink alcohol.
Buddhism	Many are vegetarians as they try to avoid intentionally killing animals. Monks and nuns are usually very strict, and some monks fast in the afternoon. Buddhists celebrate Vesak, where they eat only vegetarian food. Do not drink any alcohol.
Rastafari movement	Do not eat pork. Do not eat fish more than twelve inches long. Eat food that is natural, pure, clean or from the earth which is called 'I-tal', for example fruits, vegetables. They try to avoid food that has been chemically-modified or contain artificial additives. Do not eat food prepared with salt.
Christianity and Catholicism	Many observe Lent, a religious period where they give up certain foods for a period of 40 days and 40 nights. At Christmas and Easter, traditional foods are eaten, for example hot cross buns, Simnel cake/turkey, mince pies.

Key terms

Coronary heart disease occurs when fatty deposits build up in the coronary arteries, causing them to narrow and reducing blood flow to the heart.

Diabetes is a condition where a person's blood sugar levels are too high. It can be genetic or linked to lifestyle.

Food intolerance refers to a sensitivity to certain foods. The symptoms may include nausea, abdominal pain, joint aches and pains, tiredness and weakness.

Halal means that a food is permitted to be eaten because it is considered as 'clean' in the Islamic religion.

Kosher means that a food is permitted to be eaten because it is considered as 'clean' in the Jewish religion.

Obesity or being **obese** means being very overweight.

Osteoporosis is a condition that weakens bones, making them fragile and more likely to break.

Socio-economic

The choice of food purchased is affected by an individual's household income. Households with more than one wage earner may have more **disposable income**, meaning that they have more money to invest in the food they eat. Research suggests more money is being spent on ready-to-eat 'premium' food products and some of those who have more disposable income want higher quality food with minimal preparation. The amount of money available affects both the quantity and variety of food which can be purchased. For example, if income is limited, the house might purchase more high fat and sugary foods since these are cheaper than organic produce. Fruit and vegetables may not be purchased as they can be expensive. Most of the major food retailers offer their own brand of value ranges on key food products.

The ONS family spending survey states that 10.6 per cent of income is spent on food. The average weekly expenditure on food and non-alcoholic drinks in was £60.60. £5.50 of this was spent on bread, rice and cereals, £4.00 on fresh fruit, £4.30 on fresh vegetables and £2.20 on milk (*The office for family statistics – Family spending in the UK*).

Food choices have been affected by social changes, such as:

- Both parents being in full- or part-time employment.
- An increase in people living alone.
- People working longer hours and travelling longer distances to work.

The impact of these social changes means that people have busy lifestyles. More and more individuals are now working full-time, which can reduce the amount of time and energy they have to cook meals every evening. Working parents can find preparing meals after working all day tiring and, for convenience, choose to eat outside the home, purchase ready meals or part-prepared food products.

As the number of people living alone has increased, so has the number of single-portion ready meals purchased. These can often be processed with higher amounts of sugar or salt compared to home-cooked meals, which can have a detrimental effect on an individual's health.

Cost

The cost of food can vary from shop to shop and in different areas of the country. Supermarkets offer a wide range of food products at different costs. The popularity of value brands has grown considerably. Discount food retailers such as Aldi and Lidl can offer very competitive pricing on selected products. Foods are also often cheaper in a supermarket than in a corner shop, where you are paying for convenience. The success of own brand foods in supermarkets has meant that there are now different ranges offered at different costs ranging from value to premium.

Many people will look at how they can save money when choosing food, by:

- planning meals carefully, keeping within budget and so no food is wasted
- looking for the special offers in supermarkets
- shopping at the end of the day for reduced items, which have a shorter shelf life.

Location

Where you live can affect the choice of food. In a large city, the choice may be vast but in a rural location, it may be limited. Some larger food retailers are situated outside town centres and can be difficult to access without a car. Consumers are increasingly reliant on car ownership when making large food purchases at out-of-town shopping centres or supermarkets. In more deprived areas there may only be convenience shops where there is less choice, and often less fresh produce.

Life stage

The information regarding nutritional needs of different life stages is covered in AC1.4.

Level of activity

How active we are may influence our food choices; our energy and nutrient requirements vary according to our age, sex, body size and levels of activity. It is important that our food intake is balanced with our energy expenditure so that we maintain a healthy weight.

We can measure the level of activity an individual does by looking at their **physical activity level (PAL)**. This is a way of measuring your daily physical activity as a number. Your PAL will vary depending on how you spend your time during the day. If you are sedentary (not very active), you will have a lower PAL than someone who moves around a lot in their job, for example a personal trainer or builder.

If you eat more food than you need and you have a low PAL, any excess energy is stored as fat. If you eat less food, than you need and have a high PAL, then the fat stores in the body are used up.

Preferences

For most people, eating food is an enjoyable experience. We choose food we like to eat because food provides enjoyment as it meets an emotional need. The smell, taste, texture and appearance of food stimulates all the senses. There are some foods we enjoy eating and others we don't: everyone has unique likes and dislikes. These preferences develop over time, and are often influenced by personal experiences. For example, parents usually feed their children the food they enjoy, which can influence a child's eating preferences for the rest of their life.

Peer pressure can also have an influence on what we choose to eat. We may choose certain foods to fit in or to be liked and accepted. Peer pressure can particularly have an impact on adolescents, who may be influenced by what their friends are eating.

Information in the media will also influence food choices, such as:

- Food scares, for example the 2013 'horse meat' scandal, with the discovery of horse meat in some processed foods.

- The media using advertising techniques to persuade us to make particular food choices.

- The influence of celebrities, i.e. what they choose to eat can have an impact on our choices. Some young people may want to copy these celebrities, aspiring to look and be like them.

There are always new fashions and trends emerging that may influence our food choice. Examples of current food trends include an increase in the popularity of kale, juicing and the use of spiralisers to turn vegetables into noodle shapes.

There is an increasing demand to ethically produced food. Ethical reasons for **not** buying certain foods include when the:

- animal has been killed, for example vegetarians and vegans may share this view

- food has been **intensively farmed** in poor welfare conditions, for example battery hen farming

- food has been **genetically modified**, for example certain vegetables such as tomatoes

- food has been produced using too many chemicals

- food has high **food miles** and therefore a large **carbon footprint**.

People may prefer to follow a vegetarian diet for many different reasons, such as:

- Not enjoying the thought of eating a dead animal, fish or bird.

- Religion, i.e. it does not allow them to eat certain meats or shellfish.

- Health reasons, i.e. they might think a plant-based diet is healthier than one consisting of lots of animal products.

- Environmental reasons, i.e. they think it is wasteful to raise animals for food when the same land space could be used more economically to grow crops.

The two main types of vegetarian are:

- **Lacto-vegetarians** who will eat dairy products, for example milk, butter, cream, cheese and yoghurt, but they will not eat animal foods, for example meat, poultry, fish, eggs, and meat products, such as lard and gelatine.

- **Vegans** who will not eat anything that comes from an animal, so no food is included in their diet which involves the slaughter or the use of animals in its production, for example meat, eggs, honey. Therefore, all foods they consume are plant-based, so no dairy foods are included in their diet.

Availability

In the UK, we have access to a wide variety of foods, whereas people in developed countries might have access to a limited variety and quantity of foods.

The choice of food available in the UK has increased significantly. This is because of new developments in transport, preservation and storage of foods. We also import both foods we can grow in this country, and foods we cannot grow. This means that much of our food is available all the year round. We can buy any food we want at any time of the year but out of season it may be more expensive.

In some developing countries, there can also be a shortage of food due to drought, flooding, conflict, and failed harvests. This can also have an impact on exporting that food to other countries if, for instance, the harvest is poor or has failed.

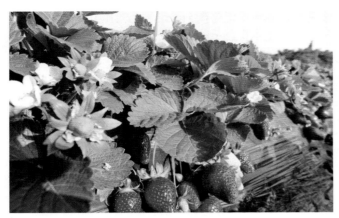

Figure 8.11 Strawberries are a seasonal food

Key terms

Carbon footprint refers to the amount of greenhouse gases produced in the production and transportation of foods.

Disposable income is the money left over for saving or spending after taxes are subtracted from income.

Food miles refers to the distance that food is transported as it travels from producer to consumer.

Genetically modified (GM) refers to foods produced from plants or animals that have had their genetic information changed by scientists.

Intensively farmed is a type of farming that aims to produce as much yield as possible, usually using chemicals and in a restricted amount of space.

Lacto-vegetarians are individuals who will eat dairy products, for example milk, butter, cream, cheese and yoghurt, but they will not eat animal foods, for example meat, poultry, fish, eggs, and meat products, such as lard and gelatine.

Physical activity level (PAL) is a way of measuring your daily physical activity as a number.

Vegan refers to a person who does not eat or use any animal or by-products of animals.

Description Activity

Develop a leaflet that will help to inform the public about the importance of a healthy diet. Describe a minimum of four factors which influence dietary intake.

2.2 The impact of dietary intake on health and well-being

Dietary intake has an impact on our health and well-being, including both long-term and short-term impacts. The correct relationship between diet, nutrition and health is a crucial one, and these will be explored in this section.

Balanced diet

A balanced diet is discussed in detail in section AC1.3 in the Department for Health section and the nutritional needs for growth and health can be found in section AC1.4.

The short-term impact of having a balanced diet is that it can make you feel and look your best, give you more energy and help you maintain a healthy weight.

The long-term impact of having a balanced diet is that it can add years to your life and reduce the risk of certain diseases including cancer, diabetes, cardiovascular disease, osteoporosis and obesity.

Growth and development
Children and adolescents require a diet which sustains their rapid growth and the development of their muscles and bones during this life stage. They require adequate quantities of foods containing protein, vitamin D, phosphorus and calcium. Children and adolescent nutritional needs are discussed in more detail in AC1.4 (nutritional needs across the life stages).

Energy
We need energy for every function and movement that our body does. Even when

you are asleep, your body needs energy for breathing, to keep your heart beating, your internal organs working and for digesting food. During the day, you need energy for walking, exercise such as running or cycling and even sitting down. You get energy from the foods that you eat, which act as a form of 'fuel' for the body.

The energy we take into our bodies by consuming food and drinks, and the energy we use, is measured in kilocalories (kcal) or kilojoules (kJ). Kilocalories are most widely used.

We get energy from the following foods:

- Starchy carbohydrates (e.g. bread, rice, pasta, potatoes, chapatis and couscous). Starchy carbohydrates should be the main source of your body's energy.

- Biscuits, nuts, most cheeses, cream, cooking oil, pastries and crisps.

- Fat is found in foods such as butter, cooking oils, cream and oily fish, and provides a concentrated source of energy.

- Protein is found in foods such as meat, fish, eggs, cheese, pulses (peas, beans and lentils) and nuts.

Your body will use carbohydrates and fats for energy first, but if there is not enough of these nutrients in your diet, it will use protein. For this reason, protein is sometimes called a **secondary source of energy**. The amount of energy you need changes throughout your life.

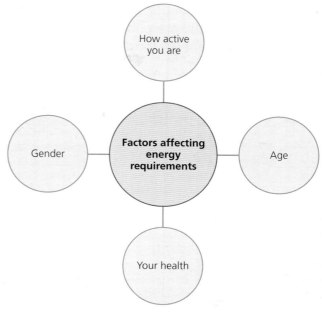

Figure 8.12 Factors affecting energy requirements

Basal metabolic rate (BMR) is the number of kilocalories you need to stay alive for 24 hours. Different people have different BMRs depending on their age, size, gender and usual levels of physical activity.

As previously mentioned, your physical activity level (PAL) is a way of measuring your daily physical activity as a number. It is calculated by the number of activities carried out during the day and how energetic these activities are. This, along with the BMR, can be used to work out how much food energy you need to consume in order to maintain your lifestyle. Most people have a PAL between 1.4 (a very inactive person) and 2.4 (a very active person).

Recommended energy sources from nutrients in the UK

Table 8.10 Recommended energy sources from nutrients in the UK

Protein	15% of total food energy from proteins.	
Fat	No more than 35% of total food energy from fats.	No more than 11% from saturated fats. Saturated fats are from animal sources, for example butter, lard and can be harmful to health as they have been linked to cardiovascular diseases.
Carbohydrate	50% of total food energy from carbohydrates.	45% from fibre-rich starchy carbohydrate and lactose (the sugar in milk) when naturally present in milk and milk products, and sugars contained within the cellular structure of fruits and vegetables. No more than 5% from free sugars.

Experts from the Scientific Advisory Committee on Nutrition (SACN) have published average requirements for energy for children and adults.

Table 8.11 Average requirements for energy for children and adults

Age	Males (kcal)	Females (kcal)
4	1,386	1,291
10	2,032	1,936
18	3,155	2,462
25–34	2,749	2,175
45–54	2,581	2,103
65–74	2,342	1,912

Young children and adolescents need more energy in relation to their size when compared with adults and the elderly. After the age of 18, energy requirements begin to fall. For those in late adulthood or the elderly (over-65s), energy needs are even lower due to a reduction in their BMR and lower physical activity levels.

Increased immunity

Some vitamins and minerals are thought to increase our immune system's ability to fight off infection and keep us healthy. See **Table 8.12** for more information.

Table 8.12 Vitamins and minerals that increase our immune system

Nutrient	Sources	How it may support our immune system
Vitamin A	Animal sources – eggs, oily fish, milk, butter, liver, cheese. Plant sources – spinach, carrots, sweet potatoes, butternut squash, cantaloupe melon, papaya.	Vitamin A helps our T-cells to find and destroy germ infected cells. T-cells are lymphocytes produced by the thymus gland and are an active part of the body's immune response.
B6 Pyridoxine	Lean meat, eggs, chicken, fish, beans, nuts, whole grains and cereals, bananas and avocados.	Vitamin B6 is involved in metabolism, the maintenance of the immune system and the formation of antibodies.
B12	Meat, eggs, milk and cheese, salmon and cod, fortified breakfast cereals.	Vitamin B12 works with vitamin B6 to make new DNA and protein, which is used to make new immune cells.
Vitamin C	Citrus fruits, blackcurrants, broccoli, red and green peppers, strawberries.	The main function of vitamin C is that is makes and maintains healthy connective tissue, helping wounds to heal.
Copper	A variety of foods.	Protects and fuels immune cells.
Vitamin D	Sunshine, milk, eggs, fortified breakfast cereals, fat spreads.	Vitamin D deficiency is associated with a reduced immune response to infection. According to the British Nutrition Foundation, about one in five of the population have low vitamin D status. This is because the action of sunlight on the skin produces vitamin D. If someone has limited exposure to the sun, then they may be deficient in vitamin D.
Folic acid	Fortified breakfast cereals, broccoli, sprouts, chick peas, spinach, and peas. Supplements, for example pregnant women are advised to take supplements of folic acid if they are planning a pregnancy, right through till they are 12 weeks pregnant.	Folic acid is needed to make new DNA and to allow the body to make immune cells in response to infection.

Nutrient	Sources	How it may increase our immune system
Iron	Meat, eggs, fortified cereals, bread, green leafy vegetables, nuts, dried fruit.	Iron helps to maintain healthy immune cells; if we don't get enough iron from the diet then our immune cells may not work as effectively.
Selenium	Nuts and seeds, eggs, liver, poultry, fish and shellfish.	Selenium maintains healthy immune cells, and can help the body make more cells as well as strengthening their response to infection.
Zinc	Zinc is found in many foods, the main sources are red meat, fish – particularly shellfish, cheese, pulses and unrefined cereals. It is easily absorbed from meat, which provides about a third of the UK population's zinc intake.	Zinc develops cells that help to fight off viruses. Research suggests that zinc is needed to make DNA, and new immune cells. Zinc is also part of an enzyme needed for developing our T-cells and for immune cell communication.

According to the British Nutrition Foundation, the interaction between diet and the gut microbiome is important to health. Emerging research suggests that there may also be potential effects for bone health and immune function.

 Key terms

Basal metabolic rate (BMR) is the number of kilocalories required for the body to function at rest. An individual's BMR will depend on factors such as age and activity levels.

Secondary source of energy is a form of energy source taken from a primary source of energy, for example food, through a transformation process. Protein is an example of a secondary source of energy, as the body prefers to use energy from carbohydrates and fats first.

Unbalanced diet

An unbalanced diet can be caused by overnutrition, i.e. eating too much food, or a certain nutrient, or undernutrition, i.e. eating too little food or a particular nutrient to meet dietary needs. In the UK, overnutrition is more of a problem than undernutrition: however, it still occurs, particularly with the micronutrients such as vitamin D, calcium and iron. The short-term impacts of overnutrition are bloating, headaches, lack of energy, acid reflux and obesity, while the long-term impacts are cardiovascular disease, increased risk of stroke and/or high blood pressure. The short-term impacts of undernutrition are usually a lack of energy, recurring illness, weakness, delayed physical and mental development, irritability, poor appetite and low weight while the long-term impacts are deficiency diseases, poor bone health and malnutrition.

Illness and disease

Your own health affects the amount of energy needed. If you are ill and cannot move around, then your energy needs will decrease. However, sometimes illnesses can increase your need for energy if your body has to repair itself.

Certain diseases have a higher risk of malnutrition, including cystic fibrosis, coeliac disease, liver disease, kidney disease and cancer. Disease can affect how the body absorbs and uses the nutrients that we eat or drink.

People may eat poorly because they are ill. People who are very ill or in pain may not eat enough to keep themselves healthy. Eating or swallowing can be difficult if an individual is unwell. Some illnesses can result in a lack of appetite and medication may decrease appetite or affect the digestion and absorption of nutrients. If food is not digested properly, the body cannot absorb the nutrients.

An unbalanced diet can also lead to a number of health-related issues and diseases.

Cardiovascular diseases

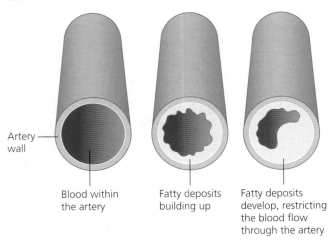

Artery wall

Blood within the artery

Fatty deposits building up

Fatty deposits develop, restricting the blood flow through the artery

Figure 8.13 How fatty deposits build up in the blood vessels

If the blood flow is reduced or stopped by a blood clot or narrowing of the blood vessels, damage may be caused to the body. If this happens in the heart it can cause a heart attack. If this happens in the brain, the person will have a stroke.

Coronary heart disease occurs when blood vessels to the heart (the coronary arteries) become blocked with fatty deposits. This can cause angina if the blood flow is restricted or a heart attack if the blood supply is cut off completely. It is the main cause of death in the UK.

A stroke occurs when the blood supply to the brain is cut off. The brain needs oxygen and nutrients to work properly. Without these, the brain cells begin to die. A stroke may lead to physical disability, brain injury or even death. It is the third largest cause of death in the UK after heart disease and cancer.

These are long-term impacts from a number of factors, diet being one of them. A diet high in cholesterol and saturated fat can cause narrowing of the blood vessels due to fatty deposits. You can reduce the risk of cardiovascular disease by following the Eatwell Guide, reducing the fat and salt in your diet and not over-eating.

Bone health

The strength of your bones depends on your diet, your exposure to sunlight and how much exercise you do. The nutrients which increase bone strength are the micronutrients, calcium and vitamin D. Vitamin D may be obtained from our diet or from exposure to sunlight.

A baby's skeleton begins to grow in the womb, so the diet of a pregnant woman is very important. During this important time in the womb and childhood, the bones are being built. Up to around the late 20s, the skeleton gets stronger as it lays down calcium aided by vitamin D.

The short-term impact is if insufficient vitamin D or calcium is eaten in the diets of children this may lead to rickets. Children with rickets have weak and soft bones. The long-term impact in adults is osteoporosis. Eating a healthy diet, including calcium and vitamin D as well as exercising, can help to prevent osteoporosis.

Tooth decay

Eating foods with high amounts of free sugars in them, such as fizzy drinks, biscuits, cakes, sweets, chocolates and desserts, can cause tooth decay.

The short-term impact is that tooth decay begins with plaque forming on your teeth and gums that contains bacteria. The long-term impact is that over time, this bacteria can interact with the sugars in the food you eat to make acid. This acid attacks your tooth enamel and can cause tooth decay. Tooth decay may lead to fillings or the loss of teeth.

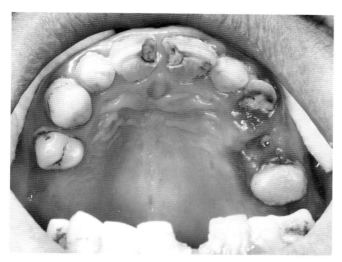

Figure 8.14 Advanced tooth decay

Iron deficiency anaemia

This occurs when there are not enough red blood cells available. The red blood cells have an important job of transporting oxygen around the body. When there are not enough red blood cells, the body becomes short of oxygen. The short-term impacts of this are pale complexion and tiredness; if left untreated the long-term impacts are breathlessness, heart palpitations and feeling very tired. If anaemia is left untreated it can make you more likely to get infections and other illnesses as the body needs iron for its immune system.

Diabetes

Type 2 diabetes is the most common type of diabetes in the UK. More and more people are developing type 2 diabetes later in life. You are more likely to develop type 2 diabetes if you:

- are overweight or obese
- are over 40 years old
- eat fatty, salty and sugary foods often
- have high blood pressure
- do not exercise regularly.

The short-term impacts of type 2 diabetes are feeling tired all the time, feeling thirsty and passing more urine than normal. If left untreated, the long-term impact is that the condition can get worse and other health problems can develop. Diabetics should follow the Eatwell Guide and make sure they eat regular meals throughout the day.

Malnutrition

Malnutrition literally means 'bad' nutrition. Malnutrition can be described as deficiency, excess or imbalance of nutrients that causes adverse effects on health and well-being. Normally, the term malnutrition is used to refer to undernutrition rather than overnutrition. Most research regards malnutrition as a deficiency or insufficiency of nutrients and as having a body mass index (BMI) of less than 18.5.

Malnutrition can affect anyone in society. A report published by the British Association for Parenteral and Enteral Nutrition (BAPEN) has estimated that malnutrition (or 'undernutrition') affects over 3 million people in the UK. Of these, about 1.3 million are over the age of 65 (**www.bapen.org.uk**).

The symptoms of malnutrition may include tiredness, slow growth in children, brittle nails, dry and scaly skin, slow wound healing and increased susceptibility to infections. Malnourished people are more likely to develop infections, visit their GP more frequently, and require longer hospital stays. Malnutrition can prevent people recovering from illness and make individuals more prone to developing health problems. Individuals can suffer reduced muscle strength and are more susceptible to hypothermia, apathy, depression and self-neglect.

It is thought that more than 3 million people are malnourished in the UK. The most vulnerable groups to suffer malnutrition are:

- Babies and children
- Individuals in late adulthood and the elderly
- Individuals with drug or alcohol addiction
- Individuals with eating disorders
- Individuals on a low income.

Obesity

As previously mentioned, obesity or being obese, means being very overweight. Body mass index (BMI) can be used to calculate whether you are in the healthy range or not. For adults, a BMI of over 30 is considered obese.

The short-term impact of obesity is that your quality of life may be impaired; you have less energy, so you may not able to participate in exercise, your joints ache, you feel tired, and you may have low self-esteem.

The long-term impacts of being obese are that you run the risk in later life of developing:

- Type 2 diabetes
- Coronary heart disease
- Stroke
- Some cancers, for example breast cancer
- Arthritis
- Depression.

Activity

Discuss the impact of vitamins and minerals in increasing our immune system.

✓ Check your understanding 2

1 Explain how vitamin A and zinc can help immunity.
2 Name two food sources of vitamin C.
3 Name a medical condition which could influence dietary intake.
4 Describe three factors other than special dietary requirements which influence dietary intake.
5 Describe the long-term impact on health of not consuming enough vitamin D or calcium throughout the life stages.

LO3 Understand how the health and social care practitioner promotes a healthy diet

3.1 How initiatives promote healthy eating

Health and social care practitioners are able to refer to a number of global, national and local initiatives that promote healthy eating and help individuals to follow a healthy diet.

Local, national and global initiatives

Local initiatives

The British Nutrition Foundation (BNF) has a range of resources for heathy eating. Annually, they have a Healthy Eating Week which is a dedicated week in the year to encourage organisations across the UK to eat more healthily. Many local groups and schools take part in a variety of fun activities.

Local hospitals, leisure centres, and doctor's surgeries often have a range of activities, resources and clinics to promote healthy eating and well-being, such as weigh-in sessions, diabetic clinics and looking after your heart sessions.

National initiatives

There are a number of national initiatives that are in place to promote healthy eating.

- National Institute for Health and Care Excellence (NICE) has developed guidelines to help hospitals identify those who are malnourished or at risk of malnutrition. NICE sets out the nutritional support that these people should receive in hospital. They recommend that the weight of a patient at risk of malnutrition is monitored closely during their stay in hospital. All hospitals should employ at least one nurse specialising in nutrition support.

- The Care Certificate is an agreed set of 15 standards that sets out the knowledge, skills and behaviours expected of specific job roles in the health and social care sectors. It was developed jointly by Skills for Care, Health Education England and Skills for Health. These standards should be covered by anyone new to the care sector. One of the standards is Standard 8: Fluids and Nutrition, which is about how to support individuals in having access to fluids, food and nutrition in accordance with their care plan (**www.skillsforcare.org.uk**).

- Change4Life is a public health programme in England. It is a campaign which aims to tackle the causes of obesity by getting families and children, exercising and eating more healthily.

- NHS School fruit and veg scheme and '5 a day'. This is aimed at children aged 4–6 years old attending a fully state-funded infant, primary or special school in England. The scheme entitles children to receive a free piece of fruit or vegetable each school day. That provides 1 of their '5 a day' portions. The scheme also helps to increase awareness of the importance of eating fruit and vegetables, and encouraging healthy eating habits that can be carried into later life.

- Sugar tax. This was introduced by the UK government in 2018. It is a tax on sugary drinks as part of an anti-obesity policy. Sugary drinks are now more expensive depending upon how much sugar has been added. This tax has been designed to reduce the consumption of sugary drinks.

Global initiatives

The World Health Organization (WHO) has developed the 'Global Action Plan for the Prevention and Control of **non-communicable diseases** (NCDs) 2013–2020'. NCDs refer to diseases such as heart attacks, strokes, cancers, respiratory diseases, asthma and diabetes. The plan is looking to achieve a 25 per cent relative reduction in premature deaths from NCDs by 2025 and stopping the rise of global obesity.

There is also the global initiate to tack childhood obesity, otherwise known as The Commission on Ending Childhood Obesity (2016). It has six recommendations to address the environment which tends to cause obesity and to tackle childhood obesity.

The six recommendations can be used by health and social care practitioners, and these are illustrated in **Figure 8.15**.

WHO also aims for a world free of all forms of malnutrition, where all people can achieve health and well-being. According to the 2016–2025 nutrition strategy, they are working towards world wide access to effective nutrition interventions and to healthy diets (**www.who.int**).

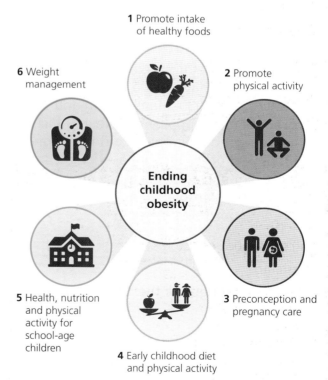

1 Promote intake of healthy foods
2 Promote physical activity
3 Preconception and pregnancy care
4 Early childhood diet and physical activity
5 Health, nutrition and physical activity for school-age children
6 Weight management

Ending childhood obesity

Figure 8.15 The six recommendations to address the environment that causes obesity and tackling childhood obesity

Current initiatives as relevant to Home Nation

The relevant initiatives currently being used in the UK (our home nation) are:

- The British Nutrition Foundation (BNF) healthy eating week
- The Change4Life public health programme in England
- The NHS School fruit and veg scheme, and '5 a day'
- The sugar tax
- The Eatwell Guide.

Description Activity

Describe how one initiative promotes healthy eating.

A minimum of two relevant and traceable references must be included and a reference list.

3.2 How the health and social care practitioner promotes a healthy diet

The social care sector employs 1.48 million people and it will have half a million extra jobs available by 2030. Many health and social care practitioners support people in their own homes, in residential accommodation or in a number of other locations, such as day centres or supported housing, by promoting a healthy diet. Examples of health and social care practitioner roles include:

- Nurse/school nurse
- Dietician
- Speech and language therapist
- Careworker
- Rehabilitation worker
- Health visitor
- Public Health Nutritionist
- Health improvement nutritionist.

They can promote a healthy diet in numerous ways, which are illustrated in **Figure 8.16**.

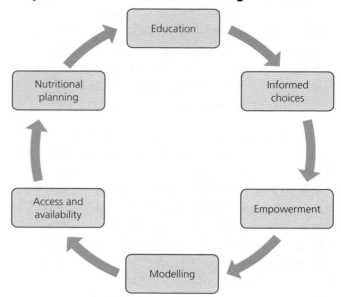

Figure 8.16 The different ways health and social care practitioners promote a healthy diet

Education

There are many practitioners that can promote a healthy diet through education. For example:

- A Public Health Nutritionist is an expert in food and nutrition. They can carry out research and use their scientific knowledge to provide advice and guidance about the positive and negative effects of food on health and well-being. They can promote health through nutrition education and training other professionals. They can promote the health benefits of good nutrition that help to support an individual's positive behaviour changes.
- A school nurse can educate students on healthy eating and give advice on diet, weight, and lifestyle.
- A health visitor can educate new mothers on the best way to feed their babies and how to introduce weaning and good eating habits for toddlers.

Informed choices

A health improvement practitioner can contribute to local programmes which can help to bring about lifestyle and behaviour change, for example stopping smoking, improving diet and promoting exercise. This can help support individuals make an informed choice about what they eat.

Change4Life is an initiative to support health and social care practitioners promote healthy eating messages. In 2018, one campaign highlights how children's snacks can be high in calories, so they advise that they should only have two snacks per day of no more than 100 kcal per snack. The website gives advice on which snacks are healthy, and primary schools can use this information to help support parents to make informed choices when preparing their children's lunchboxes.

Empowerment

Talking to a family member, nurse or doctor may help you to understand why being a healthy weight is important and help you to lose weight if you need to. They can empower people with the knowledge to make the correct choices.

For example, social care services may become involved in the case of an elderly person who is unable to shop or prepare meals. They can help empower the individual to access agencies that offer ready-made meals delivered to the home, in order to remove the pressure of shopping and preparing meals. They can also support the elderly individual in attending a local day centre that serves meals, which can help them to increase their food intake and even reduce loneliness.

Modelling

Health visitors provide a family-focused service which may be delivered in GP practices, children's centres or at home. They can act as role models to new parents. They can model and give advice on many issues including how to feed and wean babies, as well as feeding young children.

A school nurse can also model the behaviours they would like children and adolescents to follow. They promote healthy lifestyles and aim to prevent illness among school-age children.

Access and availability

Health and social care practitioners, such as a care worker or nurse, can support the treatment of malnutrition by ensuring a patient at risk gets nutrient-rich or energy dense foods in small, regular portions. They can also regularly monitor an individual who is at risk by ensuring that they are supervised or supported when eating.

A rehabilitation worker or a health improvement nutritionist can support individuals who may have social, psychological or financial issues, which are contributing to a poor diet and may help to resolve any issues that are preventing them from eating healthily. For example, they may ensure that the individual is receiving the necessary finances and that they are being used effectively to buy the right food.

Speech and language therapists also have had extra training to help those with **dysphagia**, i.e. feeding and drinking difficulties. They will often work together with other professionals, such as a dietician, health visitor and/or physiotherapist if children, adults, or the elderly have any eating and drinking difficulties. They can monitor and supervise eating habits and can prepare food accordingly if there are swallowing issues.

Nutritional planning

Dietitians are the only qualified health professionals that can assess, diagnose and treat dietary and nutritional problems of an individual. They use the most up-to-date public health and scientific research on food, health and disease and use it to guide and help people make appropriate lifestyle and food choices. They also advise and influence food and health policy in government, local communities and individuals. They create nutritional plans based on the health needs of the individual. They can provide a plan for a specific diet for an individual: it could be a diet to lose weight or just to start eating more healthy food.

Key Words

Dysphagia refers to the difficulty or discomfort in swallowing food and drink, for example coughing or choking, persistent drooling, being unable to chew food properly.

Non-communicable diseases (NCDs) are heart attacks, strokes, cancers, respiratory diseases, asthma and diabetes.

Check your understanding 3

1 Name two WHO recommendations that outline how to tackle childhood obesity.
2 Outline how a health visitor promotes a healthy diet for children.
3 Describe the recommended advice from Change4Life on children's snacks.
4 Name an initiative which could help a person who is obese.
5 Describe how a care worker could help an elderly person who is unable to shop or prepare meals.

Case scenario

William is an active 7-year-old boy. He takes snacks and packed lunches to school every day. Today, he brings the following items:
Snacks:
A packet of salt and vinegar crisps
A bar of chocolate.
Packed lunch:
Peanut butter sandwich on two slices of white bread
A high-sugar fizzy drink.

Questions

1 Do you think the food William is eating forms part of a healthy balanced diet?
2 William often complains he is hungry and thirsty at the end of the day. How could that be avoided?
3 How could William's snacks be changed to conform to the Change4Life guidelines (i.e. two snacks of less than 100 kcal each)?
4 Which of the main food groups would you say are missing from William's packed lunch and snacks?
5 Suggest a more healthy packed lunch and snacks for William, giving reasons for your choice.

Classroom Discussion

Discuss the importance of establishing healthy eating patterns in children in order to prevent obesity. Make sure your discussion includes how they can access the relevant sources of information, advice and support.

Evidence Activity

Explain how health and social care practitioners can promote a healthy diet.

Use different sources to show evidence of knowledge and understanding gained from wider reading.

Sources must be relevant and referenced using a traceable method such as Harvard referencing.

Read about it

Department of Health, 2012, *Manual of Nutrition*, 12th Edition, The Stationery Office (TSO) – this book describes the major nutrients, their roles and sources, and digestion. It outlines current food and nutrition policies and the role food plays in our health and well-being. It covers food nutrition and health, nutritional needs and health, and factors affecting food choice.

Rickus, A., Saunder, B., and Mackey, Y. (2016), *AQA GCSE Food Preparation and Nutrition*, Hodder Education

Emerging research on gut microbiota and the immune system www.nutrition.org.uk/nutritionscience/webinars/why-is-everybody-talking-about-gut-microbiota.html

Family spending in the UK: April 2017 to March 2018 – an insight into the spending habits of UK households, broken down by household characteristics and types of spending www.ons.gov.uk

For information on how to eat well, and being a healthy weight www.nhs.uk/live-well

Guidance, advice and information services for health, public health and social care professionals www.nice.org.uk

Report of the commission on ending childhood obesity www.who.int/end-childhood-obesity/final-report/en/

The care certificate, and its 15 standards. www.skillsforcare.org.uk

The Eatwell Guide www.gov.uk/government/publications/the-eatwell-guide

The Healthy Start scheme where it is possible to get free vouchers every week to spend on milk, fruit and veg, formula milk and vitamins www.healthystart.nhs.uk

The role of WHO in the development of current nutritional guideline for a healthy diet www.who.int/news-room/fact-sheets/detail/healthy-diet

Tool to calculate BMI www.nhs.uk/Tools/Pages/Healthyweightcalculator.aspx

How will I be graded?

The table below shows what learners must do to achieve each grading criterion. Learners must achieve all the criteria for a grade to be awarded. A higher grade may not be awarded before a lower grade has been achieved, although component criteria of a higher grade may have been achieved.

Grade	Assessment Criteria number	Assessment Criteria
D1	1.1	Outline the main food groups.
	1.2	Describe the components of a healthy diet. Examples may be used to support the description.
D2		A minimum of one (1) relevant and traceable reference must be included.
C1	2.1	Describe factors which influence dietary intake. A minimum of four (4) factors which influence dietary intake must be described.
C2	1.3	Summarise current nutritional guidelines for a healthy diet. A minimum of two (2) current national guidelines for a healthy diet must be summarised.
B1	1.4	Summarise nutritional needs within one (1) life stage. Examples may be used to support the summary.
B2	3.1	Describe how one (1) initiative promotes healthy eating.
B3		A minimum of two (2) relevant and traceable references must be included. A reference list must be included.
A1	2.2	Discuss the impact of dietary intake on health and well-being. Examples may be used to support the discussion.
A*1	3.2	Explain how the health and social care practitioner promotes a healthy diet. Examples may be used to support the explanation.
A*2		References must be present throughout to show evidence of knowledge and understanding gained from wider reading. References must be relevant and traceable.

Glossary

Abuse When a person is mistreated in a way that causes them pain and hurt.

Active listening A communication technique that involves understanding and interpreting what is being expressed through verbal and non-verbal communication.

Active participation An individual's involvement in all aspects of their own life, care and support.

Advocacy services Services that support individuals to speak up when they are unable to; they represent the individual's best interests.

Advocate An independent person who represents the views, needs and interests of individuals who are unable or unwilling to do so, and supports them to express their views, i.e. during a safeguarding inquiry.

Agreed ways of working The working practices that are followed in a work setting, including policies and procedures.

Aim A purpose or what is intended, for example to get fit.

Alternative and Augmentative Communication (AAC) The term used to describe various methods of communication, such as 'text-to-speech' technology, that can be used to assist people with speech difficulties.

Antioxidant Able to protect cells from harmful substances.

Aphasia A condition that affects a person's speech, understanding and use of language.

Art therapy Using art to express emotions.

Arthritis A disease that causes painful inflammation and stiffness of the joints.

Attitude The way in which an individual expresses what they think or believe through what they say or do.

Autism spectrum disorder A lifelong condition that affects how a person perceives the world and interacts with others, i.e. they may have difficulties communicating, interacting and socialising with others.

Basal metabolic rate (BMR) The number of kilocalories required for the body to function at rest. An individual's BMR will depend on factors such as age and activity levels.

Behaviours The ways in which an individual acts physically and emotionally, for example self-harming or not eating, including when interacting with others.

Beliefs Opinions that an individual accepts as true; not necessarily based on fact.

Best interests Considering an individual's circumstances and preferences before making a decision or choice on their behalf.

Binge drinking Drinking lots of alcohol in a short space of time or drinking to get drunk.

Body Mass Index (BMI) A calculation that is used to determine whether a person's weight is healthy in proportion to their height.

Body language A form of non-verbal communication in which thoughts, feelings and intentions are expressed through the movement and position of the body.

British Sign Language (BSL) The sign language used in the UK by individuals who have a hearing impairment. It uses a combination of hand gestures, facial expressions and body language. It is a different language to English with its own grammar and sentence construction.

Bureaucracy The administrative procedures that help run an organisation. Some people call bureaucracy 'red tape'.

Caldicott Principles A set of standards aimed at improving information handling in health and social care.

Capacity The ability to understand information, retain it, make and communicate decisions.

Carbon footprint The amount of greenhouse gases produced in the production and transportation of foods.

Care or support plan A personalised plan for the care and support of an individual, identifying all those involved and their responsibilities.

Care Quality Commission (CQC) The regulator of all health and social care services in England.

Cerebral palsy A group of lifelong conditions that affect movement and co-ordination, caused by a problem with the brain that occurs before, during or soon after birth.

Challenge Setting a goal that can be reached with a little effort.

Clinical Commissioning Groups (CCGs) Local public bodies made up of doctors, nurse specialists, lay people and others such as service users. They commission (buy) care services from private and NHS providers to meet the needs of their local community.

Cochlear implant Surgically implanted hearing device.

Codes of practice Standards or values that health and social care practitioners must follow to provide high-quality, safe, compassionate and effective care and support.

Coercion The action of persuading someone to do something by using force or threats.

Cognitive Referring to the development of the mind and the process of acquiring knowledge and understanding through thoughts and experiences.

Cognitive development How we understand the world and process information, perceive things and people, and learn language.

Common law The part of English law derived from previous court cases. Decisions made by judges are based on examples of similar cases. It is also called 'judge-made' law or case law.

Communication A two-way process between individuals, involving a sender and a receiver who are sending, composing, understanding and responding to a message.

Community Treatment Order As part of the Mental Health Act, some patients with mental health disorders are allowed to be discharged into the community and supervised by a community psychiatric nurse. These patients can be recalled to hospital if they stop taking their medication.

Compassion Delivering care and support with kindness, consideration, dignity and respect.

Confidential information All information that is personal or sensitive, and that is not available in the public domain.

Confidentiality Keeping something private. Protecting an individual's personal, sensitive or restricted information and only disclosing it with those who need to know it.

Consent An informed agreement to an action or decision.

Coronary heart disease A disease that occurs when fatty deposits build up in the coronary arteries, causing them to narrow and reducing blood flow to the heart.

Court of Protection A specialist court for all issues relating to people who lack the capacity to make decisions.

Creative activities Inventing and making new things. Creative means original or imaginative. Activities involve doing, not watching. Creative activities are therefore those where a person is actively involved in using their imagination to make something original.

Crisis A sudden severe onset of symptoms that can be harmful to the individual and others.

Data controller An individual who decides why and how any personal data is to be processed in an organisation.

Data processor An individual who is not an employee of the data controller, who processes the data on behalf of the data controller.

Day care centre A community-based setting, open during the day, where individuals can meet with others to socialise and participate in activities.

Dehydration When the body loses more water than it takes in.

Dementia A disorder of the mental processes caused by brain disease or injury. Examples of symptoms include memory loss and/or difficulties with thinking, problem-solving or language.

Depression A medical condition that causes low mood and that affects a person's thoughts and feelings. It usually lasts for a long time and affects their day-to-day living.

Deprivation of liberty Detaining people against their will.

Developmental milestones Key events in development, such as a baby smiling for the first time or taking its first steps.

Diabetes A condition where a person's blood sugar levels are too high. It can be genetic or linked to lifestyle.

Dignity Respecting an individual's choices, views and decisions and not making assumptions about how they want to be treated.

Direct discrimination When someone is treated unfairly because of a protected characteristic they, or someone they know, has or appears to have.

Discipline The action taken by an employer against an employee when their behaviour and/or work does not meet expected standards.

Discrimination The unfair or unequal treatment of an individual or a group.

Disposable income The money left over for saving or spending after taxes are subtracted from income.

Domiciliary care services Care and support services that are provided to individuals in their own homes.

Duty of care The health and social care practitioner's legal obligation to ensure the safety and well-being of individuals and others, such as their colleagues and visitors, while providing care and support.

Dysphagia The difficulty or discomfort in swallowing food and drink, for example coughing or choking, persistent drooling, being unable to chew food properly.

Early intervention in psychosis standards (EIP) A set of standards published by the Royal College of Psychiatrists that guide practitioners in the early treatment of people with psychosis. The standards bring together the latest research and evidence from best practice to say how people with psychosis should be cared for.

eIDAS 'Electronic identification and trust services.' These services help to verify the identity of individuals and businesses online or the authenticity of electronic documents.

Emergency protection order An order issued by the court in an emergency that enables the child to be removed from where they are living because they are at risk of physical, mental or emotional harm.

Emotional Relating to a person's feelings.

Emotional development Learning to recognise, understand, express and manage our feelings and to have empathy for others.

Empathy The ability to understand or feel what another person is experiencing from their point of view, i.e. putting oneself in another's position.

Empower Enabling and supporting individuals to be in control of their lives.

Ethnic group A group of people who share a common cultural background, such as the country they come from or the language they speak.

Exploitation Taking advantage of someone unfairly for your own benefit.

Female Genital Mutilation (FGM) A range of procedures which involve the partial or total removal of the external female genitals for non-medical reasons.

Fibre A substance found in the cell walls of vegetables, fruit, pulses and cereal grains. It is an essential component of a healthy diet.

Fine motor control The co-ordination of small muscles with the eyes, such as in movements using the hands and fingers, for example eating, cutting with scissors, buttoning clothing, etc.

Food intolerance A sensitivity to certain foods. The symptoms may include nausea, abdominal pain, joint aches and pains, tiredness and weakness.

Food miles The distance that food is transported as it travels from producer to consumer.

Fortified A food that has vitamins or minerals added to it to improve its nutritional value, for example breakfast cereals and bread.

Genetic inheritance The basic principle of genetics, explaining how characteristics are passed from one generation to the next in the form of genetic material, i.e. DNA.

Genetically modified (GM) Foods produced from plants or animals that have had their genetic information changed by scientists.

Grassroots approach Referring to the people who form the main part of an organisation or movement, rather than its leaders, for example the community in health and social care.

Gross motor control Larger movements made by the arms, legs, feet or entire body, for example crawling, running, jumping etc.

Growth Relating to size, for example getting bigger or taller.

Guardian The lead person for safeguarding an individual's confidential information.

Hacking The gaining of unauthorised access to data in a system or computer.

Halal A food is permitted to be eaten because it is considered as 'clean' in the Islamic religion.

Harassment Unwanted, intimidating or aggressive behaviour related to a protected characteristic.

Harm When someone is hurt either physically or emotionally; this may be intentional (i.e. abuse) or unintentional (i.e. an accident).

Hazards Dangers that have the potential to cause harm, such as an item (a broken chair), a situation (an individual who is distressed) or an activity (moving and positioning) that can be the cause of accidents, injuries, ill-health, deaths or damage.

Health and Well-being Boards Health and social care organisations who work together to improve the health and well-being of all those who live in the local area.

Hearing impairment A hearing loss that may occur in one or both ears. This can be partial (some loss) or a complete loss of hearing.

Hearing loops The sound systems used by individuals who use hearing aids. They provide a wireless signal that is picked up directly by the hearing aid, thus minimising any unwanted background noise.

Holistic An approach that acknowledges the whole person, rather than just one aspect of them. You should look at an individual holistically in order to meet their range of needs.

Holistic needs Involving the treatment of an individual as a whole person and therefore meeting their range of physical, emotional and social needs.

Huntington's disease An inherited disease that stops part of the brain from working properly, causing uncontrolled movements and affecting emotions and thinking abilities.

Hydration The supply of water required to maintain the correct amount of fluid in the body.

IAPT services (Improving Access to Psychological Therapies) Services that provide psychological therapies to people with anxiety disorders and depression. In many cases people can refer themselves to this service.

Impartial Being fair and objective.

Inclusive To include everyone, for example planning an activity that all can take part in whether or not they have disabilities or any other issue which may restrict them.

Inclusive practice Working in ways that involve individuals in their own care and support so that they are in control of their lives.

Independent Mental Capacity Advocate (IMCA) A person who can represent those in need when there are no family members or friends able to help.

Indicators The changes in an individual that are shown and might give cause for concern.

Indirect discrimination When a practice or system is applied without taking into account an individual's protected characteristic.

Individuals Persons accessing health and social care services.

Induction An introduction to an organisation, work setting or job role by an employer.

Inform To advise or guide.

Information Commissioner's Offices The UK's independent body that upholds information rights.

Informed choice Having all the necessary information including the options available to make choices and decisions.

Intensively farmed A type of farming that aims to produce as much yield as possible, usually using chemicals and in a restricted amount of space.

Interdependency Dependent on each other; all aspects of development, whether physical, social, emotional or cognitive, influence each other.

Interpreter A professional who converts spoken/oral or sign language communication from one language to another, such as English to British Sign Language (BSL). Interpreters must be good listeners and be able to process and memorise words and gestures while individuals are communicating.

Jargon The use of technical language or terms and abbreviations that are difficult for those not in the group or profession to understand.

Job description A document that details the purpose and responsibilities to be carried out as part of a job role.

Joined-up approach When services work together, for example a social worker from social services and a GP from primary care may support a person with addiction issues.

Kosher A food is permitted to be eaten because it is considered as 'clean' in the Jewish religion. Kosher refers to the way food is prepared, cooked and eaten under Jewish law.

Lack the capacity When an individual is unable to make a decision for themselves because of a learning disability or a condition, such as dementia, a mental health need or because they are unconscious.

Lacto-vegetarians Individuals who will eat dairy products, for example milk, butter, cream, cheese and yoghurt, but they will not eat animal foods, for example meat, poultry, fish, eggs and meat products, such as lard and gelatine.

Language acquisition device (LAD) Chomsky's theory that there is a 'tool' in the brain that helps children to quickly learn and understand language.

Lasting Power of Attorney (LPA) A way of giving someone else power to decide what is in the best interests of the person. There are two types: financial, and health and welfare.

LPAs are appointed to make decisions about an individual's personal welfare, including healthcare, property and affairs.

Learning disability A reduced ability to think and make decisions, along with difficulties coping with everyday activities, which affect a person for their whole life. For example, an individual with a learning disability may experience problems with budgeting, shopping and planning a train journey.

Legislation Laws that must be followed, for example Acts of Parliament, as well as regulations, such as the General Data Protection Regulations (GDPR).

Life skills Skills that are necessary or desirable for full participation in everyday life, such as communication or critical thinking. They are psychosocial skills, i.e. personal, social, interpersonal, cognitive, affective, and universal skills. Life skills may vary from culture to culture.

Life stages The different phases in an individual's life. Often these are classified as infancy (0–2 years), childhood (3–5 years), late childhood (6–10 years), adolescence (11–17 years), early adulthood (18–29 years), middle adulthood (30–60 years) and late adulthood (60+ years). Different areas of study focus on different stages, for example child care practitioners may subdivide the stages of childhood to look at each stage in more detail. Those working with older people may sub divide late adulthood stage into 65–80 years and 80+ years.

Local Safeguarding Children Boards Groups responsible for overseeing different organisations in each local authority. They ensure that these organisations work together to develop effective systems for safeguarding and protecting children and young people from harm and abuse.

Macronutrients Substances required by the body in large amounts, for example protein, fat and carbohydrates.

Makaton A language programme to support spoken language. It is a method of communication that uses signs and symbols with speech, following the order of spoken words, and is used by individuals who have learning disabilities.

Malnutrition A deficiency, excess, or imbalance of nutrients that causes adverse effects on health and well-being.

Medical model of health and well-being A scientific approach that sees the body as a set of systems, for example the respiratory system, the circulatory system, and focuses on the biological and physical aspects of disease.

Medium The method of transmitting a message. This may be verbal, spoken, or visual.

Mental capacity An individual's ability to make their own decisions.

Mental health Referring to 'a state of well-being in which every individual realizes his or her own potential, can cope with the normal stresses of life, can work productively and fruitfully, and is able to make a contribution to her or his community.' (WHO, 2014).

Mental ill-health An emotional or psychological disorder that hinders the individual from making the most of their abilities, and makes it difficult for them to cope with the stresses of life. It prevents them working effectively and from contributing to society.

Micronutrients Substances required by the body in small amounts, for example vitamins and minerals.

Mindfulness The ability to focus on the present moment, being aware of what is happening in your mind, body and surroundings, without judging or worrying about what might happen in the future or what has happened in the past.

Monitor To keep an overview.

Named Person A person who works with children, young people and their families to protect the interests of the child or young person.

Nature Referring to genetic, inherited characteristics and biological influences that relate to human development and behaviour.

Needs Requirements that may be social, emotional, physical or cognitive.

Need-to-know The process of sharing confidential information with others who need it, i.e. when an individual discloses that they are being harmed.

Neglect When a person's needs are not met through failure to care.

Non-communicable diseases (NCDs) Diseases such as heart attacks, strokes, cancers, respiratory diseases, asthma and diabetes.

Non-verbal communication The behaviour and elements of speech (aside from words) that convey meaning. Examples include pitch, tone, speed, volume, gestures, body language, posture, eye movements, proximity to the listener and even dress or appearance.

Nurture The environmental influences relating to human development and behaviour.

Nutrients The vital components which make up food. Each nutrient has a specific role in the body, for example the growth of bones.

Obesity Being very overweight.

Objectives Specific tasks or goals, for example to get fit enough to run 5 kilometres without stopping.

Osteoporosis A condition that weakens bones, making them fragile and more likely to break.

Others Parents/carers, family, friends, colleagues, external partners and health and social care practitioners.

Personal data Information that is personal to an individual and can identify them, such as their name or date of birth.

Person-centred care Placing the individual at the centre of working practices. The health and social care practitioner must always act in the individual's best interests to ensure that the individual remains in control of their care and support.

Person-centred practice A way of working that takes into account the individual's whole person and focuses on their unique needs, abilities, preferences and wishes.

Physical activity level (PAL) A way of measuring daily physical activity as a number.

Physical Relating to movement. A physical creative activity could be creating a dance.

Physical development How we grow and develop control over our bodies.

Picture Exchange Communication System (PECS) A non-verbal method of communication using symbols and pictures.

Pitch The quality of a vocal sound made by a person in a communication (e.g. low, high).

Policies Statements of how an organisation works based on legislation, such as a safeguarding policy. Policies outline the organisation's aims and how it works. Policies refer to an organisation's commitment, for example to data protection.

Positive personal regard Not judging another person but accepting them as they are. It is about respect for others and belief in their genuineness, even if we disagree with them.

Prejudices The negative opinions that you may have of someone, which are not based on experience of interaction.

Primary care giver The person who has the greatest responsibility for the daily care and rearing of a child.

Procedures Step-by-step guides of how to put a policy into practice.

Process (in relation to data) The process used when holding or storing data.

Professional Councils Organisations that regulate professions, such as adult social care workers who work with adults in residential care homes or day centres and who provide care in someone's home. They can provide advice and support around working with individuals who lack capacity to make decisions.

Protected characteristic The nine characteristics protected from discrimination under the Equality Act.

Puberty The physical and emotional change that marks the beginning of adulthood.

Race The common physical qualities or characteristics associated with a group of people from the same culture and/or shared history, e.g. skin colour, ethnic origin, national origin and nationality.

Reflect When a person evaluates their experiences, which can relate to their personal life and/or work to improve and change how they act, think and behave.

Register The degree of formality of language, or the language used by a group of people who share similar work or interests, for example doctors or lawyers.

Rehabilitation The process of restoring someone to health or normal life through training and therapy after addiction, or illness.

Residential short break A holiday or break where individuals can socialise and take part in activities with other people their age to give them a break from their caring responsibilities.

Resilience The ability to adapt to change.

Responsibilities Obligations that are required when carrying out your duties and care at work.

Restrictive practice Actions that deliberately limit an individual's movement or freedom. They might be used legally in, for example, an emergency, when an individual requires life-saving treatment or when escaping violent behaviour.

Risk assessment The identification of hazards, assessing the likelihood of harm from those hazards and reducing the risk of harm from them.

Risks The likelihood of harm occurring as a result of a hazard, for example an accident caused by a broken chair, damage caused by a distressed individual or a back injury caused by moving and positioning an individual.

Safeguarding Adults Reviews (SARs) An enquiry into the death or serious injury of an adult with care and support needs, where abuse or neglect is known or thought to be a factor.

They aim to provide lessons that can be learned to prevent similar incidents occurring again.

Safeguarding partners Those agencies who work together to safeguard individuals, such as the Police, the Local Authority, the NHS, health and social care organisations and education providers.

Saturated fats Fats from animal sources, for example butter and lard. They can be harmful to health as they have been linked to cardiovascular diseases.

Secondary source of energy A form of energy source taken from a primary source of energy, for example food, through a transformation process. Protein is an example of a secondary source of energy, as the body prefers to use energy from carbohydrates and fats first.

Sectioned The detention of an individual suffering from a mental disorder which needs assessment or treatment in hospital for their own health or safety and for the protection of others.

Self-awareness Being able to see yourself as others see you and being aware of your own behaviours, motivations and feelings.

Self-esteem The value or confidence a person places upon themselves.

Self-help group A group of people who provide mutual support for each other on the basis of sharing a common problem, such as isolation, an illness, disability or addiction.

Serious case reviews (SCRs) An enquiry into the death or serious injury of a child where abuse or neglect is known or thought to be a factor. SCRs provide lessons that can be learned to prevent similar incidents occurring again.

Signs Symptoms that are outwardly visible to others, for example bruises, swelling and cuts.

Skills for Care The sector skills council for people working in social work and social care for adults and children in the UK, as well as for workers in early years, children and young people's services. It sets standards and develops qualifications for those working in health and social care.

Skills for Health The sector skills council for people working in healthcare in the UK. It sets out standards and develops qualifications for those working in healthcare.

Slang A type of language that is regarded as very informal. It is more common in speech than in writing and is usually restricted to a particular context or group of people.

Social development How we interact with other people, learning the values, knowledge and skills that help us relate to others effectively.

Social model of health and well-being A holistic approach that looks at the whole person and social, physical, emotional, cultural and economic influences on health, and values individual experience.

Social How we interact with others. Some creative activities may be social, for example, practising and learning a new language as part of a group.

Special educational needs Relating to a child that has a disability or difficulties with learning that make it more difficult for them to learn than most children their age.

Stigma A mark of disgrace associated with a particular quality or characteristic, such as having mental ill-health or a disability.

Stroke A life-threatening medical condition that occurs when the blood supply to part of the brain is cut off.

Symptoms Emotional symptoms are experienced and felt by individuals, such as feeling distressed, upset and/or angry; Physical symptoms include feeling unwell, lack of sleep or poor appetite.

Therapeutic activities Those that are used as a form of treatment to restore health and are designed to reflect real-life activity.

Tone The strength of a vocal sound made by a person in a communication (e.g. quiet, loud).

Translation The process of translating words or text from one language into another.

Values Standards based on moral principles or beliefs that are important to the person.

Vegan refers to a person who does not eat or use any animal or by-products of animals.

Verbal communication The use of sounds and words to express yourself and convey meaning.

Victimisation When someone is singled out or treated unfairly. For example, for supporting or speaking up for an individual with a protected characteristic.

Vulnerable adult In the context of No Secrets, a vulnerable adult is defined as a person aged 18 years and over who is (or may be) in need of community care services, by reason of mental or other disability age or illness. They are not (or may not be) able to take care of themselves, or cannot protect themselves against significant harm or abuse.

Water intoxication A condition occurring when you drink too much water. Drinking too much water can be harmful.

Weaning The process of introducing solid foods into a baby's diet.

Well-being How a person thinks and feels about themselves, physically, mentally and emotionally. It may include aspects that are social, cultural, spiritual, intellectual and economic.

Whistleblowing When a person discloses or reports any information or activity that is deemed illegal or unethical, such as unsafe practices or abuse.

Index